DEDICATION

To Chiqui who has supported me in all my endeavors and made my life meaningful.
To my parents and family for their sacrifices, which helped me achieve my goals, and to all my teachers
who took their time to educate me so that I could provide care for others.

David

EDITOR

David A. Levy, M.D.
Department of Urology
The Everett Clinic
Everett, WA

CONTRIBUTING AUTHORS

Bolent Akduman, M.D.
Fellow, Urologic Oncology
Sunnybrook and Women's College Health
Sciences Center
Toronto, ON

Madhu Alagiri, M.D.
Assistant Professor of Surgery
University of California at San Diego
Director of Pediatric Urology
San Diego, CA

David M. Albala, M.D.
Professor of Urology and Radiology
Loyola University Medical Center
Maywood, IL.

Anthony Atala, M.D.
Department of Urology
Harvard University
Boston, MA

Marc Beaghler, M.D.
Associate Professor of Urology
Division of Urology
Loma Linda University
Loma Linda, CA

Mark Bellinger, M.D.
Associate Professor of Urology
University of Pittsburgh School of Medicine
Pittsburg, PA

Jay L. Bloch, M.D.
Urological Specialists of Southern
New Jersey, LLC
Voorhees, New Jersey

Dominick J. Carbone, Jr., M.D.
Fellow, Division of Urology
University of California School of Medicine
Los Angeles, CA

Joseph M. Carbone, M.D.
Director, Piedmont Institute for Continence
Danville Urologic Clinic
Danville, VA

John Chandler Williams, M.D.
Assistant Professor of Surgery (Urology)
University of Florida Jacksonville
Jacksonville, FL

Christopher L. Coogan, M.D.
Assistant Professor of Urology
Department of Urology
Rush-Presbyterian-St. Luke's Medical Center
Chicago, IL

Michael S. Cookson, M.D.
Assistant Professor
Department of Urologic Surgery
Vanderbilt University Medical Center
Nashville, TN

James M. Cummings, M.D., F.A.C.S.
Chief, Division of Urology/Dept. of Surgery
Univ. S. Alabama, Ste. F
Mobile, AL

John W. Davis, M.D.
American Foundation of Urologic Disease Scholar
Fellow and Instructor
Department of Urology
Eastern Virginia Medical School
Norfolk, VA

Roger E. De Filippo, M.D.
Department of Urology
Harvard University
Boston, MA

Colin P. N. Dinney, M.D., F.R.C.S.(C)
Associate Professor of Urology
and Cancer Biology
The University of Texas M.D.
Anderson Cancer Center
Houston, TX

Christopher P. Evans, M.D.
Assistant Professor
Urologic Surgery, Urologic Oncology
Department of Urology
University of California, Davis
Sacramento, CA

Matthew T. Gettman, M.D.
Resident
Department of Urology
Mayo Clinic
Rochester, MN

Reza Ghavamian, M.D.
Assistant Professor of Urology
Montefiore Medical Center
Albert Einstein College of Medicine
Bronx, NY

Gamal M. Ghoniem, M.D.
Head Section of Voiding Dysfunction Female
Urology and Reconstructive Surgery
Cleveland Clinic Florida
Ft. Lauderdale, FL

Graham F. Greene, M.D.
Assistant Professor
Head Section of Genitourinary Oncology
Department of Urology
University of Arkansas For Medical Sciences
Little Rock, Arkansas

David J. Grossklaus, M.D.
Resident Physician
Department of Urologic Surgery
Vanderbilt University Medical Center
Nashville, TN

Daniel Hoffman, M.D.
Fredericksburg, VA

Koon Ho Rha, M.D.
Fellow Department of Urology
Yonsei University
Seoul, Korea

Yves Homsy, M.D.
Children's Urology Group
Clinical Professor of Surgery and Pediatrics
Director of Pediatric Urology, Department
of Surgery
University of South Florida College of Medicine
Tampa, FL

Jonathan I. Izawa, B.Sc., M.D., F.R.C.S.(C)
Fellow in Urologic Oncology
The University of Texas
M.D. Anderson Cancer Center
Houston, Texas

Thomas W. Jarrett, M.D.
Assistant Professor of Urology
Brady Urologic Institute
Johns Hopkins University
Baltimore, MD

Evan J. Kass, M.D., F.A.A.P., F.A.C.S.
Chief Division of Pediatric Urology
William Beaumont Hospital
Royal Oak, MI

Laurence Klotz, M.D.
Professor Department of Surgery
Division of Urology
Sunnybrook and Women's College Health
Science Center
Toronto, ON

Badrinath R. Konety, M.D.
Instructor
Department of Urology
University of Pittsburgh School of Medicine
Pittsburgh, PA

Harry P. Koo, M.D.
Assistant Professor of Surgery
Pediatric Urology
University of Michigan Medical School
Ann Arbor, MN

Howard J. Korman, M.D., F.A.C.S.
William Beaumont Hospital
Royal Oak, MI

Stephen A. Kramer, M.D.
Professor of Urology
Department of Urology
Mayo Clinic
Rochester, MN

Uday Kumar, MS FRCS
Assistant Professor
Department of Urology
Section of Endourology and
Minimally Invasive Surgery
Loyola University Medical Center
Maywood, IL

Peter Langenstroer, M.D.
Medical College of Wisconsin
Milwaukee, WI

Bruce W. Lindgren, M.D.
Instructor, Departments of Urology
and Pediatrics
Loyola University Chicago Stritch School
of Medicine
Maywood, IL

Mark R. Licht, M.D.
Boca Urology, P.A.
Boca Raton, FL

Donald F. Lynch, M.D.
Professor, Department of Urology
Eastern Virginia Medical School
Norfolk, VA

James Mandell, M.D.
Dean, Albany Medical College
Professor of Surgery and Pediatrics
Albany, NY

Thomas G. Matkov, M.D.
Chief Resident
Department of Urology
Rush-Presbyterian-St. Luke's Medical Center
Chicago, IL

Badar Mian, M.D.
Fellow, Department of Urology
The University of Texas
M.D. Anderson Cancer Center
Houston, TX

Manoj Monga, M.D.
Assistant Professor of Surgery
Director of Endourology and Andrology
Division of Urology
University of California,
San Diego, CA

Nic Muruve, M.D., F.R.C.S.C.
Director of Renal Transplantation
Division of Urology
University of Missouri
Columbia, MO

Durwood E. Neal, Jr., M.D.
Professor and Chairman
Division of Urology
Southern Illinois University School of Medicine
Springfield, IL

Louis L. Pisters, M.D.
Assistant Professor of Urology
University of Texas
M.D. Anderson Cancer Center
Houston, TX

Shlomo Raz, M.D.
Professor
Division of Urology
University of California School of Medicine
Los Angeles, CA

Pramod Reddy, M.D.
Arkansas Children's Hospital
Little Rock, AR

Carlin A Ridpath, M.D.
Associate Professor of Radiology
University of Missouri-Columbia
Columbia, MO

Ramon Rodriguez, M.D.
Resident in Urology
Montefiore Medical Center
Albert Einstein College of Medicine,
Bronx, NY

Eric S. Rovner, M.D.
Assistant Professor of Urology
Division of Urology, Department of Surgery
University of Pennsylvania Health System
Philadelphia, PA

Ricardo F. Sánchez-Ortiz, M.D.
Clinical Instructor
Division of Urology
University of Pennsylvania
Philadelphia, PA

John D. Seigne, M.B.
Assistant Professor of Surgery
Division of Urology
University of South Florida
H. Lee Moffitt Cancer Center
Tampa, FL

W. Bruce Shingleton, M.D.
Associate Professor
Division of Urology
University of Mississippi Medical Center
Jackson, MI

Aseem R. Shukla, M.D.
Chief Resident
Division of Urology, Department of Surgery
University of South Florida College of Medicine
Tampa, FL

Anthony Y. Smith, M.D.
Associate Professor of Surgery/Urology
University of New Mexico School of Medicine
Albuquerque, NM

Gregory Stewart, M.D.
Resident Physician
Division of Urology
Loma Linda University
Loma Linda, CA

Steven C. Stewart, M.D.
Professor of Surgery
Division of Urology
Loma Linda University
Loma Linda, CA

Brian R. Stork, M.D.
Resident, Department of Urology
William Beaumont Hospital
Royal Oak, NH

J. Lynn Teague, M.D., FAAP
Assistant Professor of Surgery and Child Health
Division of Urology
Columbia, MO

Richard K. Valicenti, M.D.
Assistant Professor of Radiation Oncology
Thomas Jefferson University
Philadelphia, PA

Major Mark R. Wakefield, M.D.
Staff Urologist
Wright Patterson, AFB
Dayton, OH

Michael Williamson, M.D.
Professor and Vice Chair
Department of Radiology
University of New Mexico School of Medicine
Albuquerque, NM

Sang Won Han, M.D.
Associate Professor
Department of Urology
Yonsei University
Seoul, Korea

George Young, M.D.
Department of Urology
Cornell Medical Center
New York, NY

Horst Zincke, M.D.
Professor
Department of Urology
Mayo Clinic
Rochester, MN

WE APPRECIATE YOUR COMMENTS!

We appreciate your opinion and encourage you to send us any suggestions or recommendations. Please let us know if you discover any errors, or if there is any way we can make Pearls of Wisdom more helpful to you. We are also interested in recruiting new authors and editors. Please call, write, fax, or e-mail. We look forward to hearing from you.

Send comments to:

Boston Medical Publishing Corporation
237 S. 70th Street, Suite 206, Lincoln, NE, 68510

888-MBOARDS (626-2737)
402-484-6118
Fax: 402-484-6552
E-mail: bmp@emedicine.com
www.bmppearls.com

INTRODUCTION

Congratulations! Urology *Pearls of Wisdom* will help you pass urology and improve your board scores. Pearl's unique format differs from all other review and test preparation texts. Let us begin, then, with a few words on purpose, format, and use.

The primary intent of *Pearls* is to serve as a rapid review of Urology principles and serve as a study aid to improve performance on Urology written and practical examinations. With this goal in mind, the text is written in rapid-fire, question/answer format. The student receives immediate gratification with a correct answer. Questions themselves often contain a "pearl" reinforced in association with the question/answer.

Additional hooks are often attached to the answer in various forms, including mnemonics, evoked visual imagery, repetition and humor. Additional information not requested in the question may be included in the answer. The same information is often sought in several different questions. Emphasis has been placed on evoking both trivia and key facts that are easily overlooked, are quickly forgotten, and yet somehow always seem to appear on Urology exams.

Many questions have answers without explanations. This is done to enhance ease of reading and rate of learning. Explanations often occur in a later question/answer. It may happen that upon reading an answer the reader may think - "Hmm, why is that?" or, "Are you sure?" If this happens to you, GO CHECK! Truly assimilating these disparate facts into a framework of knowledge absolutely requires further reading in the surrounding concepts. Information learned, as a response to seeking an answer to a particular question is much better retained than that passively read. Take advantage of this. Use *Pearls* with your Urology text handy and open, or, if you are reviewing on train, plane, or camelback, mark questions for further investigation.

Pearls risks accuracy by aggressively pruning complex concepts down to the simplest kernel. The dynamic knowledge base and clinical practice of medicine is not like that! This text is designed to maximize your score on a test. Refer to your mentors for direction on current practice.

Pearls is designed to be used, not just read. It is an interactive text. Use a 3x5 card and cover the answers; attempt all questions. A study method we strongly recommend is oral, group study, preferably over an extended meal or pitchers. The mechanics of this method are simple and no one ever appears stupid. One person holds *Pearls*, with answers covered, and reads the question. Each person, including the reader, says "Check!" when he or she has an answer in mind. After everyone has "checked" in, someone states his or her answer. If this answer is correct, on to the next one. If not, another person states his or her answer, or the answer can be read. Usually, the person who "checks" in first gets the first shot at stating the answer. If this person is being a smarty-pants answer-hog, then others can take turns. Try it--it's almost fun! *Pearls* is also designed to be re-used several times to allow, dare we use the word, memorization. I suggest putting a check mark in each box provided every time a question is missed. Two boxes have been arbitrarily provided. If you fill all boxes on re-uses of *Pearls*, forget this question! You will get it wrong on the exam! Another suggestion is to place a check mark when the question is answered correctly once; skip all questions with check marks thereafter. Utilize whatever scheme of using the check boxes you prefer.

We welcome your comments, suggestions and criticism. Great effort has been made to verify these questions and answers. There will be answers we have provided that are at variance with the answer you would prefer. Most often this is attributable to the variance between original source . Please make us aware of any errata you find. We hope to make continuous improvements in a second edition and would greatly appreciate any input with regard to format, organization, content, presentation, or about specific questions. Please write to David A. Levy, M.D. at Dlevy17010@aol.com. We look forward to hearing from you.

Study hard and good luck!

D. A. L.

TABLE OF CONTENTS

UROGRAPHY AND CYSTOGRAPHY

Anthony Y. Smith M.D. and Michael Williamson M.D.

☐☐ **A 23-year-old man has a history of microscopic hematuria and an intravenous urogram (IVU) is planned for evaluation. The patient reports a history of an allergy to shellfish. He has not previously received IV contrast. The next step should be?**

Patients with a history of asthma, drug allergy, or allergy to shellfish have about 2x greater risk of a contrast reaction. Minor reactions include hot flashes, nausea, vomiting or urticaria while major reactions include bronchospasm, hypotension, laryngeal edema, and cardiac arrest. The overall incidence of contrast reactions is estimated to be 13% with high-osmolality agents and only 3% with low osmolality agents. The alternatives to consider in this patient include substitution of a different study (particularly had there been a severe prior reaction), the use of lower osmolality contrast agents, and pretreatment with steroids and antihistamines. A reasonable pretreatment regimen for adults consists of 50 mg prednisone at 13, 7, and 1 hour prior to the study and 50mg of diphenhydramine 1 hour before the exam.

☐☐ **A 30-year-old female is undergoing a workup for microhematuria. Her serum pregnancy test is negative. The 15 minute film from the IVU is shown. The next step should be?**

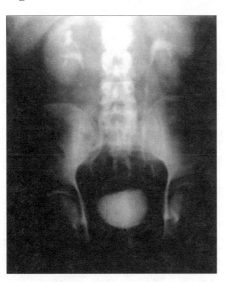

The patient should have a cystoscopy to complete the workup. The IVU is normal. It is not uncommon to have a normal study appear on a board exam. In a normal IVU, a KUB or scout film is obtained, following which approximately 1cc/kg of intravenous contrast is administered. A 30 seconds film shows the nephrogram phase of the IVU and is regarded as the best film to assess renal masses and renal contour. During the excretion phase, 5, 10 and 15 minute films are generally taken. There should be symmetric excretion. The left kidney should be no more than 2-cm longer than the right kidney. Kidneys should be roughly 3- 5 vertebral bodies in length. Forniceal angles should be sharp. Blunting of the forniceal angles is said to be the earliest radiographic sign of hydronephrosis on IVU. Three major infundibulae should be visualized along with roughly 13-14 calyces. The ureter should not show a standing column and the bladder contour, best seen on the 15 minute film, should be smooth. While the film as shown is normal, it is important to point out that the top of the left kidney is "cropped". The entire kidney should be visible on an IVU.

❑❑ **A 70-year-old man presents with microhematuria and a portion of the initial KUB done for the IVU is shown. The next step should be?**

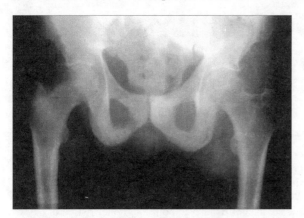

The four things to look for on the scout film are "masses, gasses, bones and stones". Each time you look at a scout film review those four things and comment about whether they are normal or abnormal. Symmetry is also important. In this case, there is asymmetry on either side of the pubic symphysis with sclerosis evident on the left. There is a somewhat moth eaten appearance to the periosteum on the left as well. Sclerotic bone lesions are found in patients with breast and prostate cancer. In this elderly man, the next step should be a prostate specific antigen and a prostate exam.

❑❑ **A child with multiple birth defects had a renal ultrasound suggestive of duplication and hydronephrosis. An IVU was performed to further evaluate the finding. The KUB obtained prior to the study is shown. The radiographic finding demonstrated is?**

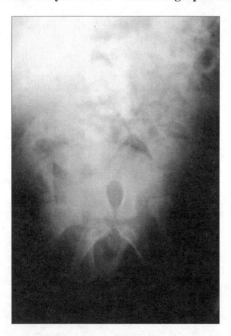

The radiograph is a classic picture of complete sacral agenesis. The sacrum is absent causing the pelvic ring to look like an inverted teardrop. Incomplete agenesis may be more difficult to diagnose. The diagnosis may be delayed until failed attempts at toilet training prompt urologic evaluation for neurogenic bladder. Sacral agenesis may be one component of the VACTERL syndrome (V=vertebral, A=imperforate anus, C=cardiac, TE=tracheoesophageal fistula, R=renal, and L=limb anomalies).

❑❑ **This plain radiograph accompanied the IVU done for evaluation of congenital urologic problems in a child. The radiographic diagnosis is?**

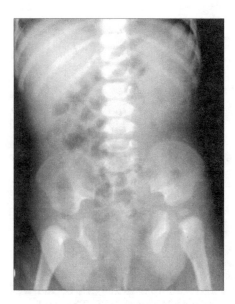

The three conditions which are associated with widening of the symphysis pubis include pregnancy, trauma and the congenital condition of exstrophy/epispadias of which this is an example. The femurs are rotated laterally. There is no separation of the SI joint to suggest trauma. This abnormality is thought to occur as a result of failed mesodermal ingrowth and consequent failure of descent of the cloacal membrane, which produces eventration of the bladder onto the abdominal wall. The spectrum ranges from pure epispadias with a dorsal penile meatus and urethra to cloacal exstrophy with eventration of both bowel and bladder.

❑❑ **A 35-year-old female presents many years after a sterility procedure in which silicone was injected into the fallopian tubes. She has had significant microscopic hematuria. The likely diagnosis is?**

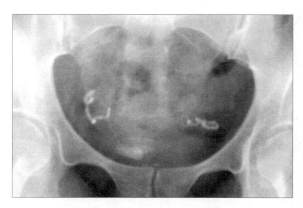

The diagnosis is a bladder stone secondary to foreign body, which in this case was the silicone, which eroded through the bladder wall producing a nidus for stone formation. It is important to consider the possibility of outlet obstruction or foreign body when treating a patient with a bladder stone.

❑❑ **This plain film was obtained in a patient undergoing a workup for microhematuria and pyuria. A routine urine submitted for culture was negative. The likely diagnosis is?**

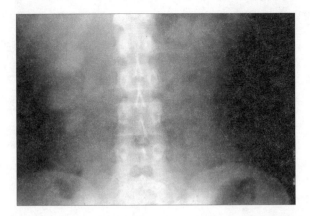

This film shows the classic "paste" stones of genitourinary tuberculosis. The stones are faint on plain film and represent dystrophic calcification of the caseating granulomas that infiltrate the parenchyma of the kidney. The tissue sloughs into the collecting system giving rise to these stones.

❑❑ **A 20-year-old diabetic female presents to the emergency room with fever to 104 degrees and a white count of 33000 associated with a left shift. The scout film from an IVU is shown. The most likely diagnosis is?**

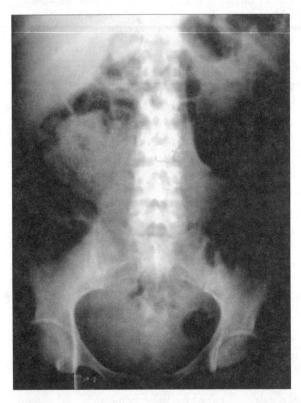

There is gas essentially replacing the left renal outline in a classic case of emphysematous pyelonephritis. The treatment is broad spectrum antibiotics and nephrectomy. A CT scan, if the patient is stable enough to tolerate the procedure, may help to distinguish a perinephric abscess due to a gas forming organism. Gas may outline the kidney in cases of duodenal trauma as well.

❑❑ **An elderly man presents with obstructive voiding symptoms, microhematuria, and an abdominal mass. A plain film was obtained prior to the IVU. The next step should be?**

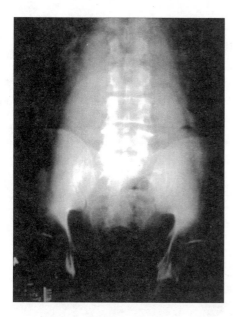

The plain film while overpenetrated shows a midline abdominal mass extending from the pelvis to well above the presumed umbilicus. The next step should be to place a Foley catheter, which in this case resulted in resolution of the mass. This is a bad case of urinary retention.

❏❏ **A patient undergoing a workup for microhematuria has the following scout film obtained prior to the study. What is the radiologic finding and what are the top three possible diagnoses?**

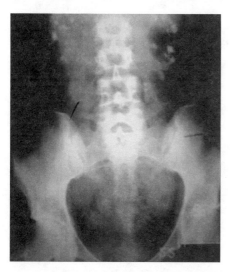

The film shows medullary nephrocalcinosis. Cortical nephrocalcinosis is seen rarely in the present era. It typically was seen as a consequence of postpartum hypotension and renal infarction that produced atrophic kidneys with calcified cortices. Medullary nephrocalcinosis on the other hand can be seen in association most commonly with medullary sponge kidney, type I renal tubular acidosis and hyperparathyroidism.

❏❏ **This scout film was obtained to evaluate left flank pain and fever. The urine pH is >7.2 and loaded with gram negative rods.   The significant findings on the film are? The likely organism cultured from the urine would be? In addition to antibiotics, what immediate procedure is likely necessary?**

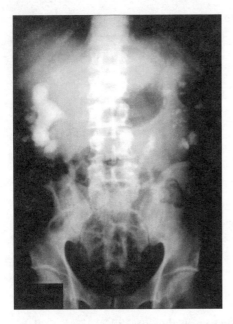

This film shows a large staghorn calculus on the right and multiple stones in both kidneys. To be classified as a staghorn calculus, the stone should fill and outline at least one calyx and infundibulum. In addition, there appears to be a large calcification medial to the left kidney which could represent ureterolithiasis. These are likely magnesium amonium phosphate (struvite) stones associated with urea splitting organisms such as a *proteus* species accounting for the alkaline urine pH. Subsequent films confirmed obstruction on the left and a left nephrostomy was placed.

❏❏   **A 30-year-old female involved in a motor vehicle accident underwent an IVU to evaluate the kidneys for a history of gross hematuria. The significant finding on the IVU is?**

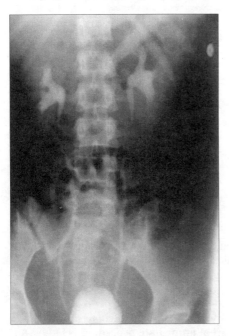

The IVU shows a pelvic fracture with obvious displacement of the SI joint on the right. It is important on any film presented to look at surrounding structures. In this case the Foley catheter has already been successfully placed. A cystogram and drainage film did not show evidence of bladder rupture.

❏❏   **A 75-year-old female is evaluated for an episode of gross painless hematuria. The IVU obtained is significant for 2 abnormalities. These are? (Figure #13)**

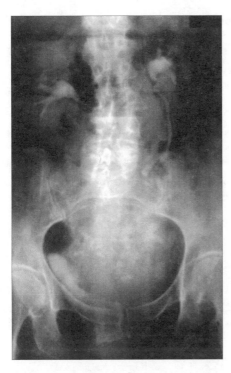

In elderly patients it is especially important to look for associated findings. In this film the left ureter deviates laterally in the upper third. There is a fine rim of calcification and a suggestion of a midline mass. On the left side, these findings are suspicious for an aortic aneurysm, which this proved to be. In addition, there is a large calcified pelvic mass displacing the bladder, which ultimately proved to be a Brenner tumor of the ovary. Not well seen is the invasive transitional cell carcinoma of the bladder, which was diagnosed by cystoscopy.

❏❏ **A 40-year-old man undergoes an IVU to evaluate microhematuria. The 15-minute film is shown. The abnormality shown is? (Figure #14)**

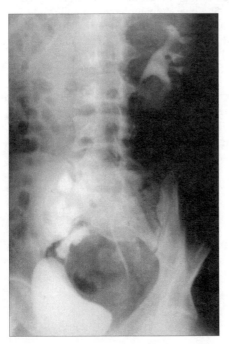

Close inspection of the IVU shows a portion of a calyceal system just below the right pelvic brim and overlying the sacrum. This is an example of an ectopic kidney. The plain film in this case did demonstrate a stone in the pelvic kidney. Up to 50% of pelvic kidneys will have hydronephrosis or reflux.

❑❑ **A 42-year-old man who presented with a history of a febrile UTI was evaluated with an IVU. The likely diagnosis is? (Figure #15)**

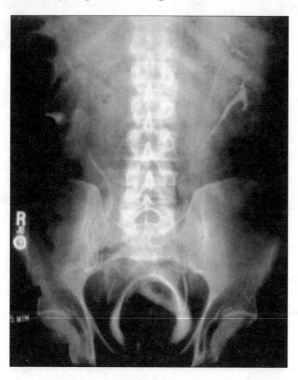

This is an IVU that we don't often see in adults. There is duplication of the collecting system on the left. Duplication of one collecting system should immediately raise suspicion about duplication in the other kidney. The right collecting system is notable for only 2 major infundibula and tilts gracefully to the right like a "drooping lilly". The collecting system is missing the upper pole calyx, which often bears close resemblance to a "ball ping hammer". Additionally, there is a large lucent smooth filling defect in the bladder, which could be confused with a tumor or BPH. However putting the whole picture together it is clear that this must be an ectopic ureterocoele with obstruction of an upper pole duplication on the right. Ectopic refers to the location of the ureteral orifice, which is likely to be outside the trigone. The Weigert-Meyer rule governing the configuration of duplicate orifices is "the upper is lower and lower is lateral". The lower pole orifice is located more laterally on the trigone and is therefore more prone to reflux while the upper pole orifice enters more medially and is more often obstructed, ectopic, or associated with a ureterocoele.

❑❑ **A 27-year-old man presents with right flank pain. His urinalysis shows 0 RBC's/hpf, 2-4 WBC's/hpf, and no bacteria. An IVU is ordered. A delayed film of the IVU is shown. The left kidney was normal on the earlier films. The radiographic diagnosis is most likely? (Figure #16)**

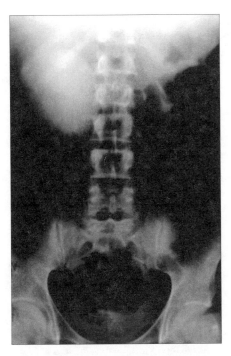

The IVU shows massive hydronephrosis on the right side with an appearance consistent with a ureteropelvic junction obstruction. A distal adynamic ureteral segment is a possibility, which could be ruled out with a retrograde pyelogram performed immediately prior to repair. A lasix renogram may give a better estimate of relative function and degree of obstruction but more importantly, may give a more sensitive test to use to assess outcome after repair. A cystogram may be helpful to rule out reflux.

❏❏ **A retrograde pyelogram was attempted in a patient with intermittent flank pain and hydronephrosis on ultrasound . The ureter is incompletely filled. The diagnosis is? (Figure #17)**

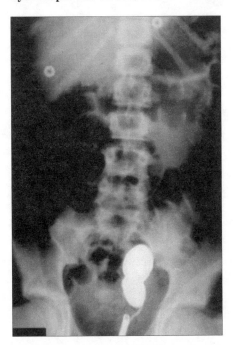

This film shows the classic appearance for a distal adynamic segment associated with a primary obstructed megaureter. The pathology is believed to be due to disordered smooth muscle in the distal segment of the ureter associated with increased collagen deposition. This segment fails to conduct the peristaltic wave and creates a functional obstruction. A similar mechanism is postulated for the majority of UPJ obstructions.

❑❑ **A 30-year-old man presented with right-sided flank pain. His urinalysis showed 0 RBC's/hpf. An IVU was obtained. A 10-minute film is shown. The two likely diagnoses are?**

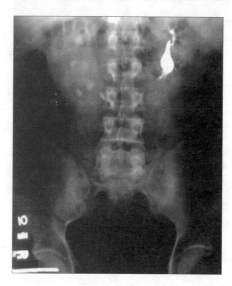

The lower pole of the left kidney has a medially based calyx which is pathognomonic for horseshoe kidney. In addition, the renal axis is shifted laterally. About 1/3 of horseshoe kidneys may have a contralateral ureteropelvic junction obstruction. The renal pelves are oriented anteriorly so the pyeloplasty is performed transabdominally. Ureterolithiasis with hydronephrosis is a possibility but no stone is seen and the patient had no significant hematuria making this diagnosis less likely. A retrograde pyelogram at the time of surgery would confirm the diagnosis and rule out a stone or distal adynamic segment.

❑❑ **An IVU was obtained to evaluate microhematuria in a young man. The radiographic diagnosis is?**

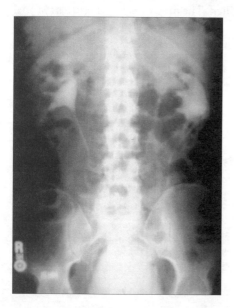

While a medially based calyx is pathognomonic for horseshoe kidney, here is the exception. The left kidney has medial calyces but the right does not. This is a malrotated left kidney. The renal pelvis is oriented anteriorly during renal ascent and the kidney then rotates medially. Most malrotated kidneys rotate laterally instead so the vessels cross anteriorly.

❑❑ **A retrograde pyelogram was obtained to evaluate an abnormality seen on IVU for microhematuria. A representative film is shown. The abnormality is?**

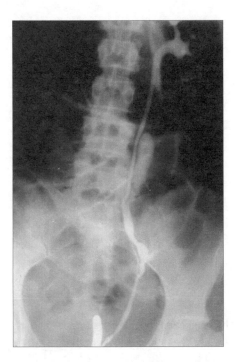

The abnormality is a blind ending ureter on the left. Blind ending ureters are two times longer than they are wide and may occur as a though there was an aborted complete or incomplete duplication. They are histologically identical to normal ureters. Ureteral diverticula fail to meet these criteria. The management is individualized but may include excision where either symptoms or infection supervene.

❑❑ **A 19-year-old male had an IVU performed for intermittent right flank pain. He has had a prior left nephrectomy. The IVU suggested obstruction of the upper 1/3 of the ureter. A representative film from a retrograde pyelogram is shown. The diagnosis is?**

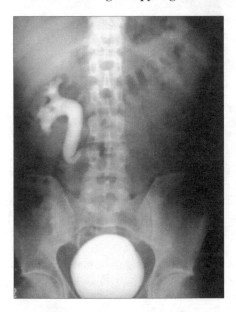

The film is classic for retrocaval ureter with medial deviation of the upper-third of the right ureter.   The embryologic derivation of the condition is best remembered by referring to the condition as persistent subcardinal vein. The first description of dismembered pyeloplasty was performed for this condition by Andersen and Hynes.

❑❑ **A 45-year-old man presented with left flank pain and gross hematuria. A representative film from the IVU is shown.   The likely diagnosis is?**

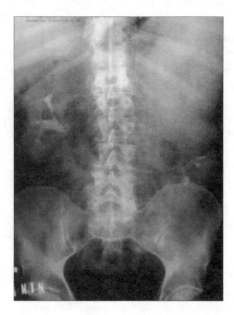

This film shows a different kind of "drooping lilly" on the left. There appear to be three major infundibulae suggesting normal collecting system architecture and arguing against a duplication. However, the " ball ping hammer" has been modified for the upper pole by compression due to a large mass. There are several densities seen in the middle of the mass and while those could represent pooling of contrast, a more likely explanation would be the presence of parenchymal calcification, which of course implies cancer. The differential would include renal cell carcinoma versus adrenal tumor but statistics favor the former. One must consider the possibility of adrenal disease when the kidney is displaced in this fashion.

❒❒ **A 50-year-old man presented with gross hematuria. The likely diagnosis is?**

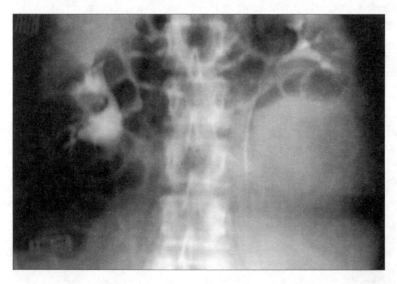

This film illustrates the principle that masses frequently stretch and distort portions of the urinary tract. The kidney is displaced cephalad and the ureter is stretched and bowed medially. These findings suggest a lower pole renal mass, which is suspicious for renal cell carcinoma.

❒❒ **A 28-year-old man presents with a history of gross hematuria. A retrograde pyelogram is undertaken to evaluate delayed function and hydronephrosis of the right kidney seen on IVU. The radiographic sign demonstrated is? The likely diagnosis is?**

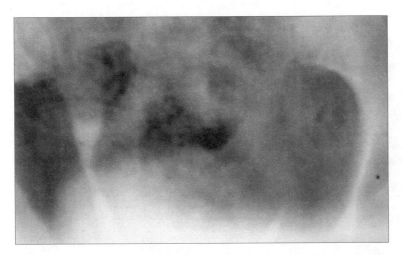

This is Bergman's sign or the "goblet sign". There is dilation of the ureter distal to a ureteral mass. The cause of this phenomenon is not well known but may be due to to and fro peristalsis of the mass. This leads to a radiographic appearance resembling a chalice or goblet on retrograde pyelogram. The likely diagnosis is transitional cell carcinoma of the ureter.

❒❒ **A 70-year-old man who has a long smoking history presents with painless gross hematuria. A retrograde pyelogram has been done to evaluate the right ureter for hydronephrosis seen on the IVU. The most likely explanation for the findings is?**

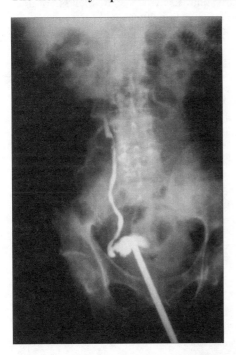

One "rat bite" guideline of film interpretation applies here. If the film looks like a rat has been at work, it is cancer until proven otherwise. The retrograde pyelogram demonstrates a filling defect in the upper third of the ureter. The initial decision is to determine whether the defect is an intraluminal or extraluminal process. Extraluminal processes tend to displace and compress the ureter. In this case a portion of the ureter appears to be "eaten" away. A rat has clearly been at work and the diagnosis is most likely transitional cell carcinoma of the ureter. Other causes of lucent filling defects would be a lucent stone, papilla, polyp, clot, or fungus ball or malakoplakia/cystitis cystica. The "rat bite" appearance however points to malignancy as the likely cause.

❒❒ **A 70-year-old man with a long smoking history presents with gross painless hematuria. An IVU is performed as part of the diagnostic evaluation. The likely diagnosis is?**

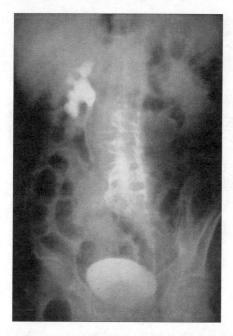

This IVU is notable for nonvisualization of the left kidney. There is a filling defect in the bladder, which could be mistaken for BPH except that it is somewhat irregular. In addition, the right kidney has a standing column of contrast to the middle third of the ureter and early hydronephrosis evidenced by blunting of the forniceal angles. Given the history, the likely diagnosis is muscle invasive transitional cell carcinoma of the bladder with obstruction of the left ureter causing nonfunction of the left kidney. In addition, the findings on the right are suspicious for transitional cell cancer of the ureter, which proved to be the case as the retrograde showed! This film makes the point that transitional cell carcinoma can be a bilateral process and the contralateral kidney must be evaluated carefully. Ureteral obstruction signals invasive cancer about 90% of the time.

❑❑ **Shown is a representative film from the IVU of a patient who presented with painless gross hematuria. The patient had a long smoking history. The two findings on the study are?**

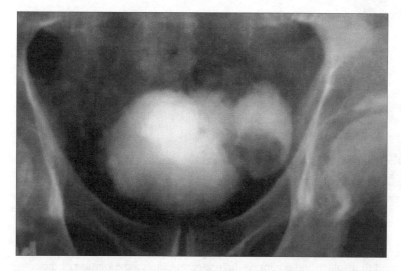

The IVU shows a bladder diverticulum with a filling defect present in the diverticulum. The filling defect is slightly irregular and given the history, the mass most likely represents a transitional cell cancer in a diverticulum, which may carry a more ominous prognosis.

❑❑ **An IVU is performed for gross hematuria and the collecting system is not well visualized. A retrograde pyelogram is performed. The likely diagnosis is?**

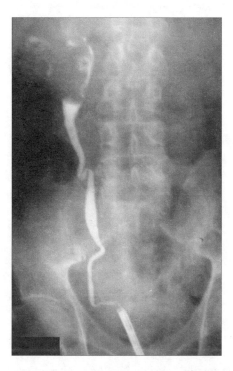

There is a nice goblet sign in the upper ureter and the collecting system architecture has been destroyed. A "rat" has been at work here and the diagnosis is most likely transitional cell carcinoma. However, the differential should also include xantho granulomatous pyelonephritis and tuberculosis.

❑❑   **A 15-year-old non-smoker presents with an episode of gross hematuria. An IVP shows delayed function of the left kidney. CT scan findings suggest a soft tissue mass in the ureter.   A retrograde pyelogram was performed. The significant findings on the study are? The two most likely diagnoses are?**

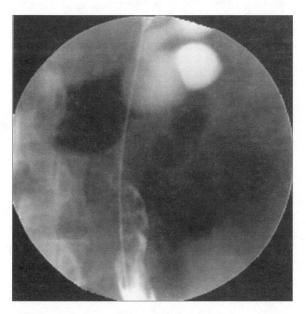

The retrograde pyelogram shows a somewhat lobulated filling defect in the upper ureter. Transitional cell carcinoma is always a possibility but in a younger patient the differential would include a fibroepithelial polyp which in fact, this turned out to be.   The CT is useful to rule out a radiolucent stone.

❑❑   **A middle aged man referred for microhematuria has 10 RBC's/hpf and 20 WBC's/hpf. A urine culture is negative. Urine cytology is negative. A representative film from the IVU is shown for the right kidney. The likely diagnosis is?**

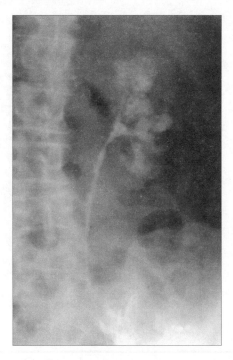

The diagnosis is tuberculosis. Most of the features of tuberculosis are illustrated in this film. Tuberculous strictures occur classically in the infundibulae, ureteropelvic junction and ureterovesical junction. In this film there are strictures of the upper pole infundibulum and UPJ with some degree of "beading" of the upper ureter. There is evidence of papillary necrosis and actual tissue slough in the film. Damage to parenchyma may progress to calyceal amputation or frank autonephrectomy. Faint amorphous calcifications were evident on the plain film.

❏❐ **This patient has a history of pyuria and vague right flank pain. Routine urine cultures have been negative. This film is the 15-minute film from an IVU. The likely diagnosis is?**

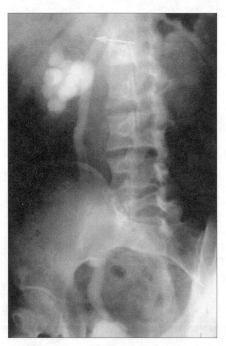

The diagnosis is again, tuberculosis. The film illustrates something that both tuberculosis and transitional cell carcinoma do and that is amputate calyces. The upper pole calyx of the right kidney is seen as just a whisp of irregular contrast (arrow). There is a distal ureteral stricture, which is not well demonstrated on the film. The bladder is contracted and the left kidney has undergone a functional autonephrectomy.

❐❑   **This film shows bilateral retrograde pyelograms obtained in a patient who had a chronic indwelling stent on the right, which had recently been removed. The radiographic finding shown is most consistent with?**

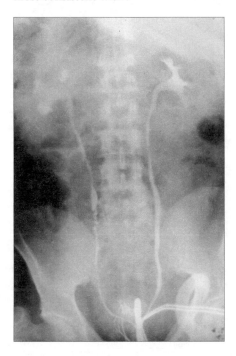

The retrograde pyelogram on the right shows extensive notching of the ureter with smooth small round filling defects. The history and radiographic findings are most consistent with ureteritis cystica. Other possibilities in the differential would be tuberculosis, malakoplakia, persistent fetal ureter or transitional cell carcinoma.

❐❑   **This patient underwent an evaluation for microhematuria and pyuria. Past history was remarkable for an extensive travel history including trips to Africa and China. An IVU was obtained and shown are a portion of the scout and 5-minute films. The most likely diagnosis is?**

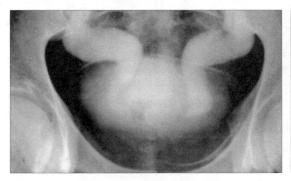 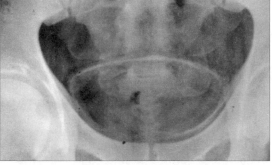

There are only a handful of things that will calcify the bladder wall, but the first one that should come to mind is shistosomiasis. Shistosomiasis is found in rivers in Africa and other parts of the world. Once in the host, the shistosoma hematobium reside in the perivesical venous plexus and lay their eggs in the bladder wall and venous tributaries of the bladder. The eggs are then shed in the urine completing its life cycle. The result of this process is an intense inflammatory reaction in the bladder. Shistosomiasis can acutely present with hematuria and inflammatory changes in the bladder wall on IVU. Late findings include calcification of the bladder and ureteral walls. Similar to tuberculosis, there may be extensive ureteral strictures. Nonfunction, stones, polypoid masses and hydronephrosis are also seen. The risk of bladder cancer is high in these patients. Consistent with the intense inflammatory reaction, there is a higher risk of squamous cell and adenocarcinoma. When there is a suspicion of an inflammatory condition involving the urinary tract, ask about the travel history.

❑❑   **A 45-year-old female presented with a history of recurrent urinary tract infection. A catheterized urine specimen grew multiple gram negative organisms. An IVU was obtained. The significant findings on the film are? The most likely diagnosis to explain the film is?**

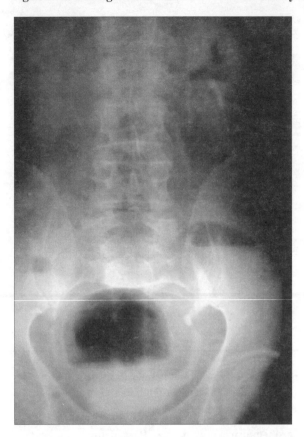

The IVU shows a large amount of gas in the bladder and outlining the left upper pole calyx. Gas can occur in the urinary tract in association with infection due to a gas forming organism. Sometimes gas will appear in the wall of the bladder in association with urinary tract infection known as emphysematous cystitis. Gas outlining the collecting system with no parenchymal gas occurring in the presence of a urinary tract infection is due to emphysematous pyelitis, which responds to antibiotics more favorably than emphysematous pyelonephritis. Renal pelvic gas can also be due to reflux of air associated with instrumentation. However, gas in amounts seen on this film should raise suspicion for a vesico-enteric fistula particularly given the history of polymicrobial infection. The most likely cause would be diverticulitis. Crohn's disease, colon cancer and other pelvic malignancies can also cause fistulas.

❑❑   **A 50-year-old female presented with a history of malaise, left sided flank pain, and low grade fever. On physical exam, a hard mass was palpable in the left upper quadrant. A urine culture grew Proteus. The IVU suggested a left renal mass associated with several calcifications, which appeared to be stones, and the kidney was essentially nonfunctional. A representative film from the retrograde pyelogram is shown. The likely diagnosis is?**

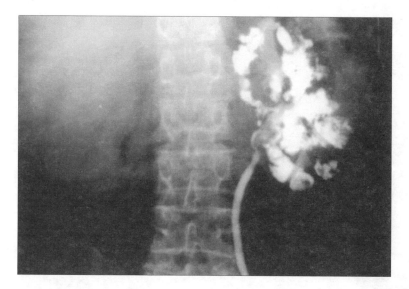

The constellation of renal mass and stones raises the differential of xanthogranulomatous pyelonephritis versus squamous cell carcinoma of the kidney. The presence of the proteus infection makes the former more likely. Renal calculi are seen in one third of cases and a mass is found in two thirds. *Proteus* is the most common organism but *E. coli* is also common. The retrograde pyelogram shows destruction of parenchyma and collecting system with multiple abscess cavities. There is a suggestion of a filling defect in the renal pelvis corresponding to the stone seen on plain film. Xanthogranulomatous pyelonephritis and tuberculosis can both violate the "rat bite" rule.

❑❑ **A middle-aged female presented with a history of recurrent urinary tract infection. The infections have all been characterized by dysuria and frequency but without fever. A post-void film from the IVU is seen. The likely diagnosis is?**

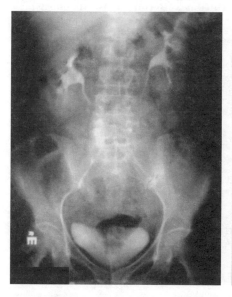

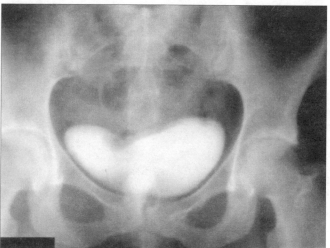

The film shows a relatively smooth double contrast density at or just distal to the bladder neck. In a female, the likely diagnosis is a urethral diverticulum. Urethral diverticula may be a cause of recurrent UTI. They may be difficult to diagnose. The diagnosis should begin with a good physical exam, which includes palpation of the urethra. An IVU and particularly the post-void bladder film may identify the diverticulum. A voiding cystogram, "double bubble' urethrogram using a special double balloon urethral catheter, and cystoscopy may also be useful.

❑❑ **A 25-year-old female presented with a history of colicky right flank pain and hematuria. A faint stone was seen overlying the right bladder shadow on plain film. Hexagonal crystals were present in the urine. The significant radiographic sign demonstrated is? The likely diagnosis is?**

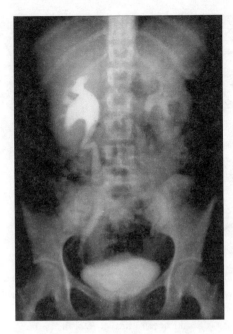

The IVU shows a "cobra head" deformity of the distal right ureter consistent with a simple orthotopic ureterocoele. The orifice is likely to be on the trigone. The faint lucency seen in the middle of the ureterocoele is likely to be a "relatively" radiolucent stone due to cystine. The crystaluria confirms this and a sodium nitroprusside test on the urine would be positive. Unlike uric acid stones, which are not seen on a plain film, cystine stones are faintly seen on the plain film but appear lucent versus contrast on the IVU.

❏❏ **This patient had an IVU performed for hematuria. A urinalysis showed numerous RBC's, no WBC's or bacteria and a pH of 5.0. The plain film did not show a stone. The significant findings and the likely diagnosis would be? What test should be performed next to confirm the diagnosis?**

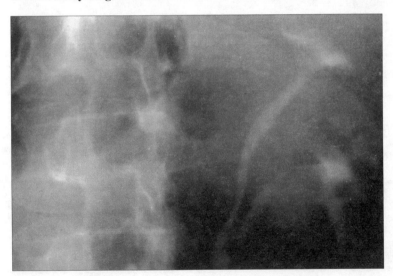

This film shows a smooth lucent filling defect in the lower pole system of a partial duplication. The surface of the defect is smooth. While the usual differential of tumor, stone, clot, papilla, and fungus ball applies, the findings are most consistent with a radiolucent uric acid stone. This could be confirmed with a noncontrasted spiral CT scan since uric acid stones appear bright white while the other possibilities would show only soft tissue.

❑❑ **This man presented with gross hematuria. The scout film from the IVU and a set of retrograde pyelograms are shown. A urine culture is sterile. The diagnosis is? The stone composition is likely to be?**

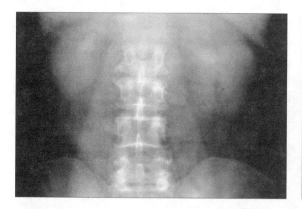 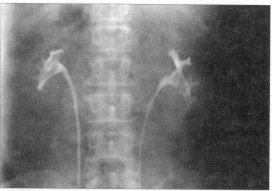

This patient has bilateral staghorn calculi. The stones are relatively radiolucent. Staghorn calculi are more often magnesium ammonium phosphate and are accompanied by infection with urea splitting organisms like *Proteus*. Struvite has a relative density of .20 while cystine is slightly lower at .15 compared to bone which has a relative radiographic density of 1. These stones are relatively radiolucent and the diagnosis in this patient was staghorn calculi due to cystine.

❑❑ **A 35-year-old man presented with a history of hypertension, gross hematuria, and abdominal masses. A representative film from the IVU and a retrograde pyelogram are shown. The diagnosis is most likely?**

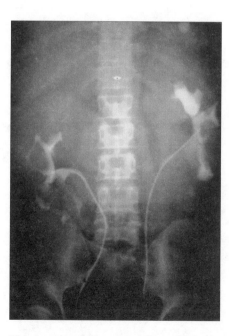 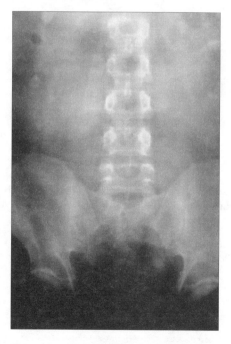

This is a set of films we don't see too often in the era of CT scanning. A normal kidney should be roughly 3 vertebral bodies in length. The IVU shows large kidneys bilaterally with diffuse splaying of both collecting systems due in this case to multiple cysts. The retrograde pyelogram confirms the IVU findings but also shows some degree of ureteral displacement due to the large kidneys. The diagnosis is autosomal dominant polycystic kidney disease. The patient may have a strong family history. Because of the risk of infecting cysts, the decision to perform retrograde pyelograms in these patients is a serious one and prophylactic antibiotics should be given. The differential diagnosis for large kidneys is long and includes; bilateral hydronephrosis, bilateral duplication, bilateral renal tumors, acute bilateral renal vein thrombosis, renal lymphoma, leukemic infiltrates, acute tubular necrosis, diuretic or contrast administration, pre-eclampsia, lupus, Wegener's, Goodpasteur's, and myeloma with amyloidosis.

❑❑ **This patient with an ileal conduit and a history of transitional cell carcinoma of the bladder had an IVU performed as part of a routine follow-up evaluation. The serum creatinine was elevated to 1.7 mg/dl. The likely diagnosis is?**

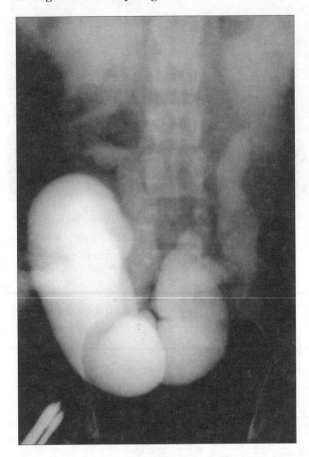

This is a classic film. The presence of bilateral hydronephrosis and a large dilated ileal loop is the conduit equivalent of bladder outlet obstruction and the diagnosis is stomal stenosis. A gentle digital exam of the stoma in the clinic would confirm this.

❑❑ **This young man sustained a gunshot wound to the abdomen and underwent a laparotomy with closure of several small bowel perforations. Two weeks later, he presented with a history of fever to 104 degrees and flank pain. An ultrasound revealed left hydronephrosis. A representative film of the IVU is shown. The likely diagnosis is?**

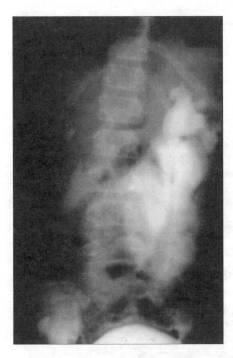

The IVU shows marked extravasation of contrast into a large urinoma. The likely diagnosis is a missed ureteral injury with an infected urinoma. Management in this case consisted of percuatneous drainage of the kidney and urinoma, antibiotics, and delayed repair. As a general radiologic principle of trauma, whether blunt or penetrating, medial extravasation of contrast should raise suspicion for ureteral injury.

❑❑ **This 20-year-old male was involved in a motor vehicle accident. He had multiple long bone fractures . His blood pressure in the field was 70 mmHg but responded quickly to fluids. He had no hematuria. A trauma IVU was performed in the trauma suite. The likely diagnosis is?**

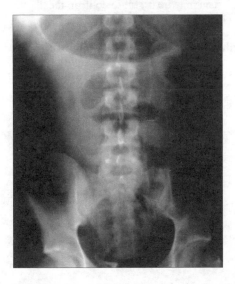

The film shows the left kidney to be functioning normally but there is absence of a nephrogram and function of the right kidney. In addition, there is a fracture of the right L1 transverse process. Fractures of transverse processes in the region of the renal hilum raise concern for a right renovascular injury. An expeditious angiogram or contrasted CT scan would confirm the diagnosis. The presence of shock, hematuria or high suspicion as with major decelerating trauma in the absence of hematuria should prompt urologic evaluation. The advent of high speed CT scanning has largely supplanted the use of IVU in the evaluation of the trauma patient. The two shot trauma IVU consists of a scout film followed by an injection of 1ml/kg of IV contrast. A second film is taken at 10 minutes post contrast injection.

❑❑ **This 50-year-old man presented with poorly localized abdominal pain and was found by ultrasound to have bilateral hydronephrosis and a serum creatinine of 6.0mg/dl. Past history is significant for migraine headaches. The prostate exam is normal and a trial of catheter drainage does not improve things. Bilateral retrograde pyelograms were obtained and the film for the right side is shown and the film on the left was nearly identical. A stent was passed easily on both sides and the creatinine responded and decreased to 2.0 mg/dl. The most likely diagnosis is?**

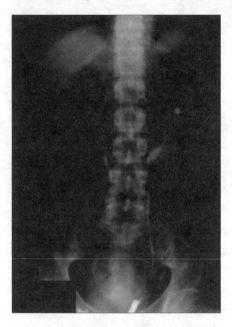 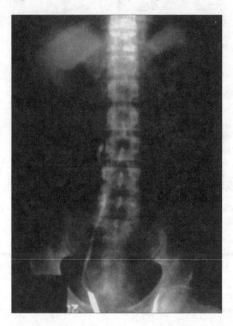

The retrograde pyelogram shows medial deviation of the ureter over the spine. The fact that a stent passed easily makes the diagnosis of stricture less likely and with medial deviation, the diagnosis is most likely retroperitoneal fibrosis. Migraine headaches provide an additional clue as the use of methysergide to treat migraines has been associated with retroperitoneal fibrosis. A CT scan may be useful to confirm the presence of a fibrous mass encircling the aorta and vena cava and encasing the ureters as well.

❑❑ **The prenatal ultrasound of a newborn male showed bilateral hydronephrosis. A follow-up study confirmed the presence of bilateral hydronephrosis. A serum creatinine was 1.7 mg/dl. 3 days post partum. A representative film of the voiding cystourethrogram is shown. The likely diagnosis is?**

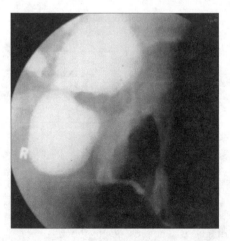

The history of bilateral hydronephrosis should prompt a look at the bladder outlet. A normal bladder outlet should be funnelled and nondilated. This film shows the three key radiographic characteristics of posterior urethral valves, which are dilation and elongation of the posterior urethra and indentation of the bladder neck. The voiding film also shows high pressure, high-grade vesicoureteral reflux, which is frequently seen with posterior urethral valves. The differential would include membranous stricture or external sphincter dysenergia, neither of which fit the history.

❑❑ **This voiding cystourethrogram was obtained in a male infant with undescended testes and bilateral hydronephrosis on ultrasound. The likely diagnosis is?**

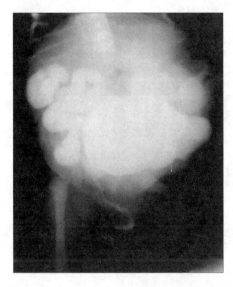

This classic film which needs little history is a case of the Eagle-Barrett or "prune belly" syndrome. The classic triad consists of a male with absent abdominal wall musculature, bilateral undescended testes and urologic anomalies. The rib cage is flared and the flanks are bulging. There is massive reflux bilaterally into tortuous and dilated ureters. In this patient, the posterior urethra is nondilated making the diagnosis of valves unlikely. However, the prostate may be hypoplastic in these patients causing the posterior urethra to appear dilated. The bladder is usually large but smooth walled as obstruction is not generally present.

❑❑ **Here is another voiding cystourethrogram performed in a male infant with hydronephrosis on antenatal ultrasound confirmed in the postnatal period by repeat ultrasound. The diagnosis is?**

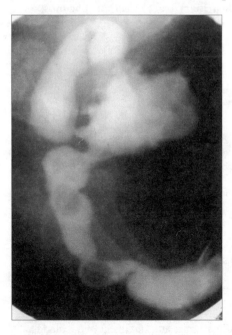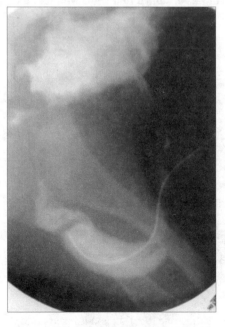

In this case, both the posterior and anterior urethra are dilated and the catheter identifies a "flap" of tissue at the distal end of a diverticulum. There is a heavily trabeculated bladder and at least unilateral massive reflux. The film is classic for anterior urethral diverticulum or anterior urethral valves as another cause of outlet obstruction in newborn males.

❑❑ **This cystogram was obtained in a young male with recurrent febrile urinary tract infections. His physical exam is normal.   The diagnosis is? What is unusual about the film?**

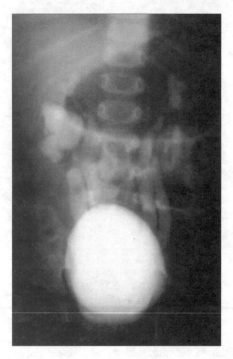

The diagnosis is bilateral vesicoureteral reflux. The cystogram shows high-grade vesicoureteral reflux into duplicate collecting systems on either side. The unusual finding on the film is the presence of reflux into both collecting systems. Because of the Weigert-Meier rule, the lower pole orifice more commonly obstructs and the upper pole system refluxes. However, reflux can occur into both segments. An alternative explanation for this film might be a low lying incomplete duplication with reflux into the solitary orifice on each side.

❑❑ **This cystogram was obtained in a child who had a febrile urinary tract infection. The most likely diagnosis is?**

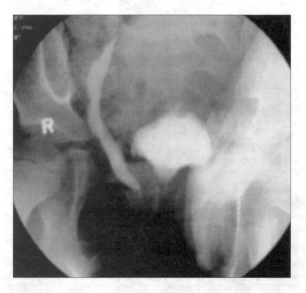

The right ureter is opacified due to reflux and it inserts into the urinary tract at a site distal to the bladder neck. The diagnosis is a refluxing ectopic ureter. In females, ectopic ureters are more often associated with the upper pole segment of duplication while in males; the ureter more commonly drains a non-duplicated system. In females, the ureter may insert into the uterus, vagina, cervix, bladder neck, vestibule or urethra while in males, insertion is most commonly in the bladder neck, prostatic urethra, seminal vesicles, vas deferens, or ejaculatory duct.

❑❑ **This child presented with umbilical discharge. A voiding cystogram was obtained. The diagnosis is?**

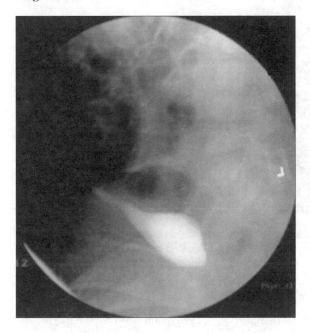

The cystogram shows a patent urachus. While persistence of the urachus has been attributed to intrauterine bladder outlet obstruction, the majority of patients with a patent urachus do not have obstruction.

❑❑ **This is a voiding cystourethrogram obtained in a child who presented with a history of voiding with two streams. The diagnosis is?**

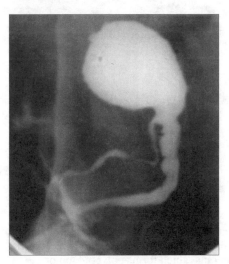

The cystogram shows a sagittal or epispadiac complete urethral duplication. Collateral or side by side duplications also exist and are more often associated with other pelvic anomalies such as imperforate anus or penile duplication. In the overwhelming majority of cases, the ventral urethra is the normal variant.

❑❑ **This cystogram was obtained in a young male who had obstructive urinary symptoms. The likely diagnosis is?**

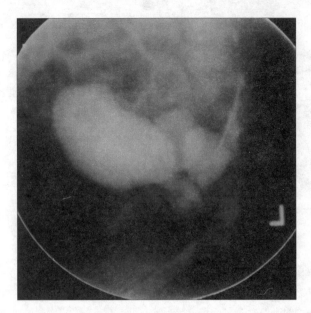

The study shows bilateral congenital bladder diverticula. While bladder diverticula may be associated with posterior urethral valves or neurogenic bladder, they may occur as an isolated entity. In this case, the posterior urethra is non-dilated and the bladder is relatively smooth making these two diagnoses less likely. Diverticula may be associated with infection but also may cause outlet obstructive symptoms. In this case, resection of the diverticulae alone relieved the symptoms.

❐❐ **This 3-year-old female had an episode of gross hematuria. A cystogram was obtained. The likely diagnosis is?**

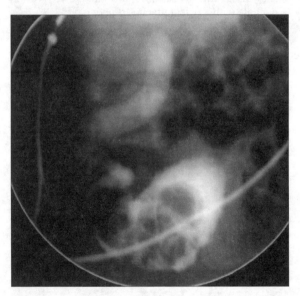

This is another classic cystogram. The classic cystographic appearance of a botryoid rhabdomyosarcoma of the bladder is that of a "cluster of grapes" which the filling defect in this cystogram certainly resembles. Sarcoma botryoides is a variant of embryonal type rhabdomyosarcoma which forms polypoid tumor masses.

❐❐ **This patient was involved in a motor vehicle trauma and had gross hematuria. The patient initially had abdominal CT scanning which was unremarkable. A cystogram was then obtained. The likely diagnosis is?**

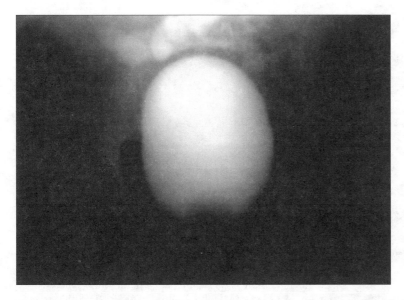

This film illustrates the importance of obtaining a scout film prior to the introduction of bladder contrast. In this case, the diagnosis is suspicious for an intraperitoneal bladder rupture. However the contour of the bladder is smooth and appears to be intact. In fact, it was subsequently proven that the contrast seen was actually oral contrast, which had been given to the patient at the time of CT scanning. Drainage films are also important since extravasation can hide behind the opacified bladder.

❏❏ **This older male had just undergone a transurethral resection of the prostate. A cystogram was obtained at the conclusion of the proceedure because of a concern about a possible bladder perforation. The diagnosis is?**

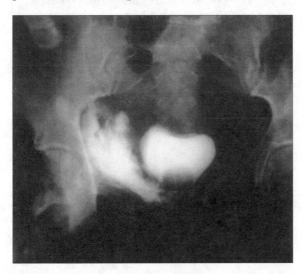

This film shows a classic extraperitoneal bladder rupture. The pattern of contrast extravasation is "flame" shaped and "whispy" in appearance and extends from the base of the bladder cephalad.

❏❏ **This patient was involved in a motor vehicle accident and sustained a pelvic fracture. A retrograde urethrogram was normal and a cystogram was performed. The likely diagnosis is?**

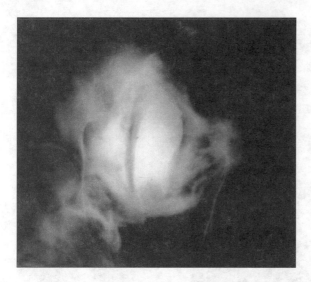

The cystogram shows a classic "teardrop" shape due to compression by the pelvic hematoma. There is "flame" shaped extravasation extending in a whispy fashion from the base of the bladder. The picture is typical for an extraperitoneal bladder rupture. Some concern for intraperitoneal rupture might be raised because of contrast located cephalad to the bladder but there is no obvious contrast outlining loops of bowel. While only 10% of pelvic fractures manifest bladder rupture, virtually 100% of extraperitoneal bladder ruptures are associated with pelvic fracture. Roughly 10% are combined intra- and extraperitoneal injuries. At least 300 cc of water soluble iodinated contrast should be instilled by gravity in order to exclude bladder rupture.

❒❒ **This patient presented following a motor vehicle accident. The patient had been drinking at the local bar prior to the accident. On presentation, he had suprapubic tenderness and a urinalysis showed gross hematuria. He did not have a pelvic fracture by plain film. An abdominal CT scan with a passive " CT cystogram" was normal. In spite of this, a standard trauma cystogram was performed. The study shows?**

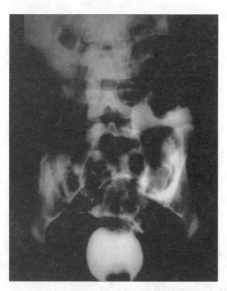

The study shows a classic intraperitoneal bladder rupture. As opposed to extraperitoneal rupture, the contrast outlines loops of bowel and the direction of extravasation is cephalad. Bladder ruptures in which there is significant contrast located cephalad to the bladder should raise suspicion for intraperitoneal rupture. A diagnostic maneuver that may help in equivocal cases is placing the patient in Trendelenberg position and repeating the film. Contrast may be seen over the liver or spleen. An active CT cystogram is usually a very sensitive test but it should be done with the standard 300 cc contrast instillation into the bladder rather than using passive filling by the IV contrast used with CT.

RADIONUCLIDE STUDIES

David M. Albala, M.D., Uday Kumar, M.S., F.R.C.S. and Pramod Reddy, M.D.,

❏❏ What are the half-lives of ^{99m}Tc, ^{123}I and ^{131}I?

The half-lives are 6 hours, 13.2 hours and 8 days respectively.

❏❏ What is a rad?

The amount of radiation energy absorbed by a patient's tissue is expressed in rad. The rad is defined as 100 ergs absorbed per gram of tissue.

❏❏ What is the difference between roentgen and rad?

Roentgen is a measure of ionization of the air by x-rays or gamma rays. Though the terms roentgen and rad are often used interchangeably, it should be remembered that roentgen is a measure of exposure, whereas the rad is a measure of energy absorbed by tissue.

❏❏ What are the most common instruments used to clinically detect ionizing radiation?

Though gas detectors such as Geiger-Muller counters are used in nuclear medicine laboratories, solid crystal detectors are most commonly employed to detect ionizing radiation. The Anger camera used in most departments uses a sodium iodide crystal.

❏❏ What isotopes are used to measure the glomerular filtration rate (GFR)?

Though ^{14}C Inulin would give an accurate measurement of GFR, it is impractical to use. ^{51}Cr EDTA and ^{99m}Tc DTPA are alternatives. In practice, ^{99m}Tc DTPA is usually used, as it also provides excellent renal images.

❏❏ Which isotopes are useful in measuring renal blood flow (RBF)?

^{131}I-Hippuran, ^{123}I-Hippuran and 99mTc-MAG3 are useful. ^{99m}Tc-MAG3 is most commonly used in the USA for these purposes.

❏❏ How is ^{99m}Tc DTPA processed in the kidney?

^{99m}Tc DTPA is filtered and concentrated in the tubules and is then excreted through the collecting system. In the normal kidney activity in the renal pelvis and ureter decrease after 5 to 10 minutes making it a useful test to detect obstruction.

❏❏ What does a DMSA scan demonstrate?

^{99m}Tc DMSA accumulates progressively in the kidneys over several hours and images the renal cortex well. It is useful to detect renal scarring, early stages of renal damage from infection and to differentiate functioning from non-functioning renal masses.

❏❏ What are the common uses of radionuclide studies after renal transplantation?

They are useful in evaluating complications such as complete renal artery occlusion, urinary obstruction or leakage. Acute tubular necrosis and rejection cause reduced perfusion and prolonged parenchymal transit times.

❏❏ **What isotopes are useful in investigating occult suppuration in the abdomen or pelvis?**

Gallium-67 citrate or indium-111 labeled leukocytes is used.

❏❏ **What is the advantage of scanning with indium-111 labeled leukocyte over Gallium-67 citrate in localizing infection?**

Studies with Indium-labeled leukocytes often can be completed in 24 hours whereas those using Gallium-67 may take 48-72 hours to complete. In addition, the latter may be taken up by certain tumors such as lymphomas and hepatomas and is taken up by kidneys and this may confuse the diagnosis.

❏❏ **How is MAG3 (Mercaptoacetylglycine) cleared by the kidney?**

MAG3 is cleared by the kidneys primarily by tubular secretion and to a lesser extent by glomerular filtration. Therefore, it is an excellent agent for estimating the effective renal plasma flow. It is used to define UPJ obstruction and differential renal function.

❏❏ **What is nuclear cystography and what is its value in ureteral reflux?**

It is the scintigraphic equivalent of conventional cystography. It is an accurate method for detecting and following reflux though it does not provide the anatomic detail of fluoroscopic studies.

❏❏ **T/F: In screening siblings for reflux, the nuclear scan is preferable to a standard voiding cystography.**

True. The radiation exposure in a nuclear scan is lower than a cystogram and when anatomic detail of VCUG is not essential, the nuclear scan is preferable.

❏❏ **What are the nuclear scan findings in testicular torsion?**

The testicle appears avascular. In cases of epididymitis hypervascularity is noted. However, in cases of intermittent torsion and late torsion hypervascularity may result from an inflammatory response. Occasional false positive and false negative results and limited availability of the nuclear scan 24 hours a day limit its usefulness in the diagnosis of torsion.

❏❏ **What is the "doughnut sign" on the nuclear scan in testicular torsion?**

In missed torsion, i.e. one that is several days old, there is often an area of hyperemia surrounding the central ischemic area of the testis. The central area appears photopenic surrounded by a rim of increased activity (doughnut).

❏❏ **What factors affect the drainage curve of the nuclear scan in patients with UPJ obstruction?**

In addition to the severity of obstruction, the size and compliance of the collecting system, the hydration of the patient, timing of diuretic and bladder drainage influence the drainage curve. A poorly functioning kidney may not respond adequately to the diuretic.

❏❏ **T/F: The advantages of the ^{99m}Tc DMSA scan over IVU in the evaluation of renal damage from pyelonephritis include: lack of study impairment by bowel gas, earlier detection of renal damage, clear visualization of kidneys despite overlying bony structures, the ability to image the kidneys in various positions to delineate specific lesions and the collecting system is clearly visualized.**

False. All are true except the visualization of the collecting system in the DMSA scan is not nearly as good as with an IVU.

❏❏ **T/F: Captopril is used to improve the accuracy of nuclear scan findings of renovascular hypertension.**

True. Captopril exaggerates the differences between the perfused and non-perfused areas of the kidney in patients with renovascular hypertension.

❑❑ What is a MIBG scan?

Metaiodobezylguanidine (MIBG) is taken up by adrenal neurons. It is labeled with iodine and used to image adrenal medulla and other active adrenergic tissues such as pheochromocytomas and neuroblastomas.

❑❑ How accurate is the MIBG scan in localizing pheochromocytomas and neuroblastomas?

^{123}I MIBG scan is 85-90% sensitive and nearly 100% specific for localizing pheochromocytomas. It is almost 100% specific and 100% sensitive for neuroblastomas.

❑❑ How are nuclear scans helpful in carcinoma of the prostate?

Bone scans with ^{99m}Tc methylenediphosphonate (MDP) are most useful in the staging of prostate cancer. They are over 95% sensitive in detecting bony metastases from carcinoma of the prostate.

❑❑ What is a "superscan" in a patient with prostate cancer?

When there is extensive involvement of the bony skeleton with metastasis in a patient with prostate cancer, the isotope is extensively taken up by the bone and the kidneys are not visualized.

❑❑ Are nuclear scans of use in renal failure?

Yes. ^{123}I and ^{131}I-hippurate and MAG3 can be concentrated even in kidneys with minimal renal function. They are of immense value in patients with renal failure or renal transplantation.

❑❑ What are the features of renal obstruction in a patient with hydronephrosis on a nuclear scan?

During the excretory phase of the scan, the renogram demonstrates increasing activity over time, even after administration of furosemide. But the test may be unreliable in patients with poorly functioning kidneys or massively dilated collecting systems.

❑❑ What is the rationale behind the performance of a Captopril Renogram in the diagnosis of obstructive uropathy?

Renin is secreted by the juxtaglomerular apparatus in renovascular hypertension and/or obstructive uropathy, as a result of poor tissue perfusion. The local vascular regulatory mechanisms of the kidney cause:
1. Release of Thromboxane, causing vasoconstriction of the afferent arteriole, causing a further decrease of renal blood flow
2. Activation of the Renin Angiotensin system (RAS), resulting in the formation of Angiotensin II, which in turn increases the efferent arteriolar tone and is primarily responsible for restoring and maintaining glomerular filtration pressure.

Use of an Angiotensin converting enzyme inhibitor i.e. Captopril can block this mechanism by preventing the vasoconstriction of the efferent arteriole, thereby causing a drop in GFR and relative renal function. This decrease is demonstrable with Captopril renography.

❑❑ What is the dose of Captopril administered for a Captopril Renogram?

0.3 mg/Kg is administered orally 1 hr prior to the radioisotope injection. A change of at least 5% (baseline scan vs. Captopril scan) is considered significant when interpreting the results.

❑❑ What constitutes a "Well-Tempered Renogram"?

The society for Fetal Urology and the Pediatric Nuclear Medicine Council, of the Society of Nuclear Medicine published guidelines for the "Well-Tempered Diuresis Renogram" in 1992.
Small field of view gamma camera is used for pediatric studies
If the child is <4 months old MAG-3 should be the radioisotope used for the study.
In children >4 months of age MAG-3 is still the preferred radioisotope, however DTPA may be substituted for it.

The patient is well hydrated. A normal saline i.v. (15 mL/Kg) over 30 minutes, begun 15 minutes prior to the administration of the radioisotope. For the remainder of the study a maintenance i.v. at 200 mL/Kg/24 hrs is administered.

The child's bladder should be catheterized to prevent any lower urinary tract dysfunction from influencing the results of the study.

Dose of diuretic (Lasix®) should be 1-2 mg/kg i.v.

❑❑ **What is an indirect radionuclide cystogram (IRC)?**

The IRC is a diagnostic test to detect vesico-ureteral reflux (VUR). It employs [^{99m}Tc] DTPA as the radionuclide tracer. It provides information about the emptying phase of the bladder and can demonstrate VUR. Since it does not provide any information about the filling phase, it will miss the 3% of VUR known to occur during this phase of the bladder cycle. The high sensitivity of the IRC combined with the advantages of lower radiation and avoidance of bladder catheterization make it a valuable alternative to the VCUG.

❑❑ **Match the following radionuclide tracers with method of action**

Tracers	Mode of secretion
1. DTPA	A. 80% tubular secretion
2. OIH	B. Both GFR dependent and tubular secretion for clearance
3. MAG-3	C. Localizes to the proximal convoluted tubules (PCT)
4. DMSA	D. Mostly tubular secretion
5. GH	E. GFR dependent for clearance

Answer: 1E, 2A, 3D, 4C, 5B.

❑❑ **What advantages does radionuclide cystography (RNC) have over a standard VCUG?**

The RNC is more sensitive and specific for the detection of vesico-ureteral reflux than a VCUG. It also has a significantly lower gonadal radiation dose (RNC = 0.001-0.005 rads vs. VCUG = 0.208 rads).

The disadvantages of RNC are:
1. Limited ability to grade reflux
2. Does not provide additional radiographic data i.e. presence of constipation or bony abnormalities etc.

❑❑ **In a child presenting with flank pain, high fever and dysuria, which radionuclide study would be appropriate to order?**

The child has features suggesting an acute pyelonephritis. DMSA renal imaging has been shown to demonstrate areas of decreased perfusion (inflammation vs. scar) in the kidneys. In order to differentiate between scar and inflammation, a renal ultrasound could be used or one could repeat DMSA scan in 6 months. Persistent cortical defects represent parenchymal scars.

❑❑ **What is the role of radionuclide imaging in the management of a duplex collecting system with an obstructed upper pole moiety?**

Radionuclide scanning (with a cortical agent) can provide information about the degree of function and amount of functioning renal tissue in each moiety of the duplex kidney. In case of an obstructed upper pole moiety, it will also serve as a diagnostic test to determine efficacy of the surgical intervention.

❑❑ **Are there any potential complications to keep in mind or to counsel the parents about, while ordering a radionuclide study?**

For the most part nuclear medicine studies are quite safe; the radiation dose involved is minimal. There is a small risk of a nosocomial UTI from urethral catheterization in radionuclide cystography. Some children may experience significant abdominal discomfort during a Lasix renogram, especially if they have intermittent obstruction and the study reproduces an obstructive episode.

❑❑ **Are there any contraindications to performing a radionuclide study on a patient?**

There are no absolute contraindications to the use of radionuclides for diagnostic purposes. A relative contraindication is pregnancy, therefore nuclear medicine scanning should not be performed on patients in the reproductive age group without first performing a pregnancy test.

❏❏ **Is there a role for radionuclide scanning in the acute evaluation of a trauma patient?**

The advent of ultra fast spiral CT scanners has changed the imaging algorithm for the evaluation of the trauma patient. There was never a clear indication for radionuclide imaging of the trauma patient. In certain select cases radionuclide scanning with a renal cortical agent might be indicated to evaluate the degree of function and amount of functioning renal tissue.

❏❏ **What is the best radionuclide agent to use in a one-month-old infant with severe hydronephrosis, suggestive of bilateral ureteropelvic junction obstruction?**

Normally it is not recommended to perform a Lasix scan on children below 3 months of age due to the relative functional immaturity of the kidneys, which limits the reliability of the results. However there are instances where the physician has to perform the test sooner, as in the above clinical case. In such instances MAG-3 is the agent of choice, as it has lower uptake in the liver and spleen and higher renal extraction providing a better target to background ratio.

❏❏ **In what clinical setting is "static" radionuclide imaging utilized?**

Static radionuclide imaging is used to evaluate vesico-ureteral reflux, urinary tract infections, hypertension and cystic diseases of the kidney. It can document renal scarring, acute pyelonephritis and differential renal function.

❏❏ **In what clinical settings is "dynamic" radionuclide imaging utilized?**

Dynamic renal functional imaging is useful for evaluating a suspected obstruction in cases of possible uretero-pelvic junction obstruction and megaureters (although the t1/2 values are of limited clinical relevance, in light of the compliance of the dilated ureter). It is also useful in evaluating renal function in cystic kidney diseases, hypertension, after a renal transplant and pyeloplasty.

❏❏ **What is "SPECT" radionuclide scanning?**

"SPECT" (Single Photon Emission Computed Tomography) is an imaging technique associated with single gamma ray emitting radiopharmaceuticals. The images are obtained using a scintillation camera, which moves around the patient to capture images from multiple angles for tomographic image reconstruction. It results in better image quality and improves the sensitivity of the test.

RETROPERITONEAL ANATOMY

Graham F. Greene, M.D.

☐☐ **When closing a flank incision, which muscle layer has an obvious free border?**

The external oblique muscle has a free border laterally that extends from the lower border of the 12th rib to its aponeurotic insertion along the iliac crest.

☐☐ **Between what 2 muscle layers do the intercostal nerves and vessels course?**

They course between the transversus abdominis and the internal oblique muscles. This is important when closing incisions to avoid entrapment of these structures.

☐☐ **What is another name for Gerota's fascia?**

Perirenal fascia or Gerota's fascia is a specialized condensation within the intermediate stratum of the retroperitoneal connective tissue. It forms a barrier to benign and malignant processes.

☐☐ **Does Gerota's fascia form a tight seal around each kidney?**

No. Gerota's fascia is weakest at its caudal aspect along the course of the gonadal vessels and ureter.

☐☐ **When resecting a large left upper pole renal mass from an anterior approach, what medial attachments need to be divided to allow reflection of the spleen, pancreas and stomach?**

Division of the phrenicocolic, splenorenal, the gastrosplenic, and the gastrophrenic ligaments, will allow reflection of the spleen, pancreas, and stomach from the craniolateral aspect of the retroperitoneum exposing the upper pole of the left kidney and adrenal gland.

☐☐ **What surgical maneuver will allow access to the intra and supra-hepatic vena cava?**

Division of the right and left triangular ligaments and continuing the incision along the cranial and caudal coronary ligaments will allow reflection of the right lobe of the liver, providing dramatic exposure to the inferior vena cava as it receives the hepatic veins and perforates the diaphragm.

☐☐ **What nerve is commonly seen coursing anterolaterally in the inguinal canal?**

The ilioinguinal nerve (L1) courses through the inguinal canal on the cord to exit the external ring and provide sensation to the pubic area.

☐☐ **What other nerve besides the ilioinguinal nerve follows the cord through the inguinal canal?**

The genital branch of the genitofemoral nerve (L1, L2). It is less conspicuous than the ilioinguinal nerve and has a dual function supplying motor innervation to the cremasteric muscle and sensation to the anterior scrotum or labia majora.

☐☐ **What nerve is clearly visualized coursing along the ventrum of the psoas muscle and proves useful in defining the lateral border for a complete pelvic lymph node dissection?**

The genitofemoral nerve (L1, L2) serves a dual purpose in supplying motor function to the cremasteric muscle and sensation to the perineum and anterior thigh.

❏❏ Define the arterial blood supply of the right adrenal gland.

The right adrenal receives its blood supply from 3 main sources. The 2 obvious ones include branches from the inferior phrenic artery as well as branches from the right renal artery. A branch that is often forgotten that passes behind the inferior vena cava is the middle adrenal artery. This can lead to significant bleeding if unrecognized and cut during a right adrenalectomy.

❏❏ Into what structures do the gonadal vessels on either side drain?

The right gonadal vein enters the inferior vena cava on its ventral lateral aspect at an oblique angle. The left gonadal vein empties into the left renal vein.

❏❏ What is the significance of a varicocele that does not diminish when examined in the supine position?

Suspect a retroperitoneal mass or process that is impairing venous drainage such as lymphoma, testicular cancer, renal cell carcinoma, or retroperitoneal fibrosis.

❏❏ What are the primary sites of lymphatic drainage from the left testis?

The most common site on the left side is the left para-aortic lymph nodes followed by the preaortic, interaortocaval, left common iliac, and left suprarenal lymph nodes in decreasing order. Left to right lymphatic drainage tends not to occur unless there is lymphatic obstruction.

❏❏ What are the primary sites of lymphatic drainage from the right testis?

The most common site on the right side is the inter-aortocaval lymph nodes followed by precaval, preaortic, right paracaval, right common iliac and left para-aortic lymph nodes in decreasing order. Lymphatic drainage proceeds from the right to left side of the retroperitoneum. Alternative routes can occur when there is lymphatic obstruction.

❏❏ Which division of the renal artery supplies the majority of the kidney?

The anterior division supplies over 75% of the kidney, including apical, upper, middle and lower vascular segments of the kidney. The posterior renal artery supplies the majority of the dorsal aspect of the kidney.

❏❏ How often can a surgeon anticipate accessory renal arteries?

In 25-40% of cases there is more than 1 renal artery arising from the lateral aorta at the level of the second lumbar vertebra. Accessory renal arteries to the right lower pole will often cross anterior to the vena cava. It becomes important to recognize such branches so that they are not divided when exposing the right renal hilum.

❏❏ Where do the renal pelvis and the upper ureter receive their arterial blood supply?

There are 3 anastomosing arteries providing the upper ureter and renal pelvis with blood supply. They include the renal artery, aorta, and gonadal artery.

❏❏ Which adrenal gland is more intimate with the cranial aspect of the kidney?

The left adrenal gland is most intimate with the cranial aspect of the left kidney. It often will drape over the ventral aspect of the upper pole. The right adrenal gland is decidedly cranial to the right kidney, and care must be given when removing it due to its short adrenal vein entering dorsolaterally into the inferior vena cava.

❏❏ What is an alternate route for venous drainage of the left adrenal gland?

The left inferior phrenic vein. The adrenal gland vein drains into the left renal vein. Close to where it enters it is joined by the inferior phrenic vein which cranially also empties into the inferior vena cava above the level of the hepatic veins. This means that you can divide the adrenal vein at the level of the renal vein without compromising its venous drainage.

❐❐ **Does ligation of the gonadal arteries at the level of the aorta compromise the gonads?**

No. The rich collateral circulation provided by the artery to the vas deferens and external spermatic artery in the male and the uterine artery in the female provide collateral blood supply to the gonad.

❐❐ **What are the first branches of the intraabdominal aorta?**

The paired inferior phrenic arteries are the first branches of the intraabdominal aorta. They give origin to the superior supraadrenal arteries.

❐❐ **What are the 3 main arterial blood supplies to the small bowel and colon?**

They include the superior mesenteric artery, inferior mesenteric artery, and the inferior and middle hemorrhoidal arteries which are branches from the internal iliac artery.

❐❐ **When is it possible to completely resect the infrahepatic vena cava for renal cell carcinoma and an IVC thrombus?**

It is possible to resect the infrahepatic vena cava when removing a large right renal mass and associated renal vein thrombus. This is due to the rich collateral venous drainage of the left kidney through the lumbar (azygos) system. The right kidney is not afforded a similar venous drainage.

❐❐ **Other than the gonadal vein, what other vein drains into the caudal aspect of the left renal vein?**

A left lumbar vein. This large lumbar vein provides collateral venous drainage as well as a potential source of bleeding when ligating the left renal vein.

❐❐ **If the inferior mesenteric artery is ligated during a retroperitoneal lymph node dissection, what artery insures blood supply to the upper rectum, sigmoid colon, descending colon, and part of the left transverse colon?**

The marginal artery of Drummond. This artery provides collateral circulation between the superior mesenteric artery and the inferior and middle hemorrhoidal vessels.

❐❐ **When assessing left para-aortic lymphadenopathy on CT scan, what clue helps you distinguish retroperitoneal structures from mesenteric structures?**

At the level of the L3 vertebra (or inferior pole of the kidneys) the inferior mesenteric artery and inferior mesenteric vein run in a cranio-caudal direction. The ureter can be seen posteriolateral to these distinct vessels. Any structures dorsomedial are in the retroperitoneal space as compared to ventrolateral structures which are in the mesentery or coelomic space.

❐❐ **In what direction does most lateral lumbar lymphatic flow proceed?**

Right to left. The lymphatics coalesce posterior to the aorta to form a localized dilation of lymphatic chain known as the cisterna chyli. This structure lies in a retrocrural position, just anterior to the first or second lumbar vertebra, and empties into the thoracic duct through the aortic hiatus of the diaphragm.

❐❐ **What is Kocher's Maneuver?**

The Kocher maneuver refers to the surgical reflection of the second and third part of the duodenum craniomedially to provide access to the right renal vessels and inferior vena cava. When combined with mobilization of the small bowel mesentery, this maneuver exposes the great vessels in anticipation of retroperitoneal dissection. It is important to recognize that the Kocher maneuver also mobilizes the head or uncinate process of the pancreas. Carefully placed retraction in this area will help prevent pancreatic injury.

❐❐ **What happens to the ipsilateral adrenal gland in cases of renal ectopia or agenesis?**

They will present in their normal anticipated location within the retroperitoneum. The adrenal glands are embryologically and functionally distinct from the kidneys. Physically they are separated from the kidneys by connective tissue septa that is in continuity with Gerota's fascia as well as varying amounts of perinephric fat.

□□ During embryological development the adrenal medulla has received what specialized cells and from where?

The adrenal medulla consists of chromaffin cells, which are derived from the neural crest and are intimately associated with the sympathetic nervous system. Chromaffin cells belong to the family of APUD (amine precursor uptake decarboxylase) cells and produce neuroactive catecholamines that are released directly into the blood stream.

□□ What zone of the adrenal cortex produces glucocorticoids?

The zona fasciculata. The adrenal gland consist of 3 zones or strata. The outermost layer of cells make up the zona glomerulosa which produce aldosterone (mineralocorticoids). The next layer is the zona fasciculata which produces glucocorticoids, and in the normal adrenal gland is usually the thickest of the 3 layers. The innermost zona reticularis is responsible for producing sex steroids.

□□ Which layer of the adrenal cortex is not regulated by pituitary release of adrenocorticotropic hormone (ACTH)?

The zona glomerulosa is not under direct pituitary regulation by ACTH. The zona glomerulosa which is the outermost layer of the adrenal cortex produces aldosterone in response to stimulation by the renin-angiotensin system.

□□ On which kidney can you find a (dromedary hump)?

Both. This normal variation of renal contour is found much more commonly on the left than the right side. It is seen as a focal bulge on the mid-lateral border of the kidney.

□□ Between what 2 layers is the para-renal (paranephric) fat located?

Between the transversalis fascia and Gerota's fascia. Within Gerota's fascia the kidney is suspended in the perirenal fat. Depending upon the body habitus of the patient, varying amounts of para-renal fat can be found external to Gerota's fascia. When surgically approaching the kidney, the transversalis fascia can sometimes be mistaken for Gerota's fascia due to the underlying para-renal fat. Failure to incise transversalis fascia impends access to the retroperitoneum.

□□ Which segmental branch of the main renal artery is most constant?

The posterior segmental artery is most constant. Prior to entering the renal hilum, the main renal artery divides into an anterior and posterior division. The posterior segmental artery supplies the majority of the dorsum of the kidney, whereas the anterior division gives rise to four anterior segmental arteries (apical, upper, middle, and lower) supplying the rest of the kidney. During nephron sparing surgery, mistaking the often long posterior segmental artery for the main renal artery can lead to incomplete arterial occlusion and blood loss.

□□ Describe intra-renal arterial anatomy.

The renal artery divides into 4 or 5 segmental branches including the posterior, apical, upper, middle and lower segmental renal arteries. The segmental arteries travel through the renal sinus and branch to give rise to lobar arteries. These lobar arteries divide again and enter the renal parenchyma as interlobar arteries and traverse the renal parenchyma through the renal columns of Bertin. At the base of the renal pyramids, the interlobar arteries branch into the arcuate arteries. In turn, the arcuate arteries branch to give rise to multiple interlobular arteries. These interlobular arteries branch within the renal cortex giving rise to the afferent arterioles of the glomerular capsule and contributing small branches to the renal capsular plexus. Blood leaves the glomerulus via the efferent arteriole and meets the venous system at the vasa recta within the renal medulla or through a capillary network within the cortex.

□□ What is implied when renal arteries are referred to as end arteries?

The renal artery and its successive branches do not have anastomosis or collateral circulation. Therefore occlusion of any of these vessels will result in ischemia and infarction of the renal parenchyma that it supplies.

❏❏ **Describe renal venous drainage.**

The capillary bed within the cortex and the vas recta drain into interlobular veins, and then into arcuate, interlobar, lobar, and segmental veins respectively. There are usually 3 to 5 segmental veins that empty into a main renal vein. Unlike renal arteries, renal parenchymal veins anastomose freely, especially in the arcuate vessels.

❏❏ **Within the kidney where are the stellate veins located?**

The stellate veins form a subcapsular venous plexus that form a communication between the interlobular veins and veins within the perinephric fat.

❏❏ **How can renal vasculature obstruct the urinary collecting system?**

Accessory lower pole arteries may cross anterior to the urinary collecting system. In that orientation they can become an extrinsic cause of ureteral pelvic junction obstruction.

❏❏ **What is the significance of the anatomical landmark along the convex border of the kidney called "Brodel's white line"?**

It is often mistaken for the relative avascular plane of the kidney used to gain access to the renal collecting system during an anatrophic nephrolithotomy. The white line of Brodel is a longitudinal crease 1-2 cm ventral to the convex border of the kidney. The actual location of the avascular longitudinal plane lies 1-2 cm dorsal to the convex border of the kidney between the posterior segmental circulation and the anterior.

❏❏ **Within the nephron of the kidney, describe the location and function of the juxtaglomerular apparatus.**

The juxtaglomerular apparatus is a specialized association between the proximal aspect of the distal convoluted tubule and the afferent renal arteriole. Specialized macula densa cells within the renal tubule detect changes with intratubular sodium concentration. They communicate with juxtaglomerular cells of the afferent arteriole which are responsible for secreting renin into the afferent arteriole and renal lymph. The juxtaglomerular cells will respond to changes in wall tension and receive input from renal nerves that can stimulate renin secretion.

❏❏ **Within the renal collecting system, what is the significance of compound papillae?**

When 2 renal pyramids fuse during their development they form a "compound" papillae. They usually occur at the renal poles. Their physiological significance lies in the fact that the configuration of the collecting ducts (of Bellini) allows for reflux of urine and potentially bacteria into the kidney. Renal parenchymal scarring secondary to infection is typically most severe overlying these compound papillae.

❏❏ **Describe the anatomy of a major calyx?**

There are usually 2 to 3 major calyces within a kidney. Each major calyx receives 2 or more infundibula, each of which drain 2 or more minor calyces.

❏❏ **Describe the muscle layers of the ureter.**

The smooth muscle layers of the ureter orient themselves in two layers: the inner longitudinal layer and an outer layer of circular and oblique muscle. The ureter's muscle wall is thickest in its pelvic portion. The circular and oblique fibers become integrated into the smooth muscle of the bladder and Waldeyer's ring. The inner longitudinal muscle fibers traverse the intramural ureter towards the ureteral orifice and trigone.

❏❏ **What are the 3 distinct narrowings normally present along the course of the ureter?**

The first of these is the ureteropelvic junction, the second is the crossing of the iliac vessels, and the third is the ureterovesical junction within the bladder.

□□ What is the nomenclature used to describe ureteral segments intraoperatively and for radiological purposes?

The ureter can be divided into an abdominal and pelvic portion. The abdominal ureter extends from the renal pelvis to the iliac vessels. The pelvic portion extends from the iliac vessels down to the bladder. For radiologic purposes the ureter can be divided into upper, middle and lower segments. The upper segment extends from the renal pelvis to the upper border of the sacrum. The mid ureter lies between the upper and lower borders of the sacrum. The lower ureteral segment extends from the lower border of the sacrum to the bladder.

□□ Describe the innervation of the kidney.

The kidney receives preganglionic sympathetic fibers from T8 (thoracic) through L1 (lumbar) spinal segments. Postganglionic fibers arise from ciliac and periaortic ganglia. Parasympathetic innervation arises from the lesser and lower splanchnic nerves as well as the vagus nerve.

□□ Describe the innervation of the ureter.

The ureter receives preganglionic sympathetic fibers from T10 through L2 spinal segments. Postganglionic fibers arise from ganglia in the aortorenal, superior and inferior hypogastric plexus. Parasympathetic input arises from the second through fourth sacral spinal segments.

□□ Does the ureter require autonomic innervation to maintain peristalsis?

Intrinsic pacemaker sites located in the minor calices of the collecting system initiate the contraction, which is then propagated down the ureter.

□□ What is necessary for any abdominal hernia (including inguinial hernias) to occur?

A defect (weakness) in the transversalis facsia which is the outer stratum of the retroperitoneal connective tissue is essential for a hernia to occur.

SURGICAL ANATOMY
OF THE PELVIS

Jonathan I. Izawa, B.Sc., M.D., F.R.C.S.(C) and Colin P. N. Dinney, M.D., F.R.C.S.(C)

❏❐ **What is the thinnest of the pelvic bones?**

The pubic bones, which are often fractured in blunt pelvic trauma and their fragments may injure the bladder, urethra and vagina.

❏❐ **T/F: The sacroiliac (SI) joint is often fractured in pelvic trauma.**

False. The synovial SI joint gains additional strength from anterior and posterior ligaments and fractures rarely involve this joint.

❏❐ **What are the origins of the muscles of the pelvic diaphragm?**

The origin of the pubococcygeus and iliococcygeus muscles is the tendinous arch of the levator ani.

❏❐ **What types of muscle fibers make up the pelvic diaphragm?**

Type I (slow-twitch) and type II (fast-twitch) fibers. These provide tonic support of the pelvic contents and allow for sudden increases in intra-abdominal pressure respectively.

❏❐ **What organs does the inner stratum cover in the pelvis and what clinical importance is related to the inner stratum?**

The inner stratum covers the rectum and the dome of the bladder. It also forms Denonvilliers' fascia, which acts as a barrier and contributes to the low rate of local extension of prostate cancer into the rectum.

❏❐ **The endopelvic fascia is continuous with what layer of the abdominal wall?**

The transversalis fascia.

❏❐ **What fascial structure extends medially from the arcus tendineus fascia in the female pelvis? What is the clinical significance of this structure?**

This structure is referred to as the periurethral, pubovesical or urethropelvic ligament and it provides support to the urethra and anterior vaginal wall. Compromise to this fascia may contribute to stress urinary incontinence, bladder neck hypermobility, cystocele or urethrocele formation.

❏❐ **T/F: The strength of the pelvic fascia can differ among individuals.**

True. Weakness in this fascia may predispose individuals to urinary incontinence or pelvic prolapse.

❏❐ **T/F: As the dorsal vein of the penis passes within the pelvis under the pubic arch it forms a venous complex and part of this complex runs within the anterior and lateral walls of the striated urinary sphincter.**

True. One must be cautious during ligation and division of the dorsal venous complex, as damage to the striated sphincter can occur.

❏❏ **What anatomic reason may account for the relatively higher incidence of axial skeletal and pelvic bone metastases in patients with metastatic prostate cancer, as opposed to lung metastases for example?**

There are numerous interconnections between the pelvic venous plexuses and the emissary veins of the pelvic bones and vertebral venous plexuses, which may be routes of dissemination of infection or tumor from the diseased prostate.

❏❏ **What accessory artery has its origin off the inferior epigastric artery and can be identified medial to the femoral vein during pelvic surgery?**

The accessory obturator artery arises from the inferior epigastric artery in 25% of patients and continues on through the obturator canal.

❏❏ **What is the most common origin of the superior vesical artery?**

The proximal portion of the obliterated umbilical artery.

❏❏ **What structures does the middle rectal artery supply?**

The middle rectal artery anastomoses with the superior and inferior rectal arteries to supply the rectum. It also gives small branches to provide additional arterial supply to the seminal vesicles and prostate.

❏❏ **What accessory vein drains into the inferior surface of the external iliac vein in at least 50% of patients?**

The accessory obturator vein. Care must be taken to not tear this vein at the time of pelvic lymph node dissection.

❏❏ **During a psoas hitch procedure, in which direction should the sutures be placed and why?**

The sutures should be placed in the direction of the muscle fibers and femoral nerve to avoid femoral nerve entrapment or damage. Caution must also be taken with retractor blades on the psoas muscle for prolonged periods, as this may also cause a femoral nerve palsy.

❏❏ **What nerve is located lateral to the psoas muscle in the iliacus fascia?**

The lateral femoral cutaneous nerve ($L_{2,3}$).

❏❏ **During a radical cystectomy in a 65-year old male for clinical T3a transitional cell carcinoma of the bladder, you notice a nerve visible on the surface of the right psoas major muscle has been damaged by an electrosurgical injury. What sensory loss do you anticipate this patient may experience if the nerve function cannot be salvaged?**

The right genitofemoral ($L_{1,2}$)nerve has been injured. Sensory loss to the anterior right thigh below the inguinal ligament and the anterior right hemi-scrotum may occur.

❏❏ **A 67-year old male three months post-radical retropubic prostatectomy, but otherwise healthy, describes difficulty in moving his left leg into the car when he is on the driver's side. He has noticed this only in the postoperative period. What nerve injury likely occurred during his surgery?**

The patient likely sustained a left obturator nerve ($L_{2,3,4}$) injury. The obturator nerve supplies the adductor muscles of the thigh.

❏❏ **Where is the obturator nerve located in relation to the obturator artery and vein?**

The obturator nerve ($L_{2,3,4}$) lies lateral and superior to the obturator vessels.

❏❏ **During a sacrospinous culposuspension, what nerve or nerve plexus is at relatively higher risk of being injured?**

The sacral plexus, as it leaves the pelvis via the greater sciatic foramen and is immediately posterior to the sacrospinous ligament. If injured, there may be sensory and motor nerve supply compromise to the posterior thigh and lower leg.

❑❑ **Where is the sacral plexus located?**

The sacral plexus is located on the surface of the piriformis muscle, deep to the endopelvic fascia and posterior to the internal iliac vessels.

❑❑ **What nerve passes through the greater sciatic foramen and supplies sensory branches to the perineum and posterior aspect of the scrotum?**

The posterior femoral cutaneous nerve ($S_{2,3}$).

❑❑ **Where is the location and anatomic orientation of the pelvic plexus?**

The pelvic plexus is rectangular, 4-5cm in length, oriented in the sagittal plane and is located at its midpoint at the tip of the seminal vesicles.

❑❑ **What are the anatomic relations of the communicating nerve fibers of the left and right components of the pelvic plexus?**

These fibers communicate posterior to the rectum, as well as anterior and posterior to the bladder neck.

❑❑ **T/F: There is no pelvic parasympathetic efferent innervation to the descending and sigmoid colon.**

False. Some pelvic parasympathetic efferent fibers travel up the hypogastric nerves to the inferior mesenteric plexus, where they will subsequently provide innervation to the descending and sigmoid colon.

❑❑ **T/F: Longitudinal smooth muscle fibers from the rectum join Denonvilliers' fascia.**

True. The fibers are located anteriorly at the inferior portion of the rectal ampulla.

❑❑ **T/F: Intramural longitudinal vessels run the length of the ureter in 75% of patients.**

True. These vessels are formed by anastomoses of segmental ureteral vessels. In the other 25% of patients, the intramural ureteral vessels form a fine interconnecting mesh with less collateral flow and renders the ureter more prone to ischemic insult. This intramural, interconnecting mesh-like vascular pattern is often found in the pelvic ureter and therefore, this portion of the ureter is less suited for ureteroureterostomy.

❑❑ **T/F: The pelvic ureter has rich adrenergic and cholinergic autonomic nerve supply and will lose its peristaltic activity if it is denervated.**

False. The ureter will continue to have peristaltic activity despite its pelvic denervation and this is driven from pacemakers in the upper urinary tract.

❑❑ **In a normal adult male, at what anatomic location are the ureters closest to each other?**

The ureters are closest and are located within 5cm of each other as they cross the iliac vessels.

❑❑ **What arteries usually supply the ureter with its largest pelvic branches?**

The inferior vesical and uterine arteries.

❑❑ **Where does the ureteral smooth muscle terminate distally?**

The verumontanum. The muscle of the trigone is made up of three distinct layers, the superficial layer, derived from the longitudinal smooth muscle of the ureter, extends down to the verumontanum.

☐☐ Where does the bulk of the lymphatic fluid from the bladder drain?

The external iliac lymph nodes. Some drainage may go to the obturator, internal iliac and common iliac lymph nodes.

☐☐ During a radical cystectomy / anterior exenteration in a 65-year-old female patient with clinical T3a transitional cell carcinoma of the bladder, what ligaments are part of the lateral and posterior bladder pedicles that will be divided.

The cardinal and uterosacral ligaments.

☐☐ T/F: The bladder wall has many post-ganglionic cell bodies.

True. The vast majority of these synapse with parasympathetic cholinergic nerve endings.

☐☐ T/F: Presacral neurectomies are effective in relieving bladder pain.

False. Afferent innervation from the bladder travels with the parasympathetic nerves, as well as the sympathetic nerves, which travel via the hypogastric nerves.

☐☐ During a radical retropubic prostatectomy the endopelvic fascia is divided lateral to the arcus tendineus fascia pelvis and is mobilized off the levator ani medially with the prostate. Is this endopelvic fascia visceral or parietal?

Parietal endopelvic fascia.

☐☐ T/F: Normal prostatic glands may be within the striated urethral sphincter.

True. There is no fibromuscular stroma or prostate capsule with these glands.

☐☐ What is the principal arterial supply to prostatic adenomas in benign prostatic hyperplasia?

The inferior vesical arteries have urethral artery branches which enter the prostate posterolaterally at its junction with the bladder and these branches are the principal arterial supply to the adenomas.

☐☐ Can a local anesthetic achieve a prostatic block?

Yes. It must be instilled into the pelvic plexus to block all afferent neurons.

☐☐ T/F: Bilateral pudendal nerve injury will always cause loss of striated external sphincter function at the level of the membranous urethra.

False. The striated sphincter has additional somatic nerve supply from a branch off the sacral plexus and it is located on the levator ani. Autonomic innervation from the cavernous nerves is also present, but this may not be significant for urinary continence.

☐☐ To what nodal location(s) do the lymphatics of the vas deferens and seminal vesicles drain?

The external and internal iliac lymph nodes.

☐☐ What structures do the uterine arteries supply?

The proximal vagina, uterus and medial two-thirds of the fallopian tubes.

☐☐ What course do the nerves from the pelvic plexus travel to reach the female pelvic viscera?

The nerves from the pelvic plexus travel through the cardinal and uterosacral ligaments. During a hysterectomy, these ligaments are divided and therefore, may result in a neurogenic bladder.

☐☐ Which nerve crosses the distal end of the external iliac artery?

The genital branch of the genitofemoral nerve.

❐❐ **What two branches of the external iliac artery are within the pelvis?**

The inferior epigastric and the deep circumflex iliac arteries.

❐❐ **At what anatomic site does the internal iliac artery branch into its anterior and posterior trunks?**

The greater sciatic foramen.

❐❐ **Where is the obturator artery origin?**

The obturator artery has a variable origin. It can arise from the anterior trunk of the internal iliac artery, the inferior epigastric artery or the inferior gluteal artery.

❐❐ **The middle sacral vein is usually a tributary of which vein?**

The left common iliac vein.

❐❐ **T/F: The external iliac lymph nodes can be further separated anatomically and functionally into three chains.**

True. The external, middle and internal chains. For example, the external chain does not receive any lymphatic drainage from organs within the pelvis and these lymph nodes are located lateral to the external iliac vessels.

❐❐ **What is unique about the Cherney incision?**

This incision involves access to the pelvic cavity and detaches the rectus muscles from the symphysis.

❐❐ **What forms the arcus tendineus fascia pelvis?**

Fusion of the visceral and parietal components of the pelvic fascia forms the arcus tendineus fascia pelvis. It appears as a white line of condensation within the pelvis that runs in a sulcus lateral to the prostate from the puboprostatic ligaments to the ischial spine.

❐❐ **Is smooth muscle present within the puboprostatic ligaments?**

Yes. There are smooth muscle fibers within the puboprostatic ligaments derived from the outer layer of detrusor musculature. Once the puboprostatic ligaments are divided during a radical retropubic prostatectomy, the ligaments contract due to their smooth muscle components and are no longer apparent.

❐❐ **T/F: In approximately 10% of patients undergoing radical retropubic prostatectomy, the superficial dorsal vein of the penis appears to be absent.**

True.

❐❐ **What areas of a normal bladder may be more prone to diverticular formation?**

The dome of the bladder where the urachus anchors the apex of the bladder to the anterior abdominal wall due to a paucity of detrusor muscle at this site. The hiatus in the detrusor where the intramural ureter passes is also more prone to diverticular formation.

❐❐ **During cystoscopic examination of a normal bladder, the urothelium over the trigone appears smooth relative to the surrounding urothelium. Why is this observation so?**

The urothelium over the trigone is usually three cells thick and the lamina propria is dense here with strongly adherent epithelial cells. Therefore, during changes in bladder volume, the trigonal epithelium remains smooth in appearance endoscopically.

❑❑ **T/F: The entire prostate is enclosed by a capsule composed of collagen, elastin and abundant smooth muscle.**

False. The prostate is devoid of a capsule at the apex and base, therefore no true capsule separates the prostate from the striated urethral sphincter or the bladder. The capsule is composed of collagen, elastin and abundant smooth muscle and is continuous with the prostatic stroma.

❑❑ **When an accessory pudendal artery is present and is supplementing or replacing penile arterial supply by the common penile artery, what is its origin and anatomic course in relation to the prostate gland?**

An accessory pudendal artery is present in about 4% of patients undergoing a radical retropubic prostatectomy and arises from the inferior vesical artery or obturator artery. It runs anterolateral to or within the prostate to reach the penis.

❑❑ **What three muscles combine to make up the pubococcygeus muscle in the female?**

The pubococcygeus muscle is a thick "U-shaped" muscle band comprised of three sections: the pubovaginalis muscle anteriorly, the puborectalis muscle and the puboanalis muscle. These muscles pull the rectum, vagina and urethra anteriorly against the pubic bone to compress the lumen of each.

❑❑ **What is the primary muscular component of urethral support in the female?**

The pubovaginalis muscle, which is the most anterior part of the levator ani.

❑❑ **While performing the incision for a radical retropubic prostatectomy, the pyrimidalis muscle is observed to be present. What is the innervation of this muscle?**

The twelfth thoracic nerve. Contraction of this muscle tenses the linea alba.

❑❑ **During a radical cystectomy and pelvic lymph node dissection, care should be taken to avoid dissection below the presacral fascia. Why?**

This dissection may disturb the presacral veins and cause unnecessary blood loss.

❑❑ **What is the lymph node of Cloquet's anatomic location?**

The lymph node of Cloquet lies within the femoral canal, medial to the external iliac vein and beneath the inguinal ligament.

❑❑ **What structure is often described as the inferolateral limit of a pelvic lymph node dissection in a radical cystectomy?**

The genitofemoral nerves. The fibroareolar tissue is divided medial to this structure in a pelvic lymph node dissection during a radical cystectomy.

❑❑ **T/F: In a nerve sparing cystoprostatectomy, the unilateral internal iliac artery should be ligated and divided to improve hemostasis and facilitate the nerve sparing procedure, thereby possibly maintaining erectile function.**

False. The internal iliac artery should be preserved and the superior vesical artery should be ligated and divided proximally in order to maintain the integrity of the internal pudendal artery and to prevent vasculogenic erectile dysfunction.

❑❑ **If the right common iliac artery is ligated, what principal vessels may contribute to collateral circulation?**

The anastomoses of the following allow collateral circulation:
1. The middle rectal branch of the internal iliac artery with the superior rectal artery from the inferior mesenteric artery.

2. The uterine, ovarian and vesical arteries of the contralateral side with the same vessels on the ligated side.
3. The lateral sacral artery from the internal iliac artery with the middle sacral artery from the aorta.
4. The inferior epigastric artery from the external iliac artery with the internal thoracic artery.
5. The lower posterior intercostal arteries with -the lumbar arteries.
6. The deep circumflex artery from the external iliac artery with the lumbar arteries from the aorta.
7. The iliolumbar artery from the internal iliac artery with the last lumbar artery.
8. The obturator artery by means of a pubic branch with the same vessel from the contralateral side. and with the inferior epigastric arteries , which also anastomose with the superior epigastric arteries.

❏❏ If the right internal iliac artery was ligated, what principal vessels may contribute to collateral circulation?

The anastomoses of the following allow collateral circulation:
1. The ovarian artery from the aorta with the uterine artery.
2. The vesical arteries of the contralateral side with the same vessels on the ligated side.
3. The middle rectal artery branches of the internal iliac artery with the superior rectal artery from the inferior mesenteric artery.
4. The obturator artery with the inferior epigastric artery and the medial femoral circumflex artery, and by means of the pubic branch of the obturator artery, with the same vessels from the contralateral side.
5. The circumflex artery with perforating branches of the deep femoral artery and the inferior gluteal artery.
6. The superior gluteal artery with the posterior branches of the lateral sacral arteries.
7. The iliolumbar artery with the last lumbar artery.
8. The lateral sacral artery with the middle sacral artery.
9. The iliac circumflex artery with the iliolumbar and the superior gluteal arteries.

❏❏ During a radical cystectomy (anterior exenteration) and an ileal conduit in a 65-year old female, the vagina is observed to have very good vascular supply when the anterior wall is resected en bloc with the specimen. What is the main arterial supply to the vagina?

The vaginal arteries, which can be represented by one, two or three arterial vessels. These include arterial branches that can arise from the uterine artery, inferior vesical artery or separate arterial branches directly from the anterior trunk of the internal iliac artery.

❏❏ What are the branches of the obturator artery within the pelvis?

The iliac, vesical and pubic arterial branches. The iliac branches ascend in the iliac fossa and supply the iliacus muscle and ilium, while anastomosing with branches of the iliolumbar artery. The vesical branch courses medially and posteriorly to help supply the bladder. The pubic branch arises from the obturator artery just before it leaves the pelvis and ascends inside the pelvis to communicate with the same vessel on the contralateral side and with the inferior epigastric vessels.

❏❏ What are the anatomic relations of the internal pudendal artery in the male?

The internal pudendal artery in the male lies anterior to the piriformis muscle, sacral plexus of nerves and the inferior gluteal artery. As it crosses the ischial spine, it is covered by the gluteus maximus muscle and overlapped by the sacrotuberous ligament. The pudendal nerve is medial to the artery and the nerve to the obturator internus muscle is lateral to the internal pudendal artery.

❏❏ What is the venous drainage of the vagina?

The venous drainage occurs by means of the vaginal plexus of veins along the lateral aspect of the vagina. These are in continuity with the uterine, vesical and rectal venous plexuses. The vaginal plexuses are drained by one or two vaginal veins on each side that flow into the internal iliac veins either directly or through the connections with the internal pudendal veins.

❏❏ How many external iliac lymph nodes are usually present in the normal adult and what is their anatomic arrangement?

There are usually eight to ten external iliac lymph nodes that lie along the external iliac vessels. They are arranged in three groups. One group is on the lateral aspect, another on the medial aspect and a third group, which is on the anterior aspect of the external iliac vessels. The third group of lymph nodes on the anterior aspect o the vessels is sometimes absent.

❑❑ **What are the origins of the arteries that supply the seminal vesicles?**

These arteries are derived from the middle vesical, inferior vesical and middle rectal arteries.

❑❑ **How does the ureteral smooth muscle change as the ureter approaches the bladder?**

The spirally oriented mural smooth muscle fibers become longitudinal. The fine longitudinal smooth muscle fibers from the ureter pass to either side of their respective orifices to join the lateral and posterior ureteral wall fibers and fan out over the base of the bladder. The fibers form the triangular and superficial muscle of the trigone.

EMBRYOLOGY OF THE GENITOURINARY TRACT

Mark Bellinger, M.D.

❏❏ **A female infant is found to have unilateral renal agenesis. Ultrasound examination of the contralateral kidney and bladder and pelvis are normal. What concern should lead the Urologist to recommend long-term monitoring of this child?**

Females with unilateral renal agenesis have a significant incidence of ipsilateral mullerian anomalies, and may present in early adolescence with a pelvic mass indicative of hydrometrocolpos due to any of a spectrum of uterine or vaginal anomalies, commonly uterus didelphys with an obstructed uterine horn.

❏❏ **Ectopic and fused kidneys often have anomalous collecting systems. What is the orientation of the renal pelvis in most anomalous kidneys.**

The renal pelvis begins development in an anterior position, and the kidneys rotate during ascent so that the pelves come to lie in a medial position. Most kidneys, which are anomalous in location, display incomplete rotation. The pelves are likely to be located in an anterior position.

❏❏ **A one month-old female has a duplex left kidney with hydroureteronephrosis of the lower pole segment, which has a thin cortex. What is the most likely explanation for the hydronephrosis?**

In a completely duplicated collecting system, the upper pole is most likely to be hydronephrotic due to ureteral obstruction (ectopic ureter, ureterocele), while hydronephrosis of the lower pole system is most likely due to vesicoureteric reflux.

❏❏ **A two month-old male is found to have a right ureteral duplication with upper pole hydroureteronephrosis and a cystic mass in the bladder. What is the first logical therapeutic intervention to consider?**

The child's most likely diagnosis is ureteral duplication with a ureterocele subtending the upper pole ureter. In most cases, transurethral incision of the ureterocele is an appropriate first therapeutic intervention.

❏❏ **A seven-year old boy is found to have a complete right ureteral duplication with hydroureteronephrosis of the upper pole system during evaluation for nocturnal enuresis. Is this anomaly likely to be a cause of his incontinence?**

No. Ectopic ureters in males insert into the lower genitourinary tract above the external sphincter, including insertion into the Wolffian duct system (vas, seminal vesicle).

❏❏ **An infant is found to have a right multicystic dysplastic kidney. What studies should be done to evaluate the left kidney?**

An ultrasound should be done to rule out hydronephrosis, and a voiding cystourethrogram should be performed since there is a greater than 30% incidence of contralateral vesicoureteric reflux.

❏❏ **An infant has drainage of clear fluid from the umbilicus. A small catheter is placed into the umbilical sinus and contrast injected is seen to pass into the gastrointestinal tract. What is the diagnosis?**

The child has persistence of the omphalomesenteric (vitelline) duct, which connects with the terminal ileum at the site at which a Meckel's diverticulum would be found.

□□ **Early rupture of the cloacal membrane may result in a spectrum of urological anomalies. List them.**

Cloacal exstrophy, exstrophy of the bladder, epispadias.

□□ **Horseshoe kidneys have an incidence of hydronephrosis that in some cases is caused by anomalous renal vasculature. Why is the incidence of this type of ureteral obstruction so high?**

Horseshoe kidneys take their vascular supply from a ladder of vessels which alternately appear and involute as the kidneys ascend toward the flank. Persistence of such "anomalous" vessels may result in ureteral obstruction, most commonly at the ureteropelvic junction obstruction.

□□ **In cases of unilateral renal agenesis, is ipsilateral adrenal agenesis likely to occur?**

No. Ipsilateral adrenal agenesis occurs in less than 10 percent of cases.

□□ **In crossed renal ectopia, are the kidneys more likely to be fused or non-fused?**

Cross-fused renal ectopia is more common.

□□ **In cross-fused renal ectopia, where does the ureter of the crossed kidney usually enter the bladder?**

The ureter draining the ectopic kidney usually crosses the midline to enter the contralateral trigone.

□□ **Explain the Meyer-Weigert law in relation to ureteral duplication.**

The law states that in complete ureteral duplication, the orifice to the lower pole ureter inserts in to the bladder in a more lateral and cranial position, while the ureter to the upper pole inserts in a more caudal and medial position.

□□ **A fourteen-year old male is found to have right ureteral obstruction secondary to retrocaval ureter. What is the embryological explanation for this anomaly?**

Retrocaval ureter is a result of persistence of (failure of involution of) the right subcardinal vein.

□□ **The fetal testis produces two hormones which are essential for the development of the internal genitalia. Name these hormones and indicate what effect they have on the developing genital structures.**

Testosterone supports the development of the wolffian duct structures (seminal vesicles, vas, etc.). Mullerian-inhibiting substance acts ipsilaterally to suppress the development of the mullerian structures (fallopian tube, uterus, upper vagina).

□□ **A one-month old male is found to have a left flank mass. What are the two most likely diagnoses, and what would be your first imaging study in this case.**

The most likely diagnoses are hydronephrosis and multicystic renal dysplasia. The primary imaging technique for infants with abdominal masses should be ultrasound.

□□ **A female neonate has a midline pelvic abdominal mass and a bulging interlabial mass. What is the most likely diagnosis?**

The most likely mass is hydrometrocolpos secondary to imperforate hymen.

□□ **Describe the various types of posterior urethral valves.**

Type 1 are sail-like paired valves which extend from the verumontanum. Type 2 valves are small mucosal folds which are urodynamically insignificant. Type 3 valves appear as an iris diaphragm.

❑❑ **A 12-year old male presents with terminal hematuria and is found to have a polyp in his posterior urethra arising from the veru montanum. What is the cause of this polyp and the most likely pathological diagnosis? Where else in the urinary tract are similar lesions occasionally found?**

The polyp is most likely a benign fibroepitheliomatous polyp of congenital origin. Similar polyps may be found in the ureter and renal pelvis.

❑❑ **A fifteen-year old male with dysuria is found to have a cystic lesion in the bulbous urethra. What is its most likely embryological origin?**

This is most likely a Cowper's Duct cyst.

❑❑ **A 12-year old boy with dysuria and bloody urethral spotting is found to have a small diverticulum on the roof of the distal urethra in the fossa navicularis. What is the correct term for this diverticulum?**

This lesion is known as a lacuna magna.

❑❑ **A one-month old female is found to have a cystic mass prolapsing through the urethral meatus, and ultrasound of the abdomen shows hydronephrosis of the upper pole of the left kidney. What is the most likely diagnosis?**

The mass is a prolapsed ureterocele, which subtends the upper ureter of a completely duplicated left collecting system.

❑❑ **A three-year old girl is found to have grade 3 left vesicoureteric reflux. What is the most likely anatomic location of the left ureteral orifice as seen at cystoscopy, and what is the embryological explanation for its position.**

The ureter will likely be positioned in the bladder in a position lateral to the normal trigonal position. This is thought to be the result of a ureteral bud arising from the mesonephric duct in a position more caudal than usual. As a result, as the caudal mesonephric duct becomes absorbed into the trigonal structure, the ureteral orifice will migrate into a dorsolateral position in the bladder base.

❑❑ **A three-year old boy is found to have a small, hydronephrotic left kidney and ureter. At cystoscopy, no left ureteral orifice can be identified. Where does the ureter most likely insert?**

The ureter most likely is inserted into the Wolffian system (seminal vesicle, vas). This anomaly represents failure of the ureteral bud to separate from its Wolffian duct origin.

❑❑ **An infant being evaluated after urinary tract infection has an intravenous urogram performed. The study shows small folds in the upper portion of the left ureter without significant hydronephrosis. What is the nature and significance of these ureteral findings?**

The IVP has demonstrated "fetal folds" in the upper ureter. These persistent fetal infoldings generally are insignificant and disappear with time.

❑❑ **What is the embryological explanation for bifid ureters?**

Bifid ureters are thought to be the result of bifurcation of the ureteral bud during its ascent toward the renal mesenchyme.

❑❑ **What is the most proximal extent of the ureteral bud in the renal collecting system?**

The ureteral bud ascends to join the metanephric blastema and unite with the glomerular structures. The collecting ducts of the kidney are the most proximal extent of the ureteral bud.

❑❑ **Explain the differences in embryogenesis between multicystic renal dysplasia and autosomal-dominant polycystic disease.**

The cysts in multicystic renal dysplasia are a reflection of failure of normal organogenesis, Immature renal parenchyma and cystic dysplasia are found. In Polycystic disease, the normal architecture of the nephron is destroyed by obstruction of the nephron and resulting cystic deformation.

❏❏ **At what stage of fetal development does the kidney begin to produce urine.**

At approximately nine to twelve weeks.

❏❏ **Congenital spinal anomalies may be associated with what urinary tract anomaly?**

Congenital spinal anomalies may be found in association with renal anomaly, in particular unilateral renal agenesis.

❏❏ **Describe the syndrome in which urethral valves may be associated with unilateral renal dysplasia.**

In the VURD syndrome (vesicoureteric reflux, renal dysplasia), a dysplastic kidney may be found to be associated with massive unilateral vesicoureteric reflux.

❏❏ **What ureteral anomaly is found in conjunction with multicystic renal dysplasia?**

Ureteral atresia.

❏❏ **Explain the anomalies found in the Triad syndrome.**

The Triad, or Prune-Belly syndrome is a constellation of abnormal abdominal musculature, intra-abdominal undescended testes, and an abnormal (dysmorphic) urinary tract.

❏❏ **What embryological explanations have been proposed to explain the Prune Belly Syndrome?**

The explanations offered have been primarily those of anomalous development of the mesenchyme and a transient infravesical obstruction during early embryogenesis.

❏❏ **What is the state of the prostate in boys with Prune Belly Syndrome?**

The prostate is hypoplastic.

❏❏ **It is very difficult to pass a urethral catheter into the bladder of a boy with hypospadias. What is the likely explanation for this?**

The child most likely has an enlarged prostatic utricle.

❏❏ **A one-year old male has a non-palpable right testis, At the time of exploration, the inguinal canal is empty. Where should the surgeon look to be sure that the testis is absent?**

The testis descends from a position above the internal inguinal ring. Testes above the ring are located in the abdominal cavity if they are not congenitally absent. In most cases, a testis or blind-ending vas and vessels can be found in the abdomen by laparoscopy or open exploration. Retroperitoneal dissection, as practiced in the past, may allow the surgeon to miss an abdominal testis.

❏❏ **At the time of exploration, an undescended testis is found outside of the external inguinal ring. The cord structures are long enough to reach the scrotum easily. Should the tunica vaginalis overlying the testis be opened?**

Yes, since most undescended testes have a persistently patent processus vaginalis which does not close after the testis descends into the inguinal canal. This processus should be ligated at the internal inguinal ring.

❏❏ **At exploration for an undescended testis, a blind-ending vascular structure is noted in the inguinal canal. Is exploration complete?**

No. To be sure that a testis is not present, the vas deferens should be identified. The vas and vessels may, in a small number of cases, be separate.

❑❑ **At the time of inguinal herniorrhaphy in a two-year old boy, a bright yellow circular nodule approximately 3mm. in diameter is noted in the inguinal canal attached to the cord structures. What does this represent?**

This is an adrenal rest. No therapy is necessary. It represents the common anlage of the genitourinary ridge in early development.

❑❑ **A 30-week gestation neonate is noted to have bilateral canalicular testes. Is there any chance that descent will occur after birth?**

Yes. The incidence of cryptorchidism in premature infants is approximately 30%, while it is about 3% in full-term neonates and less than 1% at a year of age.

❑❑ **In the classical literature of urology, what is the embryological importance of epididymitis in a prepubescent male.**

The worry is that the boy may have an ectopic ureter draining into the vas deferens or seminal vesicle. Renal ultrasound examination is warranted in these cases.

❑❑ **Describe the anatomy of the exstrophic tissue seen in cloacal exstrophy.**

The exstrophic tissue classically consists of a midline segment of hindgut, frequently with a prolapsed ileum and one or more openings to at least one appendix. The bladder is split into two hemi-bladders by the hind gut. Widely separated genital tubercles are seen as a hemi-scrotum and hemi-penis on each side, or a hemi-clitoris on each side. The anus is imperforate. Most children also have a myelomeningocele and an omphalocele.

❑❑ **Primary obstructive megaureter is most commonly caused by what anatomic entity?**

Obstructive megaureter is thought in most cases to be due to an adynamic distal ureteral segment.

❑❑ **Vaginal atresia may be associated with anomalies of the urinary tract. What is the most commonly recognized urinary tract anomaly seen?**

Unilateral renal agenesis.

❑❑ **What is the embryological origin of the vagina?**

The upper portion of the vagina originates from the mullerian duct. The lower portion (distal to the hymen) originates from the urogenital sinus.

❑❑ **The appendix testis is an embryological remnant of what structure?**

The mullerian duct.

❑❑ **A neonate with imperforate anus is seen to pass meconium per urethra. What is the most likely site of the connection between the urinary and gastrointestinal tracts?**

Embryologically, the most likely site of the fistula is the posterior urethra, although fistulization may occur in the base of the bladder.

❑❑ **List at least three mechanisms that have been proposed to explain why testicles descend from the abdomen into the scrotum .**

The first is the abdominal pressure theory, which proposes than intra-abdominal pressure forces the testis out of the abdomen. The second is that the process is entirely controlled by hormonal influence. Another theory is that the gubernaculum pulls the testis into the scrotum.

❑❑ What is the embryological origin of the appendix epididymis?

The Wolffian duct.

❑❑ What is the embryological explanation for uterus didelphys?

The mullerian ducts are paired structures, which fuse distally to form the upper portion of the vagina and the uterus, the cranial unfused portions forming the fallopian tubes. Failure of fusion may result in one of several anomalies of the uterus, including uterus didelphys and bicornuate uterus.

❑❑ Explain the embryological cause of midshaft hypospadias.

Hypospadias is a result of incomplete formation of the urethra. If the urethral folds fail to fuse in the midline, hypospadias may result.

❑❑ In cloacal exstrophy, how can an anomaly such as hemiscrotum with hemiphallus come to exist?

If the cloacal membrane ruptures early, this acts as a wedge to keep the genital tubercles and genital folds widely separate, so each component of the hemiscrotum and hemiphallus develops widely separate from its contralateral mate.

❑❑ At what stage in gestation is nephron formation completed?

Nephron formation is usually complete by approximately 36 weeks.

❑❑ What is the embryological explanation for communicating hydrocele?

The explanation is that the processus vaginalis fails to obliterate (persistence of a patent processus vaginalis).

❑❑ Glomerular filtration rate progressively increases during fetal development. At what postnatal age does GFR reach its peak?

At approximately four months.

❑❑ A male neonate is found to have bilateral hydroureteronephrosis, echogenic renal parenchyma, and bilateral pneumothorax. What is the most likely diagnosis?

This child is likely to have urethral obstruction secondary to posterior urethral valves.

❑❑ What is the mechanism of neonatal testicular torsion?

The mechanism of this type of torsion, extravaginal torsion, is thought to be different from intravaginal torsion seen in adolescents and adults. In extravaginal torsion, the entire spermatic cord and its coverings appears to twist.

❑❑ In Potter's syndrome (bilateral renal agenesis), are the adrenal glands usually absent?

No. The adrenals are usually normal.

❑❑ What is the renal anatomic defect found in association with megacalycosis?

Under development of the renal medulla.

❑❑ What is the likely location of a ureter which originates from a higher than normal site on the mesonephric duct ?

According to Mackie and Stephens, the ureter will come to lie more caudal and medial in the bladder than a normal ureteral orifice.

❏❏ **What is the importance of the mesonephric kidney to normal embryonic development of the genitourinary tract?**

The mesonephric kidney never functions in the human, but the mesonephric (Wolffian) duct is key to the genital ducts in the male and to the development of the ureteral bud, and thus the kidney,

❏❏ **Explain one theory for the development of ureteroceles.**

Failure of normal perforation of Chawalla's membrane, which separates the ureter from the bladder is thought to result in the formation of ureteroceles.

❏❏ **What are the anatomic correlates of the Mullerian tubercle in both male and female?**

The verumontanum and the hymen, respectively.

❏❏ **In patients with a thoracic kidney, is a diaphragmatic hernia necessarily present?**

No.

❏❏ **In crossed renal ectopia, is fusion or non-fusion of the kidneys more common?**

Most crossed ectopic kidneys are fused.

❏❏ **What is a proposed etiology for the formation of calyceal diverticula?**

It is proposed that failure of involution of third and fourth-order branches of the ureteral bud may result in formation of calyceal diverticula.

❏❏ **Infundibulopelvic stenosis may represent an embryological midpoint between which two congenital renal anomalies?**

Ureteropelvic junction obstruction and multicystic renal dysplasia.

❏❏ **What is the embryological origin of the seminal vesicle?**

The Wolffian duct.

❏❏ **What is the mechanism by which the cloaca becomes divided into the urogenital sinus and rectum?**

The urorectal septum grows to meet the cloacal membrane, forming the perineal body as it fuses with the cloacal membrane. This divides the cloacal membrane into an anterior urogenital membrane and a posterior anal membrane.

❏❏ **Which portions of the male urethra have their embryological origin from the urogenital sinus?**

The prostatic and membranous urethra.

❏❏ **As a horseshoe kidney ascends from the pelvis, which vessel may prevent its ascent into the flank?**

The inferior mesenteric artery.

❏❏ **Which embryonic structure, extending from the bladder to the umbilicus, may remain patent and result in urinary drainage?**

The allantois.

❏❏ **For normal gonadal development, the primary germ cells must migrate from the wall of the yolk sac to paired structures along the dorsal portion of the embryo between the dorsal mesentery and the mesonephros. What are these paired structures that will develop into the primitive gonad?**

They are the genital ridges.

❑❑ There have been two general theories to explain the formation of the glanular urethra. Explain each theory.

The first is that the urethral folds, which fuse to form the pendulous urethra, fuse all the way to the glans. The second theory holds that the pendulous urethra is formed in this manner, while a solid core of ectoderm burrows into the glans to unite with the proximal urethra, and then canalize.

❑❑ Explain the embryological origins of the labia minora and labia majora.

The labia minora are formed from the urethral folds, while the labia majora are derived from the genital swellings.

❑❑ Explain the proposed etiology for exstrophy of the urinary bladder.

Exstrophy occurs when early rupture of the cloacal membrane causes failure of mesenchymal migration into the area.

CONGENITAL DISORDERS OF THE LOWER URINARY TRACT

Anthony Atala, M.D. and Roger E. De Filippo, M.D.

❑❑ **Describe the normal embryonic development of the bladder.**

The body of the bladder is derived primarily from the anterior portion of the cloaca, following separation of the cloaca into anterior and posterior sections by the uro-rectal septum. The base of the bladder and trigone are derived from the distal ends of the wolffian duct, which is also known as the common excretory duct.

❑❑ **Anomalies of the bladder are most likely to occur during what stage of embryonic development?**

Anomalies of bladder formation occur during the fifth to seventh weeks of gestation, corresponding to the early stages of bladder development.

❑❑ **Explain the theory behind embryonic maldevelopment resulting in extstrophy of the bladder.**

The theory of embryonic maldevelopment in exstrophy is based on theories and experiments held by Marshall and Muecke (1964). Abnormal overdevelopment of the cloacal membrane prevents medial migration of the mesenchymal tissue and proper lower abdominal wall development. The timing and premature rupture of this defective cloacal membrane determines the variant of exstrophy-epispadias complex that results.

❑❑ **What is the incidence of classic bladder exstrophy?**

The incidence is estimated to be between one in 10,000 and one in 50,000 live births.

❑❑ **Is there an increased incidence of recurrence in a given family affected with exstrophy of the bladder?**

Yes. The incidence is approximately one in 100.

❑❑ **Is there an increased risk of bladder exstrophy in offspring of individuals with bladder exstrophy?**

Yes. The incidence is one in 70 live births, a 500-fold greater incidence than in the general population.

❑❑ **How do mothers of infants with exstrophy differ primarily from mothers of children with other congenital birth defects.**

Bladder exstrophy tends to occur in infants of younger mothers and mothers of higher parity.

❑❑ **What is the most common skeletal defect associated with bladder exstrophy?**

Widening of the symphysis pubis.

❑❑ **Describe the bony pelvic deformity associated with bladder exstrophy.**

Twelve degree outward rotation of the posterior pelvis on each side, retroversion of the acetabuli, 15-degree external rotation and 30% shortening of the pubic rami, and progressive diastasis of the symphysis pubis.

❏❏ List the various entities in the exstrophy-epispadias syndrome.

Classical exstrophy, cloacal exstrophy, supra vesical fissure, duplicate exstrophy, and covered exstrophy.

❏❏ The surgeon is called to the neonatal ICU to evaluate a child less than 5 hours post-partum. He notices that in addition to a classic bladder exstrophy the child also has a large omphalocele. Which should the surgeon close first?

Usually small omphaloceles can be closed with the bladder. However, in cases where a large omphalocele is associated with bladder exstrophy, the omphalocele is closed first and the treatment of the exstrophy defect is postponed until circumstances allow for bladder closure.

❏❏ What some of the recommendations the surgeon can make regarding nursery management of the bladder exstrophy while the child awaits bladder closure?

The umbilical cord should be tied with Dexon sutures close to the abdominal wall and the umbilical clamp removed so as not to traumatize the bladder mucosa and cause excoriation of the bladder surface.

The bladder must be covered with a nonadherent film wrap or other plastic film to prevent the mucosa from sticking to clothing or diapers.

The surface of the bladder should be irrigated free of debris by sterile saline gently squirted on the bladder surface and the plastic film should be reapplied with each diaper change.

Vaseline gauze should never be used to cover the bladder because it lifts off the delicate mucosa when it is removed.

❏❏ In male patients with classic exstrophy, what is the orientation of the autonomic nerves responsible for potency?

Autonomic innervation of the corpus cavernosum is provided by the cavernous nerves which normally course along the posterolateral aspect of the prostate, traversing the urogenital diaphragm and coursing within the membranous urethra. In patients with exstrophy, these nerves are displaced laterally.

❏❏ Is the need for sexual reassignment common in cases of male exstrophy?

No.

❏❏ What are the five characteristics associated with bladder exstrophy that are identified on prenatal ultrasound?

(1) a bladder that can not be demonstrated, (2) a lower abdominal bulge that represents the exstrophied bladder, (3)a very diminuitive penis with an anteriorly placed scrotum, (4) a low-set umbilicus, and (5) abnormal widening of the iliac crests.

❏❏ What determines a useful size and capacity following successful closure of an exstrohied bladder at birth?

A bladder that demonstrates good elasticity and contractility, as well as an estimated volume of 3 ml or more can be expected to develop a useful size and capacity following successful closure.

❏❏ The surgeon plans to perform primary closure of a bladder exstrophy on a child 24 hours postnatally. Will bilateral iliac osteotomies be necessary?

Not usually. When patients are seen within the first 48 hours of life, the bladder and pelvic ring closure can usually be carried out without osteotomies because of the malleability of the pelvic ring. After 72 hours, osteotomies are necessary.

❏❏ What is the primary argument against performing osteotomies?

Osteotomies can cause retraction of the penis toward the pubic bones, resulting in apparent shortening.

❏❏ **What determines successful acquisition of continence after a classic Young-Dees-Leadbetter reconstruction in a patient with bladder exstrophy?**

The most important predictor of continence is adequate bladder capacity (approximately 60 ml) under anesthesia prior to bladder neck reconstruction. This usually occurs when the child is between 3 and 4 years of age.

❏❏ **How should the surgeon counsel the parents as to when to expect significant urinary continence after successful bladder neck reconstruction?**

Most children gain significant dry intervals on average approximately 100 days after surgery, and the time to complete dryness averages just over 1 year.

❏❏ **What is the most common urologic defect that is usually associated with closure of an exstrophied bladder?**

Vesicoureteral reflux in the closed exstrophied bladder occurs nearly in 100% of cases and requires subsequent surgery.

❏❏ **What is the most common complication after bladder exstrophy closure?**

Bladder prolapse.

❏❏ **What is the most appropriate treatment of bladder prolapse or dehisence after initial closure?**

The bladder should be left extruded and re-closure should be postponed for 4 to 6 months until inflammation from the primary closure has subsided.

❏❏ **Approximately 4 weeks postoperatively, the surgeon is preparing to remove the child's suprapubic tube. What important maneuver must the surgeon perform prior to removal of the suprapubic tube?**

Prior to removal of the suprapubic tube, the bladder outlet is calibrated by a urethral catheter, urethral sound, or cystoscopy to ensure adequate outlet drainage.

❏❏ **In the classic exstrophy-epispadias complex, should penile and urethral reconstruction be performed before or after bladder neck reconstruction?**

Penile and urethral reconstruction can be performed either at the time of initial bladder closure (one stage repair) or 2 to 3 years after bladder closure, depending on the surgeons preference.

❏❏ **What are the 4 key concerns that must be considered to ensure a functional and cosmetically acceptable penis?**

Correcting dorsal chordee, (2) uretheral reconstruction, (3) glandular reconstruction, and (4) penile skin closure.

❏❏ **What is the most common complication in exstrophy patients after urethral reconstruction?**

Urethrocutaneous fistula. The incidence is approximately 12%.

❏❏ **Of carcinomas identified among exstrophied bladders, what is the most prevalent histologic type?**

Of carcinomas identified in exstophied bladders, 80% are adenocarcinomas. Squamous cell carcinoma, undifferentiated carcinoma, and rhabdomyosarcoma make up the remaining 20%.

❏❏ **What is the most serious long-term complication of ureterosigmoidostomy diversion?**

Adenocarcinoma of the colon.

❐❐ **What is the incidence of cloacal exstrophy?**

The incidence of cloacal exstrophy is one in 200,000 to 400,000 live births.

❐❐ **What are the two main theories regarding the embryology behind cloacal exstrophy?**

Patten and Barry (1952) proposed that the paired primordia of the genital tubercles are displaced caudally. This permits persistence of the more cephalad cloacal membrane. If there is incomplete urorectal septal division and disintergration of the unstable cloacal membrane, then both the exstrophied bladder and bowel would be on the ventral abdominal surface.

Marshall and Muecke (1964) suggested that the cloacal membrane is overly developed. This prevents medial migration of the mesenchymal layer between the inner endodermal and outer ectodermal layers. If the cloaca membrane ruptures before fusion of the genital tubercles and prior to caudal movement of the urorectal septum, the ventral abdominal defect occurs (Gearhart and Jeffs, 1992).

❐❐ **It is important for the surgeon to decide whether to perform a one- or two-stage closure during the neonatal period. What are the three most important factors determining a one-stage closure of cloacal exstrophy?**

(1) The overall status of the infant, (2) the size of the omphalocele, and (3) the presence of other severe anomalies.

❐❐ **What are the principles guiding management of the bowel in cloacal exstrophy?**

All efforts must be taken to conserve all bowel segments, to minimize fluid and electrolyte loss, and to make bowel available for later urinary tract and vaginal reconstruction .

❐❐ **What is the most common vertebral anomaly associated with cloacal exstrophy?**

Myelomeningocele.

❐❐ **What are the most common upper urinary tract anomalies associated with cloacal exstrophy?**

The most common upper urinary tract anomalies encountered are pelvic kidney or renal agenesis, in up to 1/3 of patients.

❐❐ **What genital anomaly leads to the possible rearing of XY cloacal exstrophy patients as females?**

A rudimentary bifid phallus.

❐❐ **What is the incidence of complete epispadias?**

The incidence of complete epispadias is one in 117,000 males and one in 484,000 females.

❐❐ **What is the classic appearance of the internal genitalia in female epispadias?**

Normal internal genitalia.

❐❐ **What is the most important factor prior to bladder neck reconstruction in the child born with complete male epispadias?**

Bladder capacity, as in the classic exstrophy patient.

❐❐ **What is the most common cause of neurogenic bladder dysfunction in children?**

Abnormal spinal column development.

❐❐ **What is the incidence of myelodysplasia in the United States?**

1 per 1000 births.

❏❏ **Is there a higher incidence of myelodysplasia in affected families?**

Yes. If spina bifida is already present in one member of a family, there is a 2% to 5% chance that a second sibling will be born with the same condition. The incidence doubles when more than one family member has a neurospinal dysraphism.

❏❏ **A young woman with a family history of spina bifida is interested in getting pregnant and asks her urologist what she can do to reduce the risk of having a child with myelodysplasia? What suggestions can her urologist make?**

Folate deficiency can lead to myelodysplastic abnormalities. Maternal ingestion of 400 ug of folate per day can reduce the incidence of spina bifida by 50%.

❏❏ **What are the cutaneous lesions that may occur with various occult dysraphic states that can be identified on physical exam?**

These lesions include (1) lipomeningocele, (2) hair patch, (3) a dermal vascular malformation, (4) a dimple, and (5) an abnormal gluteal cleft.

❏❏ **What are the different types of occult spinal dysraphisms?**

(1) lipomeningocele, (2) intradural lipoma, (3) diastematomyelia, (4) tight filum terminale, (5) dermoid cyst/sinus, (6) aberrant nerve roots, (7) anterior sacral meningocele, and (8) cauda equina tumor.

❏❏ **A four year child is referred to the urologist after failed attempts at toilet training. The urologists notices sacral agenesis on a plain x-ray of the abdomen and pelvis. What should the urologist expect to find during physical examination with regards to the child's sensation?**

Sensation in the perianal dermatomes, is usually intact, and lower extremity function is normal in children with sacral agenesis.

❏❏ **What type of xray most easily confirms the diagnosis of sacral agenesis?**

A lateral film of the lower spine confirms the diagnosis of sacral agenesis. Recently MRI has also been used, and a sharp termination of the conus seems to be the consistent finding.

❏❏ **Most spinal defects occur at what vertebral level?**

Most spinal defects occur at the level of the lumbosacral and lumbar vertebrae, with the sacral, thoracic, and cervical areas affected in decreasing order.

❏❏ **A urology resident notices that an infant born with myelomeningocele is difficult to arouse and obtunded. He orders a head CT immediately. What may he expect to find on CT that is often associated with the child's diagnosis?**

In 85% of affected children with myelomeningocele, there is an associated Arnold-Chiari malformation, in which the cerebelar tonsils have herniated down through the foramen magnum, obstructing the fourth ventricle and preventing the cerebrospinal fluid from entering the subarachnoid space surrounding the brain and spinal cord and causing hydrocephallus.

❏❏ **What is a major contraindication to the Credé maneuver for management of an infant's bladder with myelodysplasia?**

Credé voiding should be avoided in children with vesicoureteral reflux, especially those with reactive external sphincters. Credé maneuver results in a reflex response in the external sphincter and increases urethral resistance and intravesical pressure, aggravating the degree of reflux and damage to the kidneys.

❏❏ **When is it appropriate to perform urodynamic studies on a child born with myelomeningocele?**

Ideally, urodynamic studies should be performed immediately after the baby is born; however, the risk of spinal infection and the urgency for spinal closure has not made this a viable alternative. Therefore, urodynamic studies are delayed until it is safe to transport the child to the urodyamic suite and place him on his back or side for the test. Urodynamic studies must be an integral part of the newborn assessment along with radiologic evaluation of the upper and lower urinary tract.

❑❑ **What do you expect the radiologic appearance of the urinary tract to be in a newborn with myelodysplasia?**

The urinary tract has a normal radiologic appearance in 90% of newborns.

❑❑ **What specifically on urodynamic studies will the urologist try to identify in order to determine whether clean intermittent catheterization alone or in combination with anticholinergic medicine is indicated?**

Detrussor filling pressures greater than 40 cm H_2O, and voiding pressures higher than 80 to 100 cm H_2O.

❑❑ **At what age can clean intermittent catheterization be started?**

If indicated CIC should begin in the newborn period. When CIC is begun as a newborn, it is easier for parents to master, and for children to accept as they grow older. Complications rarely occur and urinary tract infections occur in less than 30%.

❑❑ **A 5 year old boy born with myelomeningocele and non compliant with CIC undergoes bilateral vesicoureteral reimplant for bilateral grade II/III vesicoureteral reflux. One year after surgery the reflux has recurred. What is the most likely reason for failure of his antireflux surgery?**

Since this child has a history of noncompliance with CIC, failure to empty his bladder is the most likely reason for his recurrent reflux.

❑❑ **A 6 year-old boy with a history of high imperforate anus which was corrected in infancy is referred to the urologist for recurrent urinary tract infections. Urine culture demonstrates multiple organisms. What is the most likely source of infection in this child?**

The incidence of rectourinary fistula is high (80%) in infants with supralevator lesions, or high imperforate anus. Bacteriuria is a common presenting symptom.

❑❑ **What is the most common urinary tract abnormality noted in infants born with imperforate anus?**

The most common abnormality is vesicoureteral reflux followed by renal agenesis.

❑❑ **Which type of imperforate anus is at greater risk of having bony and/or urologic abnormalities associated with it, high or low imperforate anus?**

High imperforate anus.

❑❑ **When are urodynamic studies indicated in the evaluation of a child born with imperforate anus?**

If radiologic studies indicate vertebral bony anomalies then urodynamic studies are performed in the first few months of life. Urodynamic studies are also indicated prior to repair in the child with a high imperforate anus who has undergone an initial colostomy.

❑❑ **What is the incidence of neurogenic bladder in infants with imperforate anus?**

18 to 30%.

CONGENITAL DISORDERS OF THE UPPER URINARY TRACT

Evan J. Kass M.D. and Brian R. Stork M.D.

❏❏ **What is the etiology of Potter's syndrome?**

Oligohydramnios secondary to inadequate urine production is believed to be the causative mechanism for the characteristic facial findings as well as the pulmonary hypoplasia and orthopedic abnormalities that accompany Potter's syndrome.

❏❏ **T/F: Potter's syndrome is pathognomonic for bilateral renal agenesis?**

False. The findings that accompany Potter's syndrome can be found in other conditions in which fetal oligohydramnios is present including autosomal recessive polycystic kidney disease, posterior urethral valves, and prune-belly syndrome.

❏❏ **What is the embryological basis for the characteristic findings of the Mayer-Rokitansky-Kuster-Hauser Syndrome?**

During fetal development the mullerian ducts are adjacent to the wolffian ducts. Mullerian duct abnormalities may result in vaginal agenesis as well as malformation of the ipsilateral uterine horn or fallopian tube. The close proximity of the wolffian duct structures to the Mullerian duct structures may result in renal agenesis or ectopia.

❏❏ **Patients found to have a missing vas deferens during an infertility workup should been screened for what abnormality?**

Ipsilateral renal agenesis.

❏❏ **What is the long-term prognosis for a baby born with a solitary kidney?**

The patient is at increased risk for developing proteinuria, hypertension, and renal insufficiency over the course of his or her lifetime, however, the patient's life expectancy is normal.

❏❏ **Is ureteropelvic junction obstruction a common finding in a patient with a horseshoe kindey?**

Yes. Up to 33% of patients with a horseshoe kidney will have evidence of ureteropelvic junction obstruction.

❏❏ **The cephalad migration of a horseshoe kidney is limited by what structure?**

The inferior mesenteric artery.

❏❏ **What is the normal direction of rotation of the human kidney as it ascends out of the pelvis?**

The kidney normally rotates 90 degrees ventromedially during ascent, therefore, the renal pelvis which was originally directed anteriorly becomes directed medially.

❏❏ **T/F: Most crossed ectopic kidneys are fused with their mate?**

True. Approximately 90% of crossed ectopic kidneys are fused with a normally placed mate.

❏❏ **What is the most common cause of hydronephrosis in the fetal kidney?**

Ureteropelvic junction obstructions are the etiology of up to 80% of cases of fetal hydronephrosis.

❏❏ T/F: Most cases of prenatally diagnosed ureteropelvic junction obstruction require urgent surgical intervention following delivery?

False. Debate continues surrounding the management of prenatally diagnosed ureteropelvic junction obstructions. Most often surgery is not necessary or can be performed on an elective basis after an appropriate evaluation and period of observation.

❏❏ In what percent of patients with ureteropelvic junction obstruction does the contralateral kindey demonstrate evidence of ureteropelvic junction obstruction?

In patients found to have ureteropelvic junction obstruction evidence for bilateral obstruction exists in 10% to 40% of cases.

❏❏ In what percentage of patients with ureteropelvic junction obstruction does vesicoureteral reflux coexist?

Severe vesicourereral reflux coexists in 10% of cases whereas minor degrees of vesicoureteral reflux have been documented in as many as 40% of cases.

❏❏ Define the terms dysplasia, aplastic dysplasia, and familial adysplasia.

Dysplasia refers to the histologic findings of focal, diffuse, or segmentally arranged primitive structures that result from abnormal metanephric differentiation. Aplastic dysplasia is a small quantity of tissue that is nonfunctional and dysplastic by histologic criteria. Familial adysplasia is a term, which identifies multiple persons in a single family with renal agenesis, renal dysplasia, multicystic dysplasia, or renal aplasia.

❏❏ What is the most common type of renal cystic disease?

Multicystic dysplasia.

❏❏ A child is discovered to have a multicystic dysplastic kidney. This patient's contralateral kidney should be screened for what abnormalities?

The contralateral collecting system should been screened for vesicoureteral reflux which is present in 18-43% of cases and for ureteropelvic junction obstruction which has been demonstrated in 3-12% of cases.

❏❏ What is the average amount of renal parenchyma drained by the upper pole of a duplicated collecting system?

About one-third of total renal parenchyma is drained by the upper pole of a duplicated collecting system.

❏❏ A ureteric bud arising on the mesonephric duct in an abnormally caudal location predisposes to what abnormality?

The ureteral orifice will ultimately reside in a more cranial and lateral position within the bladder and be predisposed to vesicoureteral reflux.

❏❏ The upper pole ureter of a duplicated collecting system is predisposed to what abnormality?

Obstruction with subsequent hydronephrosis.

❏❏ What is the Weigert-Meyer rule?

The inferior and medial ureteral orifice in a duplicated collecting system drains the upper pole collecting system, whereas, the superior and lateral ureteral orifice drains the lower pole collecting system.

❏❏ T/F: Ectopic ureteral orifices in female patients are often associated with duplicated collecting systems?

True. More than 80% of ectopic ureters in female patients are associated with duplicated collecting systems.

☐☐ **Do male patients with ectopic ureteral orifices tend to have duplicated collecting systems?**

No. Ectopic ureteral orifices in boys drain single collecting systems in the majority of cases.

☐☐ **A boy with a duplicated collecting system is found to have an ectopic ureter. Where will the terminal portion of the ectopic ureter most likely be found?**

Ectopic ureters in males terminate in the posterior urethra in approximately 50% of cases and the seminal vesicles in about 30% of cases.

☐☐ **T/F: In a girl with continuous urinary incontinence found to have an ectopic ureter the ectopic ureteral orifice will most likely be found within the vagina?**

False. The ectopic ureteral orifice will most often be found within the urethra or at the vestibule.

☐☐ **What is Chawalla's membrane?**

Chawalla's membrane is a two-layered cell structure that transiently divides the ureteral bud from the urogenital sinus at approximately 37 days gestation. Many investigators believe that incomplete dissolution of this membrane is the etiology of ureterocele formation.

☐☐ **Ureteroceles tend to occur in patients of what race and sex?**

Ureteroceles are significantly more common in Caucasians and occur four times more frequently in females than males.

☐☐ **What is a pseudoureterocele?**

A radiographic finding in which a dilated ectopic ureter coursing behind the bladder impinges on the bladder wall giving the appearance of a ureterocele.

☐☐ **What is the most common cause of urethral obstruction in a young girl?**

A prolapsing ureterocele.

☐☐ **What is the length to diameter ratio in a normal non-refluxing pediatric ureter?**

5:1

☐☐ **What is the embryology of a circumcaval ureter or preureteral vena cava?**

The inferior vena cava develops from a plexus of fetal veins. Normally the inferior vena cava forms from the right supracardial vein as the right subcardial vein atrophies. If the right subcardial vein fails to atrophy and becomes the inferior vena cava, a segment of ureter becomes trapped behind the vena cava.

☐☐ **What is the most common etiology of renal calculi in children?**

Hypercalciuria as a side effect of furosemide or glucocorticoid therapy

☐☐ **What is a pseudotumor of the kidney?**

A hypertrophied column of Bertin which may be sufficiently large to compress and deform the adjacent collecting system.

☐☐ **What is the clinical course of classic congenital mesoblastic nephroma?**

Classic congenital mesoblastic nephroma is a benign tumor and treatment is limited to surgical excision.

❏❏ **What is a nephrogenic rest?**

A nephrogenic rest is an abnormal focus of nephrogenic cells. Although these cells can be induced to form Wilm's tumor, the majority of nephrogenic rests involute and do not result in tumor formation.

❏❏ **What hepatic abnormality is associated with Autosomal Recessive Polycystic Kidney Disease?**

Congenital hepatic fibrosis.

❏❏ **What are the ultrasound characteristics of Autosomal Recessive Polycystic Kidney disease?**

As a result of the enormous number of interfaces created by the tightly compacted, dilated collecting ducts, the kidneys appear large and homogeneously hyperechogenic.

❏❏ **What neurological, gastrointestinal, and cardiac anomalies are associated with autosomal dominant polycystic kidney disease?**

Berry aneurysms, colonic diverticula, and mitral valve prolapse.

❏❏ **Juvenile nephronophthisis and medullary cystic disease are transmitted by what modes of inheritance?**

Juvenile nephronophthisis is usually transmitted as an autosomal recessive trait whereas medullary cystic disease is transmitted as an autosomal dominent trait.

❏❏ **What are the characteristics of Alport's Syndrome?**

Hereditary nephritis, high frequency hearing loss, ocular abnormalities, microhematuria, and proteinuria.

PRUNE BELLY SYNDROME

J. Lynn Teague, M.D., F.A.A.P. and Major Mark R. Wakefield, M.D.

❏❏ **What are alternate, perhaps less stigmatizing, names for the Prune Belly Syndrome?**

Prune Belly vividly describes the clinical appearance of most patients with the syndrome. However, many clinicians consider the negative connotations to be stigmatizing and socially undesirable. Thus, several alternatives have been proposed. Eagle-Barrett Syndrome recognizes one of the original descriptions of a series of 9 patients in 1950. Abdominal Wall Deficiency Syndrome is a descriptive nomenclature. Mesenchymal Dysplasia Syndrome alludes to a suspected but unproven etiology. Triad Syndrome emphasizes the three components of the classic syndrome. Nonetheless, Prune Belly Syndrome remains the common terminology, in part because of its intensely descriptive nature.

❏❏ **What are the three classic features that characterize Prune Belly Syndrome?**

Triad syndrome refers to three specific features of Prune Belly Syndrome. Urinary tract dilation, specifically megaureters, abdominal wall deficiency, and cryptorchidism. The defective abdominal musculature gives the typical appearance of a wrinkled prune, with laxity of the anterior abdominal wall. The testes are both nonpalpable. The urinary tract dilation includes tortuous, dilated ureters, as well as varying degrees of an enlarged smooth walled bladder and dilated prostatic urethra.

❏❏ **What is the approximate incidence of Prune Belly Syndrome in males?**

The true incidence of Prune Belly Syndrome is not well known. The estimated incidence is similar to that of bladder exstrophy. The reported range is 1 per 35,000 to 50,000 live births. The classic Triad syndrome only occurs in males. However, variations, which include two of the three features of the classic triad, can occur in males or females. The incidence is uncertain for patients with incomplete Prune Belly Syndrome, but probably is one fourth as common as the classic syndrome. Furthermore, approximately 15% of patients in one series of patients with incomplete Prune Belly Syndrome were female.

❏❏ **To whom does Pseudo Prune Belly Syndrome refer?**

Incomplete Prune Belly Syndrome refers to patients with two of the three classic findings of the triad. For females, this would include the dilation of the urinary tract and lax abdominal musculature, but not the undescended testes, although other genital anomalies do occur. Pseudo Prune Belly Syndrome refers to those male patients with incomplete Prune Belly Syndrome with typical genitourinary findings of ureteral dilation and undescended testes but with a normal abdominal wall.

❏❏ **What percentage of patients will have an atypical presentation of Prune Belly Syndrome?**

As many as 25% in some series of patients will have an incomplete form of Prune Belly Syndrome. Most of these patients will have the typical urinary tract finding of dilated ureters, but will have either normal abdominal wall musculature (the Pseudo Prune Belly Syndrome) or descended testicles. Females with incomplete Prune Belly Syndrome are even less common, affecting less than 5% of patients with the Syndrome. In females, the upper tact dilation may be less severe.

❏❏ **What are some of the proposed embryologic etiologies of Prune Belly Syndrome?**

There are several theories explaining the embryogenesis of prune Belly Syndrome. Each theory has both supporting experimental and empiric evidence, but none have been proven to be true or false. These theories are not necessarily mutually exclusive.

Urinary tract obstruction may result from a transient urethral membrane at a critical phase of development. Abdominal wall laxity then results from outward compression from the dilated urinary tract. The migration of the testicles is blocked by the enlarged bladder. Primary prostatic maldevelopment with hypolasia of the prostatic urethra is another possible cause of urinary tract obstruction. In either case fetal urinary ascites may or may not play a critical role.

Primary mesodermal maldevelopment may also explain Prune Belly Syndrome. Failure of myoblast precursors to differentiate and / or migrate appropriately may explain the abnormal development of the abdominal wall. The laxity of the abdominal wall may then be the primary event. The urinary tract dilation and undescended testicles then result from decreased intraabdominal pressures. However, if the developmental defect occurs early enough (third week of gestation), then all of the abnormalities may be explained by a common event in the mesenchymal tissues.

Persistence of the yolk sac has been implicated in the abdominal wall abnormalities, resulting in redundant tissues.

☐☐ What is the role of prenatal diagnosis with fetal ultrasound in Prune Belly Syndrome?

In general, prenatal diagnosis of Prune Belly Syndrome has not been reliable. There are high false positive and false negative rates of prenatal detection. The typical intra-uterine appearance of Prune Belly Syndrome is bilateral hydronephrosis with an enlarged, non-cycling bladder. Earlier fetal ascites and oligohydramnious may also be suggestive of Prune Belly Syndrome. However, the differential diagnosis of these findings includes posterior uretheral valves, vesico-ureteral reflux, bilateral uretero-pelvic junction obstruction, neurogenic bladder, and megacystis / megalourethra syndromes.

☐☐ Late presentations of Prune Belly Syndrome are typified by what characteristics?

Although the typical appearance of the abdomen in neonates with Prune Belly Syndrome usually leads to prompt diagnosis, some children present at a later age. These children often have less severe forms of the syndrome. These children may present with difficulty sitting from a supine position as a result of weaker abdominal muscles. Further more, walking may be delayed due to difficulty in standing and balance. Older children will have a characteristic pot-belly with a loss of wrinkling of the skin due to stretching by the abdominal viscera.

☐☐ What diagnostic evaluation in patients with Prune Belly Syndrome should be avoided?

The voiding cystourethrogram should be avoided in the early neonatal period. Instrumentation of the urinary tract puts the patient at increased risk of infection and sepsis. The diagnosis should be suspected based on the findings of physical exam. Due to the lax abdominal wall, the dilated bladder and ureters are often palpable. Although used previously to confirm the diagnosis, intravenous pyelogram does not image the urinary tract well due to poor concentrating ability of the neonatal kidneys and dilution of contrast in the dilated urinary tract. Abdominal ultrasound can be useful in assessing the degree of urinary tract dilation. Serial assessment of serum electrolytes, renal function, and urine culture are important diagnostic tests.

☐☐ What is the most common non-genitourinary anomaly in patients with Prune Belly Syndrome?

Thoracic Cage malformations, including the mildest forms of pectus excavatum and pectus carinatum, occur in more than 75% of patients with Prune Belly Syndrome. The chest wall malformations are likely due to the restrictive effects of oligohydramnios. In the most severe form pulmonary hypoplasia may occur, with associated pneumothorax and a high neonatal mortality rate. Most patients, however, have only mild pulmonary dysfunction, often only evident on formal pulmonary function testing. Furthermore, these patients will have a less forceful cough due to weaker abdominal musculature. Thus, patients with Prune Belly Syndrome are at an increased risk for post-operative respiratory distress, pneumonia, and bronchitis. Other common anomalies associated with Prune Belly Syndrome include cardiac, gastrointestinal, and orthopedic deformities.

☐☐ What is the most common anomaly of the muscleskeletal system in patients with Prune Belly Syndrome?

Skin dimples on the knee or elbow are the most common abnormality of the muscleskeletal system, excluding the typical abdominal wall defects. The skin dimples occur in 45% of patients. More severe anomalies include varus deformity of the feet (club foot), which occurs in 25% of patients, congenital hip dislocation (5%), spinal dysmorphism (5%), and rarely severe lower extremity hypoplasia. These dimples are likely the result of compression from oligohydramnios. Other etiologies have been proposed: ischemia from compressed iliac vessels and a common defect in mesenchymal development at 3 weeks of gestation. Cardiac anomalies occur in 10% of patients with Prune Belly Syndrome. The most common cardiac abnomalities, which occur more commonly than in the general population, include patent ductus arteriosus, ventricular septal defect, atrial septal defect, and Tetrology of Fallot.

Malrotation of the midgut occurs more frequently in patients with the severe form of Prune Belly Syndrome. Other gastrointestinal anomalies, including gastroschisis and omphalocele, have been described in patients with Prune Belly Syndrome.

❑❑ **In addition to the classic triad of findings, what are the common anomalies of the urinary system in Prune Belly patients?**

The penile urethra is usually normal, though scaphoid megalourethra is associated with Prune Belly Syndrome. The prostatic urethra is hypoplastic in most patients with Prune Belly Syndrome. The bladder neck is wide open and tapers to the normal membranous urethra. The prostatic urethra appears dilated as a result of the prostatic hypoplasia. The prostatic utricle and ejaculatory ducts are often dilated. The bladder is enlarged but usually does not have trabeculation. The patent urachus may persist, especially if there is urethral atresia. The ureters are involved, with the proximal ureters typically being less dilated. The kidneys are aflicted by varying degrees of hydronephrosis and renal dysplasia.

❑❑ **What is the likelihood of renal failure among patients with Prune Belly Syndrome?**

Despite recent improvements in the treatment of patients with Prune Belly Syndrome, approximately one-third of patients will progress to end stage renal disease.

❑❑ **What causes renal failure in patients with Prune Belly Syndrome?**

Renal failure in patients with Prune Belly Syndrome results from the reflux of infected urine and subsequent chronic pyelonephritis. High-grade obstruction or high pressure reflux may result in severe renal dysplasia at birth, as seen in some neonatal autopsy studies. However, most patients with Prune Belly Syndrome have low pressure vesicoureteral reflux. As long as the urine remains sterile, the risk of renal failure appears to be low, despite the high incidence reflux and dilation of the urinary tract.

❑❑ **What is the role of renal transplantation in patients with Prune Belly Syndrome?**

Renal transplantation in patients with Prune Belly Syndrome is as successful as transplantation for other indications in children. Special attention must be directed towards management of the urinary tract prior to transplantation. Adequate bladder emptying with clean intermittent catheterization is often necessary and is favorable to urinary diversion.

❑❑ **How common is vesicoureteral reflux in patients with Prune Belly Syndrome?**

Vesicoureteral reflux occurs in as many as 85% of the patients with Prune Belly Sydrome. The reflux tends to be low pressure. Most children with Prune Belly Sundrome do not outgrow the reflux. Nonetheless, surgery to correct the reflux is usually reserved for those patients with recurrent pyelonephritis, whose reflux is refractory to more conservative therapies such as vesicostomy. Ureteroneocystotomy is associated with a high risk of ureterovesical obstruction and recurrence of reflux in patients with Prune Belly Syndrome.

❑❑ **What are the typical characteristics of the ureters in patients with Prune Belly Syndrome?**

The ureters in patients with Prune Belly Syndrome are dilated. The proximal ureters tend to be spared, with increased dilation and tortuousity in the distal segments. The ureters may have decreased smooth muscle and an altered collagen matrix, which leads to a loss of lumenal coaptation and ineffective peristalsis. The proximal ureters are more suitable for reimplantation when indicated because of improved proximal peristalsis.

❑❑ **What are the typical characteristics of the bladder in patients with Prune Belly Syndrome?**

The bladder in patients with Prune Belly Syndrome is enlarged. The bladder is thick walled, but it is typically smooth with minimal trabeculation or diverticula. Dilation of the urachus may result in a pseudodiverticulum at the dome of the bladder. The intertrigonal ridge is wide with laterally placed ureteral orifices. The bladder neck is open and funnels into the prostatic urethra.

❏❏ What does cystometrogram evaluation in patients with Prune Belly Syndrome typically demonstrate?

Bladder function in patients with Prune Belly Syndrome is variable. Initial urodynamic evaluation with cystomerogram will usually demonstrate a high capacity bladder with normal compliance, decreased sensation, and poor contractility. Bladder pressures during voiding are low. Emptying is often incomplete.

❏❏ Where is the typical location of the undescended testes in patients with Prune Belly Syndrome?

The testicles are usually located at the pelvic brim. Early orchiopexy is often possible. The Fowler-Stephens technique is often necessary for the testicles to reach the scrotum. Testicular autotransplantation with micovascular anastamosis has also been performed.

❏❏ What is the cause of infertility in patients with Prune Belly Syndrome?

Infertility in patients with Prune Belly Syndrome is multifactorial. Failure of emission is common. Prostatic and seminal fluids may be insufficient. Spermatogenesis may also be altered. Early orchiopexy, electroejacualtion, and intracytoplasmic sperm injection may allow for fertility is some patients with Prune Belly Syndrome.

❏❏ What are the growth characteristics of patients with Prune Belly Sydrome?

In general, the growth of children with Prune Belly Syndrome depends upon their renal function. With impaired renal function, there is significant growth delay. Nonetheless, growth retardation occurs in more than one third of those patients with normal renal function.

❏❏ What is the initial management of Prune Belly Syndrome?

The initial management of patients with Prune Belly Syndrome has evolved and now relies upon the recognition of the syndrome and generally involves noninvasive therapies. Stabilization of the associated cardiopulmonary complications is paramount, as they are often more serious in the neonatal period. Usually the child is able to spontaneously void, but this may be facilitated by bladder massage. Prophylactic antibiotics are indicated, as vesicoureteral reflux can be assumed to exist. Catheter drainage or other instrumentation (e.g. during a VCUG) should be avoided, as the possibility of urinary tract infection is a significant risk. If the patient has persistent azotemia or acidosis urinary tract diversion may be indicated. Cutaneous vesicotmy is the primary form of diversion. Stomal stenosis appears to be more common in children with Prune Belly Syndrome, therefore, a large caliber (28 French) vesicostomy is advisable. Occasionally, percutaneous nephrostomies are needed in the setting of sepsis. Cutaneous ureterostomies may be necessary if the ureters are obstructed distally due to extreme tortuosity. Urethrotomy to improve urinary drainage is now limited to the few patients with anatomic urethral obstruction.

❏❏ What are the long-term treatment options for patients with Prune Belly Syndrome?

The treatment of patients with Prune Belly Syndrome must be individualized. However, in general, most patients can be treated conservatively with delayed surgical reconstruction. Prophylactic antibiotics are indicated for the initial treatment of vesicoureteral reflux, which is present in more than 85% of patients. If recurrent pyelonephritis ensues, ureteral reimplantation may be needed. The proximal ureters are utilized as their function is less impaired than the distal ureter. If tapering of a redundant ureter is needed, imbrication may be advantageous, in order to preserve the ureteric blood supply. Reduction cystoplasty is usually limited to excision of urachal remnants. Orchiopexy should be performed early, often with a transabdominal approach. A staged procedure such as Stephen Fowlers orchiopexy may be needed in order for the testicles to reach the scrotum in some patients. Microvascular autotransplantation has also been employed.

There have been significant improvements in the surgical approaches to abdominal wall reconstruction. Although primarily a cosmetic procedure, improved pulmonary function may result from abdominal wall reconstruction.

□□ **What is the prognosis for patients with Prune Belly Syndrome?**

The prognosis for patients with Prune Belly Syndrome has improved. Some infants are stillborn, and as many as 25% of patients in some series died in the neonatal period due to urospepsis, renal failure or most commonly concomitant cardiopulmonary disease. With improvement in neonatal intensive care, the neonatal mortality rate is less than 10%, and death is more often due to renal failure as a result of severe renal dysplasia.

Despite avoidance of urinary tract instrumentation and the use of suppressive antibiotics, urinary tract infection is common. More than 75% of patients will develop urinary tract infections; however, febrile infections and pyelonephritis is unusual, especially in those patients with good renal function.
Renal failure occurs in 25-30% of patients with Prune Belly Syndrome. The presence of early renal insufficiency and urospesis predict progression to renal failure. A nadir serum creatinine greater than 0.7 mg/dl predicts the development of renal failure. When needed, renal transplantation can be performed safely.

CRYPTORCHIDISM/ DIAGNOSIS AND MANAGEMENT

Harry P. Koo, M.D.

❑❑ **What region of the Y chromosome is the gene that is thought to encode for human testis-determining factor (TDF) localized?**

The region thought to encode the human testis-determining factor (TDF) has been localized to the short arm of the Y chromosome between the centromere and the pseudoautosomal region.

❑❑ **During the sexual differentiation of the gonad into a testis, what are the first cells to differentiate in the testis?**

The Sertoli cells.

❑❑ **What is the primordial hormone of the fetal testis?**

Around the seventh week of gestation, mullerian-inhibiting substance is produced by the Sertoli cells.

❑❑ **What is the mullerian-inhibiting substance?**

The mullerian-inhibiting substance is a hormone produced by the testis, which suppresses the mullerian ducts. In the male, the mullerian duct regresses to the appendix testis and the prostatic utricle.

❑❑ **When does testosterone production begin in utero?**

By the ninth week of gestation, Leydig cells produce testosterone.

❑❑ **What are the crucial periods of testosterone surge in the developing male from fetus to young adulthood?**

The initial surge of testosterone occurs between 11 and 16 weeks gestation. After birth, the decrease in circulating maternal estrogens stimulates pituitary gonadotropins to produce a second surge of testosterone, with the levels peaking between 60 to 90 days of life. The Leydig cells then remain dormant until puberty when increasing levels of gonadotropin-releasing hormone (GnRH) produce a pulse-synchronized increase in LH and testosterone.

❑❑ **What is the incidence of cryptorchidism in premature infants, term infants and adults, respectively?**

The incidence of cryptorchidism in premature infants is 30%; in term infants 3%; in adults 0.8%.

❑❑ **By one year of age, what percent of cryptorchid testes spontaneously descend in premature infants, and in term infants?**

Approximately 95% of premature cryptorchid testis and 75% of term cryptorchid testis spontaneously descend by 1 year of age. The majority of the testes that descend usually will do so in the first 3-months of life.

❑❑ **What is the incidence of bilateral cryptorchidism?**

Approximately 10 per cent of children with cryptorchidism have bilateral undescended testes.

❏❏ **What mechanisms are involved in promoting testicular descent?**

Normal testicular descent may be multifactorial. Of the many theories, the most commonly proposed factors include: (1) Endocrine factors play the major role in promoting testicular descent. The process is androgen mediated and regulated by pituitary gonadotropin. (2) The traction theory is based on the concept that there is downward traction on the testis by the gubernaculum. (3) In the differential growth theory, the testis is pulled into the scrotum by the relatively immobile gubernaculum as a result of the rapid growth of the body wall. (4) Intraabdominal pressure theory is based on the belief that increased intraabdominal pressure pushes the testis through the internal ring. (5) The epididymal theory postulates that the differentiation and maturation of the epididymis induces testicular descent.

❏❏ **When does testicular descent occur in utero?**

Testicular descent occurs in the third trimester. Prenatal ultrasonography typically shows no testicular descent before 28 weeks gestation.

❏❏ **What is the difference between a cryptorchid and an ectopic testis?**

A cryptorchid testis is a testis that is located along the normal path of descent but has failed to reach a dependent position in the scrotum. Ectopic testes descend normally through the external ring but then migrate away from its normal pathway. Testicular ectopia is believed to be directly related to the development of the gubernaculum.

❏❏ **What is the most common location for a cryptorchid testis?**

Cryptorchid testis may be intraabdominal or canalicular. The most common location is in the inguinal canal.

❏❏ **What is the most common location for an ectopic testis?**

Possible locations for ectopic testes include the superficial inguinal pouch, perineum, femoral canal, suprapubic, and transverse scrotal. The most common ectopic location is the superificial inguinal pouch.

❏❏ **What options are available for hormonal therapy?**

Medical therapy for cryptorchidism involves hormonal administration. Currently human chorionic gonadotropin (hCG) and gonadotropin releasing hormone (GnRH) are utilized in hormonal therapy.

❏❏ **What is the mechanism of action and dosage for hCG?**

The role of hCG for management of cryptorchidism is presumably via stimulation of Leydig cells, resulting in increased plasma testosterone levels and thus promoting testicular descent. hCG is administered parenterally in doses varying from 5,000 I.U to more than 40,000 I.U. Injections are given over a period of 2 to 4 weeks.

❏❏ **What are the potential side effects of hCG?**

At doses above 15,000 I.U. significant side effects have been reported including: changes in testicular histology, alterations in bone age, and transient increased in penile size.

❏❏ **What is the mechanism of action and dosage for GnRH?**

GnRH therapy is based on the premise that children with cryptorchidism have an abnormal hypothalamic-pituitary axis. Thus, GnRH stimulation to increase LH levels will promote testicular descent. GnRH is administered transnasally at a dose of 1.2 mg per day for 4 weeks. Although GnRH nasal spray has been used in Europe, it is not approved for use in the United States.

❏❏ **How successful is hormonal therapy?**

There is a wide range of reported success rates for hormonal therapy. Those series reporting higher success rates probably include a large number of patients with retractile testes. Success rates with hCG vary between 14% and 50%. Success rates with GnRH therapy vary from 6% to 70%. There is approximately 10% relapse rate with GnRH therapy.

❏❏ **What percentage of cryptorchid testes is nonpalpable?**

Nonpalpable testes comprise 5% to 28% of undescended testes in various series.

❏❏ **What are the roles of ultrasound, CT, and MRI in localizing a nonpalpable testis?**

Generally, a good physical examination by a urologist is more valuable and reliable than are ultrasonography, CT scanning and MR imaging. CT scans and MR imaging may discern gonads in older children. However, due to the significant false-negative rate with each of these studies, failure to demonstrate a testis does not prove that it is absent.

❏❏ **What is (are) the best option(s) for locating a nonpalpable testis?**

Surgical exploration is the gold standard. However, with the advancement in laparoscopic technology, most pediatric urologists consider laparoscopy as the best initial step in localizing a nonpalpable testis or proving its absence. The accuracy of laparoscopy as a diagnostic modality for nonpalpable testis exceeds 95%.

❏❏ **What are the increased risks of an undescended testis?**

(1) Infertility – has been reported in up to 50% of patients with unilateral cryptorchidism and up to 75% of men with a history of bilateral cryptorchidism.
(2) Testicular cancer – is approximately 10 times more common in undescended testes. The risk of tumor is up to six times higher than in a cryptorchid testis in another location.
(3) A patent processus vaginalis (hernia) – is present in approximately 90% of all cryptorchid testis.
(4) Testicular torsion – is more common in undescended testes.

❏❏ **What factors contribute to decreased fertility in cryptorchidism?**

(1) Prolonged extrascrotal location of the testis from untreated cryptorchidism results in decreased testicular volume and progressive histologic deterioration.
(2) Increased incidence of abnormal ductal structures (epididymal abnormalities, vasal abnormalities) in cryptorchid testis may affect sperm transport.
(3) Testicular abnormalities are present even in the contralateral testis in patients with unilateral cryptorchidism.

❏❏ **What is the most common tumor in cryptorchid testis?**

Seminoma.

❏❏ **A nine-year-old boy has a solitary right testis on physical examination for youth hockey league. Laparoscopy as a toddler had revealed blind ending spermatic vessels on the left. What is the preferred recommendation for this boy regarding any further medical evaluation, and regarding participating in contact sports?**

The prior documentation of blind ending spermatic vessels confirms absence of the left testis so no further evaluation is necessary. Advice about possible torsion of solitary testis and testicular self-examination should be discussed. The Committee on Sports Medicine of the American Academy of Pediatrics recommends that patients with a solitary testis be allowed to participate in contacts sports if they wear a protective cup.

❏❏ **What are the three likely findings at laparoscopy for nonpalpable testis?**

(1) Blind ending vessels above the internal inguinal ring. (2) Cord structures (vas deferens and spermatic vessel leash) entering the internal ring. (3) An intra-abdominal testis.

❏❏ **During laparoscopy for a nonpalpable left testis, the spermatic vessels and vas deferens could be visualized coursing distal to the internal inguinal ring. What is the next course of action?**

Following the removal of the laparoscope, left inguinal exploration should be performed to find a potentially viable testis, which may have been missed on the physical examination. The most likely finding in this situation would be the presence of a testicular remnant. Since there is the risk of potential malignant degeneration of the dysplastic remnant, excision should be performed.

❑❑ If a confirmation of solitary descended testis is made at the time of inguinal exploration or laparoscopy, how should the normally descended testis be managed?

There is controversy regarding the management of solitary descended testis. In order to prevent testicular torsion in the remaining testis, prophylactic scrotal orchidopexy could be performed at the time of surgery. The opponents to this approach express concerns about possible compromise to the fertility potential of the testis by having sutures placed through testicular tissue. Until there are data showing clear benefit of one approach over the other, the individual surgeon should decide on the appropriate management following an informed discussion with the family.

❑❑ During an inguinal exploration for nonpalpable right testis, the vas deferens was present but no testicular tissue could be identified. What is the next course of action?

The most important point here is that one cannot confirm an absence of testis by finding a blind ending vas deferens. In this situation, depending on the comfort of the surgeon and the availability of surgical equipment, either laparoscopy or abdominal exploration should be performed to look for an intraabdominal testis or blind ending spermatic vessels. Blind ending spermatic vessels confirm absence of testis.

❑❑ A five-year-old boy is referred from his primary care physician for bilateral undescended testes. As part of the evaluation by the primary care physician, ultrasound and CT scans were performed which revealed a normal sized right testis in the inguinal region and an absent left testis. Physical examination by the consulting urologist revealed a normal right testis located in the superficial inguinal pouch and a nonpalpable left testis. What should be done at the time of surgery?

Right inguinal orchidopexy should be performed. One cannot rely on ultrasound and CT to confirm absence of left testis. Laparoscopy or inguinal (with possible abdominal) exploration should be performed for the nonpalpable left testis.

❑❑ During laparoscopy for a nonpalpable right testis in an 18-month-old toddler, an intra-abdominal testis is identified. What are the various options for management?

The desired goal is to place the testis in the scrotum without vascular compromise. A variety of techniques are applicable for intra-abdominal testis, including single or two-stage orchidopexy. Single-stage orchidopexy techniques include Fowler-Stephens orchidopexy, abdominal extraperitoneal approach (Jones technique), laparoscopic orchidopexy, and microsurgical autotransplantation. Two-stage orchidopexy is performed by initially ligating the spermatic vessels laparoscopically followed by open or laparoscopic Fowler-Stephens orchidopexy.

❑❑ During an inguinal orchidopexy, a hernia sac is noted to be present with the undescended testis. As the hernia sac is being dissected off the cord, a tear is made in the sac extending proximal to the internal inguinal ring. What is the next course of action?

The internal ring should be opened with the use of electrocautery to gain exposure to the peritoneum. The hernia sac can be dissected in an antegrade (from the peritoneum) fashion to obtain sound closure of the peritoneum.

❑❑ What are the important elements in obtaining adequate spermatic cord length for inguinal orchidopexy?

The important elements include: mobilization to the internal inguinal ring, division of lateral spermatic fascia, division of the hernia sac and dissection of the cord off the posterior peritoneum.

❑❑ During an inguinal orchidopexy for an undescended testis located in the inguinal canal, the testis could only be mobilized to the upper scrotum using the standard orchiopexy techniques. What other maneuver could be performed to gain some additional length for orchidopexy?

When the standard orchidopexy maneuvers still do not provide adequate spermatic cord length for successful placement of the testis, the floor of the internal ring may be taken down, dividing the inferior epigastric vessels and transversalis fascia, thereby allowing the testis and cord to make a direct path to the pubic tubercle (Prentiss technique). The floor of the inguinal canal is then closed over the cord, superimposing the internal and external inguinal rings.

❏❏ **A newborn with severe scrotal hypospadias and chordee is noted to have a left nonpalpable testis. What possible intersex condition should be considered in the differential diagnosis?**

Mixed gonadal dysgenesis should be evaluated in babies with ambiguous genitalia and unilateral undescended gonad. Most of these patients have a mosaic 46,XY/ 45,XO karyotype. Their gonadal composition is characterized by testicular tissue on one side, and a dysgenetic gonad (streak) on the other. There is often a remnant of a fallopian tube and uterus present with the streak gonad.

❏❏ **A newborn is being evaluated for proximal hypospadias and bilateral nonpalpable testes. What potentially life-threatening condition needs to be considered and urgently evaluated?**

Congenital adrenal hyperplasia (CAH) from 21-hydroxylase deficiency, must be ruled out in newborns with bilateral cryptorchidism and ambiguous genitalia. The deficiency of biologically active mineralocorticoid in type II CAH results in electrolyte imbalances with salt and water loss. There are rare instances of congenital adrenal hyperplasia where the infant may appear fully virilized.

❏❏ **How should the newborn be evaluated for possible congenital adrenal hyperplasia (CAH)?**

(1) A rectal examination, pelvic ultrasound or retrograde genitogram should be performed to detect a cervix and uterus. (2) Karyotyping can be done within 48-hours with activated T-lymphocytes. (3) Raised plasma 17-OH progesterone level is diagnostic of CAH. (4) Electrolytes should be drawn to identify newborns with potential electrolyte imbalance.

❏❏ **In an otherwise normal 46,XY phenotypic male with bilateral nonpalpable testes, how can anorchidism (also called "vanishing testis" or "testicular regression syndrome") be diagnosed nonsurgically?**

Markedly elevated luteinizing hormone (LH) and follicle stimulating hormone (FSH) levels and absent testosterone response to human chorionic gonadotropin (hCG) stimulation indicate absent testes bilaterally with considerable certainty. Elevated levels of serum gonadotropins do not establish the diagnosis of bilateral anorchia after nine years of age. The recent availability of mullerian inhibiting substance assay may permit even more accurate determination of anorchia.

❏❏ **A five-year-old boy presents with retraction of the testis following previous inguinal orchidopexy performed at two years of age. Physical examination confirms a normal sized testis at the level of the right external inguinal ring. How should the reoperative orchidopexy be approached?**

A successful approach to reoperative orchidopexy entails the en bloc mobilization of the testis with a strip of the external oblique fascia attached to the underlying vas deferens and spermatic vessels. This technique minimizes potential injury to the spermatic cord structures that may be adherent to the undersurface of the external oblique fascia.

MEGAURETER, ECTOPIC URETER, VESICOURETERAL REFLUX, AND URETEROCELE

Madhu Alagiri, M.D.

❏❏ **What is the definition of a megaureter?**

A Megaureter is a generic term referring to an enlarged ureter and does not imply a specific etiology. In the pediatric population, a megaureter typically has a diameter of greater than 7 mm.

❏❏ **What are the four primary classifications of megaureter?**

The classification of a megaureter is based upon the respective pathology. For example, a primary obstructed megaureter is a dilated ureter that is obstructed at the ureterovesical junction. Currently, there are four accepted subtypes of megaureter as follows:

1. Non-refluxing, obstructed (primary obstructed megaureter)
2. Refluxing, non-obstructed megaureter
3. Non-refluxing, non-obstructed megaureter
4. Refluxing, obstructed megaureter

❏❏ **T/F: A primary obstructed megaureter is more common in males than females.**

True. A primary obstructed megaureter is four times more common in males than females.

❏❏ **T/F: The ureteral orifice of a primary obstructed megaureter is usually ectopic.**

False. The ureteral orifice of a primary obstructed megaureter is typically normal in appearance and location.

❏❏ **What is the histopathologic defect found in a primary obstructed megaureter?**

Several detailed histopathologic reviews have demonstrated that there is an abnormal proliferation of both collagen and circular muscle fibers in the terminal segment of a primary obstructed megaureter. This defect prevents normal peristalsis and results in an adynamic distal ureter.

❏❏ **T/F: Next to a ureteropelvic junction obstruction, a megaureter is the second most common cause of pathologic hydronephrosis in the newborn.**

True. With the advent of antenatal ultrasound, the incidence of neonatal hydronephrosis has increased dramatically. Both ureteropelvic junction obstruction and megaureter are diagnosed much more frequently.

❏❏ **In a neonate with a suspected megaureter based on an antenatal ultrasound, what is the initial study of choice?**

Ultrasound after the first 48 - hours of life is the ideal study. It is non-invasive, painless, and does not involve radiation exposure. Furthermore, it can easily identify a dilated ureter as well as indicate possible causes of hydronephrosis such as a ureteropelvic junction obstruction or a ureterocele.

❏❏ **T/F: A voiding cystourethrogram is not indicated if the ultrasound shows a dilated ureter and kidney but a normal bladder.**

False. A voiding cystourethrogram is an essential element in the evaluation of a megaureter. Approximately 5% of patients will have co-existing reflux in the presence of an obstructing megaureter. Furthermore, high-grade reflux alone can result in a megaureter.

❏❏ In the imaging evaluation of a megaureter, what is the next step after an ultrasound and a voiding cystourethrogram?

A diuretic renogram is the next step in the evaluation and classification of a suspected megaureter. By calculating the half-time clearance of the radioisotope in the kidney and ureter, the location and severity of the obstruction can be determined. A half-time clearance of greater than 20 minutes is consistent with obstruction. Renal scans also measure relative renal function, which can have a significant bearing on treatment.

❏❏ Define the pressure-perfusion test (Whitaker test) in determining ureteral obstruction.

The pressure-perfusion or Whitaker test refers to an invasive procedure that measures intrapelvic and intravesical pressures during infusion of fluids via a percutaneous nephrostomy. Obstruction is implied when the pressure gradient between the kidney and bladder exceeds 15-cm H_2O when infusing at a rate of 10 ml / minute. While useful in cases where obstruction is not readily apparent, the Whitaker test is not universally accepted as a diagnostic modality.

❏❏ Based on imaging studies, the diagnosis of a primary obstructed megaureter is suspected. What is the initial treatment?

Once a primary obstructed megaureter is suspected or confirmed, initial therapy should be antibiotic prophylaxis. Urinary infections in the presence of an obstruction can have devastating consequences. This is particularly true for infants, who are more susceptible to renal damage with concomitant infection than adults.

❏❏ T/F: An imaging evaluation of a megaureter shows that it is neither obstructed nor refluxing, and both kidneys have relatively equal renal function. The next step, in the management of this patient, is observation and serial ultrasounds.

True. Even though the ureter is not obstructed at present, follow-up ultrasounds will be required for several years to ensure that the hydronephrosis decreases or disappears. Repeat renal scans may also be required to ensure that obstruction does not develop.

❏❏ What diuretic renogram criteria would constitute a strong indication to surgically correct a primary obstructed megaureter?

A renal scan that involves a lasix-induced diuretic phase is called a diuretic renogram. Induced diuresis is important to rule-out a false-positive obstruction. With a diuretic renogram, a relative decrease in renal function (< 35%) and a delayed half-time clearance of the radioisotope (T1/2>20 min) are strong indications for surgical correction.

❏❏ Why is ureteral tailoring or tapering an important tool in the surgical management of a megaureter?

An important element in successful reimplantation surgery is preservation of an adequate submucosal tunnel in comparison to ureteral diameter. Ureteral tapering techniques can reduce the diameter of a megaureter allowing for a shorter reimplant tunnel. A tunnel to diameter ratio of 5:1 is generally accepted as necessary to reduce the possibility of post-operative reflux. In addition, narrowing the ureteral lumen can enhance efficient peristalsis.

❏❏ Name three prominent ureteral tapering techniques used in the repair of megaureter.

Hendren repair: excision of the excess ureter with suture approximation of the remaining ureter.
Kalicinski repair: folding of the excess ureter over onto itself to narrow the ureteral lumen.
Starr repair: plication of the ureteral wall to narrow the lumen.

❑❑ **List four recognized complications of a megaureter repair.**

Ischemic ureteral stricture or fistula.
Urinary extravasation.
Ureteral kinking and obstruction.
Vesicoureteral reflux.

❑❑ **Describe the post-operative evaluation for patients who have undergone repair of a primary obstructed megaureter.**

Post-operatively, patients should remain on prophylactic antibiotic therapy until repeat studies have confirmed resolution of the obstruction. An ultrasound, voiding cystourethrogram, and diuretic renogram should be performed approximately 3-months after surgery. If these studies show persistent obstruction or reflux, antibiotics should be continued. The patient should be restudied periodically over the next few years to determine if a revision procedure is necessary.

❑❑ **What is the most common congenital anomaly found in the urinary tract?**

Ureteral duplication, either partial or complete, is the most common congenital anomaly found in the urinary tract. Ureteral duplication has no clinical significance.

❑❑ **Define the Weigert-Meyer law.**

The Weigert-Meyer law pertains to complete ureteral duplication. It states that the ureteral orifice draining the upper moiety occupies a position inferior and medial to the orifice draining the lower moiety.

❑❑ **What is the definition and etiology of an ectopic ureter?**

An ectopic ureter has an orifice that is not in its proper location on the trigone of the bladder. The ectopic orifice is thought to result from improper development of the terminal mesonephric duct. During fetal development, ureteral budding is further cephalad than normal. This delays ureteral absorption into the bladder resulting in ureteral ectopia.

❑❑ **T/F: An ectopic ureter is found more frequently in males.**

False. An ectopic ureter is six times more common in females than males.

❑❑ **T/F: An ectopic ureter is associated with complete ureteral duplication.**

True. Most ectopic ureters (70%) are associated with complete ureteral duplication.

❑❑ **What is the classic presentation of an ectopic ureter in a female?**

In a female, the classic presentation is a patient with continuous dampness or wetness who otherwise voids normally. The continuous urine leak is due to the ectopic positioning of the orifice distal to the bladder neck and urethral sphincter mechanism.

❑❑ **T/F: In males, an ectopic ureter can sometimes be associated with incontinence.**

False. In males, an ectopic ureter will not drain distal to the urethral sphincter mechanism and will not present as continuous incontinence.

❑❑ **In the male, name four primary urologic structures into which an ectopic ureter can drain.**

An ectopic ureter can drain into other mesonephric duct structures including the seminal vesicles, vas deferens, epididymis, and prostatic urethra / ejaculatory duct.

❑❑ **In the female, list three gynecologic structures that an ectopic ureter can drain into.**

In a female, an ectopic ureter typically drains into the bladder neck, urethra, or vaginal vestibule. However, an ectopic orifice can also be found in the vagina, uterus, or fallopian tubes.

❏❏ What is the embryological origin of the bladder and trigone?

The bladder is of endodermal origin while the trigone is of mesodermal origin.

❏❏ What vestigial structures are remnants of the mesonephric duct in the female?

In the female, the vestigial mesonephric remnants are Gartner's ducts. Segments of these ducts can become clinically significant cystic masses and are referred to as Gartner's duct cysts.

❏❏ What would be the most likely cause of post-natal demise in a neonate with bilateral ureteral ectopia, renal dysplasia, and oligohydramnios?

An adequate amount of fetal urine is necessary for proper pulmonary development. Rather than succumb to renal failure, the newborn infant is more likely to be at immediate risk from pulmonary dysplasia as a result of the oligohydramnios.

❏❏ T/F: In males, single-system ectopia is more common than duplex-system ectopia.

True. While ureteral ectopia is much more common in females than males, males have a higher incidence of an ectopic ureter involving a non-duplicated collecting system.

❏❏ An otherwise normal, 5-year-old child presents with epididymo-orchitis. Besides treating the infection, what is the next step in evaluating this patient?

It is unusual for a pre-pubertal child to have epididymo-orchitis. An ultrasound is required to rule out an ectopic ureteral insertion contiguous with the epididymis.

❏❏ On a screening ultrasound, a child is noted to have a duplex collecting system and a suspected ectopic ureter. A voiding cystourethrogram is performed and shows no evidence of reflux. Antibiotic prophylaxis has been started. What is the next step in evaluating this patient?

A diuretic renal scan is the next step in evaluating this patient. This study is important since it measures both obstruction and function. The renal moiety associated with an ectopic ureter is typically dysplastic and demonstrates poor renal function.

❏❏ A 3-year-old male patient underwent a voiding cystourethrogram for a urinary tract infection evaluation. The catheter was inserted per urethra and contrast was instilled. The fluoroscopic picture showed a dilated ureter and renal pelvis but no bladder. How is this scenario possible?

An ectopic ureter can have a patulous orifice entering at the prostatic urethra. During insertion, the urethral catheter can inadvertently bypass the bladder and enter the ectopic orifice. This would explain the above scenario. Cystoscopy of the patient will often reveal a large ureteral orifice and dilated ureter.

❏❏ A 3-year-old girl is found to have a left ectopic ureter draining an upper moiety. She has an otherwise normal left lower moiety. An ultrasound shows poor parenchymal preservation and severe hydroureteronephrosis of the upper moiety. A voiding cystourethrogram is normal. A renal scan shows no function in the affected segment. She has had recurrent febrile urinary tract infections requiring hospitalization. What is the best course of action for this patient?

Surgical management of an ectopic ureter can be controversial. However, in a child with a non-functioning hydronephrotic, symptomatic moiety, the best course of action is a heminephroureterectomy. The distal ureter is usually left in place to avoid damage to the urethral sphincter complex.

❏❏ What is the function of the vesicoureteral junction?

The vesicoureteral junction connects the terminal ureter to the bladder. It is surrounded by a fascial sheath (Waldeyer's sheath), which accompanies it through the ureteral hiatus to the trigone. The function of the vesicoureteral junction is to allow urine to drain freely while preventing reflux by closing firmly when the bladder distends.

⬜⬜ **What percentage of children with UTIs have vesicoureteral reflux?**

The percentage of children with a UTI who have reflux is significant and ranges between 30% to 50%.

⬜⬜ **T/F: Vesicoureteral reflux does not have a genetic component, and risk of reflux in siblings is minimal.**

False. Vesicoureteral reflux does have a genetic component. Approximately 33% of siblings and up to 66% of offspring can be affected. Controversy exists as to who should undergo screening with either a voiding cystourethrogram or an isotope cystogram.

⬜⬜ **Describe the international classification for grading vesicoureteral reflux.**

The international classification for vesicoureteral reflux is based on the appearance of the urinary tract during a voiding cystourethrogram. The classification is divided into five grades as described below.

Grade I.   Reflux into a non-dilated ureter.
Grade II.   Reflux into the renal collecting system without dilation.
Grade III. Reflux into the collecting system with dilation of the calyces.
Grade IV.   Same as grade III with dilation of the pelvis and moderate tortuosity of the ureter.
Grade V.   Reflux into the collecting system with gross dilation and tortuosity of the ureter, gross dilation of the collecting system, and loss of calyceal architecture.

⬜⬜ **What is the prevalence of vesicoureteral reflux in the general pediatric population?**

The prevalence of reflux in the pediatric population is less than 1%. The majority of patients are identified when they undergo imaging studies as part of a UTI evaluation.

⬜⬜ **T/F: Vesicoureteral reflux is uncommon in the African-American population.**

True. Vesicoureteral reflux is approximately tens times more likely in Caucasians than in African-Americans.

⬜⬜ **What is the cause of primary vesicoureteral reflux?**

Primary reflux is due to an inadequate length of intramural ureter. Lack of submucosal or intramural ureteral length prevents the terminal ureter from closing like a flap valve when the bladder fills.

⬜⬜ **How do anatomic and functional obstructive processes contribute to the severity of vesicoureteral reflux and make it refractory to surgical correction?**

Anatomic obstructions such as posterior urethral valves or strictures increase intravesical voiding pressures and contribute to the failure of the proper function of the vesicoureteral junction. Functional obstruction such as a neurogenic bladder or detrusor sphincter dyssynergia can also contribute to poor bladder compliance. Surgical repair will be more likely to fail if the obstructive processes are not ameliorated first.

⬜⬜ **What is the best initial therapy for a 4-year-old girl with newly identified grade II left vesicoureteral reflux?**

Because low and moderate grade reflux (I-III) has a good chance for spontaneous resolution, antibiotic prophylaxis and observation is the best initial therapy for this child. Approximately 80% of patients with low-grade reflux will have spontaneous resolution, and more than 50% of patients with grade III reflux will have resolution. Grade IV reflux has a 10% chance of resolution, and grade V reflux rarely resolves spontaneously.

⬜⬜ **List three strong indications for considering surgical correction in a child with low-grade vesicoureteral reflux.**

Breakthrough infections or persistently positive urine cultures indicate that antibiotic prophylaxis is not working and surgical correction should be considered.
Non-compliance with medical therapy is another strong indication for surgical consideration.

Anatomic issues such as a periureteral diverticulum or grade V vesicoureteral reflux deserve surgical consideration due to the low likelihood of spontaneous resolution.

Less stringent indications for surgical repair include: failure of renal growth, new scarring seen on imaging studies, persistent reflux followed for several years, and reflux persisting into puberty.

❑❑ T/F: The Glenn-Anderson repair for ureteral reimplantation involves an intravesical approach and placement of the submucosal tunnel and neo-orifice on the contralateral trigone.

False. Intravesical reimplantation of the ureter on the contralateral trigone is known as the Cohen or cross-trigonal procedure. The Glenn-Anderson repair refers to the placement of the submucosal ureter and orifice on the ipsilateral trigone. One theoretical advantage of the Glenn-Anderson repair is that it would allow easy endoscopic access to the ureter in the post-operative period.

❑❑ T/F: The Lich-Gregoir repair refers to a repair that is done extravesically for vesicoureteral reflux.

True. The Lich-Gregoir is an extravesical repair. An adequate intravesical tunnel is created by incising the detrusor muscle and laying the ureter in the submucosal trough. Since this approach can decrease patient morbidity, it has enjoyed popularity among both urologists and transplant surgeons.

❑❑ T/F: Endoscopic bulking agents have achieved the same success rate as open ureteral reimplantation in treating vesicoureteral reflux.

False. Open ureteral reimplantation has an approximate success rate of 95%. Use of collagen as a bulking agent has a success rate approaching 80%. Durability of endoscopic bulking agents has also been an issue.

❑❑ Besides general surgical concerns, list three complications specific to ureteral reimplantation surgery.

Besides bleeding and infection, ureteral reimplantation surgery can be complicated by persistent reflux, ureteral obstruction, bladder diverticulum, and contralateral reflux.

❑❑ T/F: If a post-reimplantation voiding cystogram shows persistent reflux, the most appropriate management is to proceed to surgery to revise the ureteral reimplantation.

False. It may take several months for the ureter to heal and the flap-valve mechanism to become competent. If post-operative reflux is noted, antibiotic prophylaxis should be continued, and the study should be repeated in a few months. Occasionally, patients will need a revision procedure, and the re-operation rate ranges from 1 to 3%.

❑❑ T/F: If a patient had bilateral reflux in the past but now only has unilateral left vesicoureteral reflux, the most appropriate surgical repair is bilateral ureteral reimplantation.

True. Contralateral reflux as a complication in an otherwise normal ureter can be as high as 20%. If the ureter has been noted to reflux in the past, the incidence of post-operative reflux approaches 45%. Therefore, in the above scenario, the most appropriate repair is bilateral ureteral reimplantation.

❑❑ Define a ureterocele.

A ureterocele refers to a cystic dilation of the terminal, intravesical ureter. In the pediatric population, it is typically associated with obstruction.

❑❑ What is Chwalla's membrane?

Chwalla's membrane refers to an embryological, one-cell-layer membrane that is found between the primitive ureteral orifice and the urogenital sinus. Persistence of Chwalla's membrane is thought to be a possible precursor to a ureterocele.

❑❑ T/F: A single-system ureterocele is more likely in a male.

True. Although the embryological cause is unknown, a single-system ureterocele is much more common in males than females.

❏❏ **T/F: A duplex-system ureterocele usually involves the upper moiety.**

True. A ureterocele, in a completely duplicated urinary system, usually involves the upper moiety and its orifice tends to be ectopic. Also, a duplex-system ureterocele is four times more common than a single-system ureterocele, and it is more prevalent in females.

❏❏ **T/F: A voiding cystourethrogram is the most sensitive test to identify a ureterocele.**

False. A voiding cystourethrogram is an important study in the evaluation of a ureterocele. However, a bladder ultrasound should be the initial study when a ureterocele is suspected. Ultrasound imaging can readily identify the cystic mass (ureterocele) within the bladder.

❏❏ **T/F: A ureterocele can cause bladder outlet obstruction and urinary retention.**

True. A large ureterocele can displace the ureter and encompass the entire bladder trigone. In females, a ureterocele may prolapse through the urethra and present as a cystic introital mass causing urinary retention.

❏❏ **Define a cecoureterocele.**

A cecoureterocele refers to a large ureterocele that has progressed submucosally beyond the ureteral orifice. It typically involves the distal trigone and urethra and can cause bladder outlet obstruction.

❏❏ **In a 4-year-old male with a single-system ureterocele and a functioning kidney, what is the best initial course of action to correct the ureterocele?**

A single-system ureterocele tends to drain a functioning renal unit. This is especially true if the ureterocele is orthotopic. While there are conflicting opinions regarding management, endoscopic incision of the ureterocele is the preferred approach. This minimally invasive technique can successfully alleviate obstruction, but it can also create a refluxing ureter. Post-incision reflux can be managed by observation, antibiotic prophylaxis, and surgical correction if necessary.

❏❏ **In a-3-year old girl with an upper moiety ureterocele and an associated dysplastic renal segment, what is the best course of action?**

A renal scan can objectively measure renal function and obstruction. If the affected renal segment functions poorly, a heminephrectomy and subtotal ureterectomy is warranted. Ablation of the distal ureter is usually not necessary but may be required as a secondary procedure if infections develop.

❏❏ **T/F: In patients with a ureterocele, a common contralateral congenital anomaly is ureteral duplication.**

True. Patients with a ureterocele have several associated congenital urologic anomalies. Approximately 50% will have contralateral ureteral duplication. Other associated anomalies include renal segment dysplasia, renal fusion, ectopia, and reflux.

UROLOGICAL EMERGENCIES IN THE NEWBORN

Yves L. Homsy, M.D. and Aseem R. Shukla, M.D.

❏❏ **A 23-year-old pregnant female presents for evaluation of prenatally detected unilateral hydronephrosis. There is no oligohydramnios. What would be your consideration and recommendation to the patient?**

Prenatal fetal hydronephrosis is the most commonly diagnosed fetal urologic abnormality (incidence 1 in 5000). With normal amniotic fluid levels, close follow-up throughout the pregnancy and in the neonatal/newborn period as well as through the first year of life are required. The majority of cases of prenatal low-grade hydronephrosis may stabilize and resolve within the first year of life.

❏❏ **This woman delivered a 7 lb. 3 oz. otherwise healthy male infant. Postnatal ultrasonography confirms the presence of unilateral hydronephrosis. What further evaluation do you recommend?**

Careful physical examination with an emphasis on observing the infant's active voiding is an important first step. The infant should be started on antibiotic prophylaxis as the incidence of urinary tract infection is approximately 3% in the first six months of life. A voiding cystourethogram (VCUG) and nuclear renogram (DTPA or MAG 3) should also be scheduled.

❏❏ **A 32-week prenatal ultrasound of a male fetus followed for hydronephrosis reveals increasing bilateral hydronephrosis, a dilated bladder, and new-onset marked oligohydramnios. What is your recommendation?**

Posterior urethral valves leading to bilateral hydronephrosis with oligohydramnios is the most likely etiology, and this situation represents a rare urologic indication for induction of labor or fetal intervention. Fetal lung maturity should be evaluated with a lecithin/sphingomyelin amniotic fluid ratio prior to a final recommendation. If fetal surgical intervention is considered then fetal renal function should be estimated by the urinary sodium and osmolality obtained by fetal bladder aspiration. A high-grade obstruction of a single system also requires a similarly rapid response.

❏❏ **Consultation is requested for an otherwise healthy term infant with a palpable right-sided abdominal mass. Prenatal sonography was not performed. How do you proceed with your physical examination?**

A general exam must begin with initial attention to subcutaneous nodules (neuroblastoma) or dehydration, particularly with hematuria (as seen in renal vein thrombosis). The patient should be placed in the lateral decubitus position for kidney palpation by supporting the flank with one hand and palpating the upper quadrant subcostally with the opposite hand. Care should be taken to avoid extensive abdominal manipulation after the initial examination to prevent the rare occurrence of rupture as seen in cases of Wilm's tumor/mesoblastic nephroma. Transillumination of the flank mass may distinguish cystic from solid lesions. Following a complete physical exam, including careful blood pressure measurements, ultrasonography is indicated.

❏❏ **What are causes of non-obstructive fetal hydronephrosis?**

Vesicoureteral reflux (incidence of 15 to 20% in white and less than 1% in black patients with prenatal hydronephrosis) and fetal ureteral folds are common causes of mild or transient ureteral dilatation noted in prenatal ultrasounds.

❏❏ A prenatal ultrasound detects oligohydramnios and the presence of multiple small cysts (1-2 mm in diameter). Liver sonography demonstrates periportal fibrosis. What are the most likely diagnosis and prognosis?

Hepatic fibrosis with a polycystic kidney is consistent with autosomal recessive polcysystic kidney disease of the infantile form. After birth, contrast urography will reveal severely delayed function and a nephrogram with an alternating radially oriented sunray pattern. While an occasional child will survive beyond infancy, most infants are stillborn or die with the first few weeks.

❏❏ What is the most likely cause of an abdominal mass in a healthy appearing male infant and how can it be differentiated from the second most common cause of neonatal abdominal masses?

Hydronephrosis due to UPJ is the most common cause of neonatal abdominal mass. Multicystic dysplastic kidney (MCDK) is the second most common cause of the neonatal abdominal mass and can be distinguished from UPJ obstruction by the technetium^{99m} DMSA renal scan. The renal scan usually demonstrates some function in the hydronephrotic kidney and non-function of the MCDK.

❏❏ An infant is diagnosed with a multicystic dysplastic kidney on the right side based on the "cluster of grapes" appearance on ultrasound and lack of function by DMSA renal scan. What is of concern regarding the contralateral kidney?

The contralateral kidney and collecting system must be carefully studied in cases of MCDK. Contralateral vesicoureteral reflux is the most commonly encountered abnormality with an incidence of 20-40%. Contralateral hydronephrosis due to ureteropelvic junction obstruction occurs in approximately 10% of infants with multicystic kidney disease.

❏❏ A one-month-old female infant is admitted to the neonatal intensive care unit with failure to thrive and respiratory distress. Physical exam reveals a large right-sided abdominal mass. Ultrasonography reveals an enlarged right kidney with multiple non-communicating cystic structures. A renal scan reveals no perfusion to the affected side and normal function of the left kidney. What treatment would you recommend?

This clinical scenario is consistent with the findings of multicystic kidney disease (MCKD). Symptoms including respiratory distress, failure to thrive, hypertension, or hemorrhage are clear indications for immediate nephrectomy in certain cases of MCKD. There is no role for observation in these circumstances.

❏❏ A clinically stable, otherwise healthy term neonate is diagnosed with left MCDK by ultrasound. The right kidney is noted to be free of reflux with intact renal function. Is there a role for observation? Must a nephrectomy be performed?

In the absence of hypertension, feeding or developmental problems due to mechanical or obstructive complications, immediate surgical excision is unnecessary. Concern for onset of hypertension, malignant degeneration of the MCDK to Wilm's tumor, or less commonly, renal cell carcinoma remains an argument for prophylactic removal of these non-functioning moieties. The minimal morbidity of a procedure accomplished through a small incision and the freedom from regular follow-ups or ultrasonography are additional factors favoring nephrectomy. Non-interventional follow-up and the ability to sonographically follow MCDK's, as well as the high incidence of near complete involution favor observation in these cases. One must remember, however, that while the cystic fluid found within MCDK's may be resorbed, the cyst wall is a persistent remnant.

❏❏ A term infant is noted to have a fixed, unilateral mass extending to the midline. Also noted are multiple bluish skin nodules. What is the most likely diagnosis and treatment?

This clinical picture most likely represents neuroblastoma, an embryonal tumor of neural crest origin. Neuroblastoma is the most common solid abdominal mass and the most common malignant tumor in infancy. For low stage tumors, (I-II) surgical excision remains the treatment of choice. For stage III and higher disease, chemotherapy and radiation therapy are employed as multimodal therapies. As an exception for higher stage disease, surgical excision is often the standard of care without irradiation or chemotherapy in cases of stage IV-S disease (hepatic metastases, skin nodules and bone marrow involvement).

❏❏ **A lower abdominal mass is palpated in a newborn female. Examination of the perineum reveals a mass in the introitus. The mass persists following placement of a urethral catheter. What is the most likely diagnosis?**

A lower abdominal mass in an otherwise healthy female patient is most likely due to hydometrocolpos, or distension of the vagina and uterus.

❏❏ **What anatomical abnormalities most commonly lead to hydrometrocolpos?**

An imperforate hymen is the most common cause of hydrometrocolpos. A less common etiology is a high transverse vaginal septum, which can be associated with a persistent urogenital sinus. In cases of a high transverse vaginal septum, the external anatomy may appear deceptively normal but ultrasonography of the abdominal mass will reveal a cystic midline structure posterior to the bladder without septation.

❏❏ **Three days following Gomco clamp circumcision, an newborn infant develops brisk bleeding from the incision. What is the risk of hemorrhage and how should it be treated following circumcision?**

Hemorrhage occurs in approximately 1% of cases. The incidence is highest at 3 days after birth due to the physiologic depression of plasma levels of vitamin K – dependent clotting factor. If conservative measures such as compression with an epinephrine soaked gauze sponge or thrombin application fails, hemostatic suture placement is required.

❏❏ **Consultation is requested approximately seven days following a neonatal circumcision. Examination of the penis reveals dehiscence of the incision line with complete exposure of the ventral penile shaft. Treatment options include?**

Healing by secondary intention is the preferred approach following such a dehiscence. In rare cases, extensive denudation of skin may require skin grafting to prevent secondary chordee or scarring.

❏❏ **A 9-day-old infant undergoing a sepsis workup is noted to have a palpable right- sided abdominal mass with associated gross hematuria. What is the most likely diagnosis?**

The most likely diagnosis is renal vein thrombosis (RVT). Sixty percent – 70% of patients with renal vein thrombosis have findings of a palpable mass, with associated gross hematuria and proteinuria.

❏❏ **A 2-day-old infant born to a diabetic mother has polyuria (10ml/kg/hr). Is the child at risk for compromised renal function?**

Yes. Infants of diabetic mothers experiencing an osmotic diuresis as well as infants with profuse diarrhea, sepsis, acute hypoxia and hypotension are at risk for RVT. Renal vein thrombosis often occurs due to low renal perfusion pressures and increased blood viscosity secondary to extracellular volume contraction with resultant sludging of blood in renal venules.

❏❏ **A 4-day-old infant with a palpable abdominal mass, gross hematuria and thrombocytopenia undergoes an abdominal Doppler ultrasound that confirms the diagnosis of unilateral RVT without caval thrombus. Appropriate treatment includes?**

Vigorous hydration, electrolyte management and treatment of underlying cause are critical for patient well being. Aggressive anticoagulation and thrombolytic therapy are employed in certain situations. Thrombolytic agents such as urokinase, streptokinase and tissue plasminogen activator are utilized for bilateral RVT.

❏❏ **Following successful treatment of RVT, what sequellae may develop?**

Fibrosis of the kidney, renovascular hypertension, nephrotic syndrome and chronic pyelonephritis are all possible sequelae of RVT. Hypertension in association with an atrophic kidney is often renin-mediated and a nephrectomy is curative.

❏❏ **A 35-week gestation newborn is anuric for 36-hours following birth. Physical examination is unremarkable. Should a workup for acute renal failure commence?**

No. 92% and 99.4% of term newborns void within 24-hours and 48-hours of birth, respectively. Acute renal failure is suspected only if anuria persists more than 48 hours.

❏❏ **The same infant persists with urine output of 0.7 ml/kg/hr and a serum creatinine of 1.1 mg/dl at 72-hours. There is no history of oligohydramnios. What is the most common cause of oliguria in the newborn and how is it treated?**

Prerenal renal failure secondary to inadequate perfusion is the most common cause of oliguria in the newborn. Hypotension from sepsis, maternal antepartum hemorrhage or surgical bleeding may lead to renal hypoperfusion. Similarly, congestive heart failure due to cardiac anomalies or dehydration may also lead to renal ischemia. Neonatal intensive care admission with volume expansion will rapidly reverse prerenal renal failure. Oligohydramnios is usually present in infants with anuria or oliguria due to postrenal causes.

❏❏ **A term infant in the neonatal intensive unit has multiple unsucessful attempts at umbilical artery catheterization. Consultation is requested 24 hours later for apparent new onset neonatal ascites. What is the likely diagnosis?**

Urachal laceration due to attempted umbilical arterial catheterization is the most common cause of neonatal intraperitoneal bladder rupture. Evaluation should consist of a VCUG and possibly a diagnostic paracentesis. While management may be conservative for most cases of neonatal ascites, initial operative management is recommended in cases of intraperitoneal bladder rupture.

❏❏ **A term male infant is admitted the intensive care unit immediately postpartum with hypotension, and tachycardia. Physical exam is remarkable for a penis of only 1.5 cm stretched penile length. The external genitalia are otherwise normal. Electrolyte studies reveal hyponatremia, hyperkalemia and hypoglycemia. What is the most likely diagnosis and how must the infant be treated?**

This critically ill infant with clear micropenis (penile length 2.5 standard deviations below the mean) must be evaluated for panhypopituitarism. Following intravenous glucose and electrolyte replacement, serial serum glucose, sodium, and potassium evaluations are necessary. Serial gonadotropin and testosterone measurements from birth through three months of age will eventually document a neonatal luteinizing hormone (LH) surge in normal infants.

❏❏ **A 1300-gram pre-term infant is being treated for respiratory distress syndrome (RDS) in the neonatal intensive care unit (NICU). Abdominal x-rays reveal bilateral 0.7 mm renal stones on a abdominal x-ray. The etiology of this condition includes?**

Furosemide, commonly used in the treatment of RDS and other conditions common to premature infants in the NICU setting is associated with nephrolithiasis. Furosemide causes a hypercalciuric state with a secondary increased resorption of calcium in the proximal tubule and subsequent renal stone formation. Excessive calcium and glucose intake in specialized formulas for premature infants is another recognized cause of neonatal nephrolithiasis.

❏❏ **A premature infant in the NICU with patent ductus arteriosus receives furosemide at 2 mg/kg/day for 4-weeks. An abdominal x-ray reveals bilateral nephrocalcinosis. What is the most appropriate treatment?**

Furosemide induced renal parenchymal stone disease rarely requires surgical intervention. The administration of hydrochlorothiazide, reduced calcium intake, and cessation of furosemide therapy often results in resolution of nephrolithiasis. In cases of discrete, massive calculus formation, shock wave lithotripsy or open surgical intervention may be warranted.

❏❏ **Umbilical artery catheterization is performed on a premature infant in the neonatal intensive care unit (NICU). Twenty-four hours later the infant has gross hematuria and hypertension. The hypertension is refractory to aggressive medical management. What is the diagnosis and the most appropriate treatment?**

A recognized complication of umbilical artery catheterization is renal artery thrombosis, either alone or as part of an extensive aorto-iliac thrombus. The clinical diagnosis can be confirmed by Doppler ultrasonography and radionuclide imaging, if necessary. While aggressive medical therapy combined with thrombolyis has a role in the treatement of many cases of renal artery thrombosis, nephrectomy would be indicated in this life-threatening case.

❏❏ **A 38-week gestational age male infant is delivered following prolonged labor with meconium aspiration. Aggressive resuscitation efforts are successfull. On day 3 of life an abdominal mass is palpated on the right side. What is the likely sonographic finding and what is your diagnosis?**

Sudden increases in intra-abdominal pressure during prolonged labor may result in adrenal hemorrhage with the observed physical findings. Adrenal hemorrhage typically involves the right adrenal gland and sonographic findings initially demonstrate a hyperechoic or solid mass over the superior pole of the kidney. With time, the lesion may become hypoechoic and decreases in size. This finding should not be confused with neuroblastoma, the most common adrenal malignancy of infancy which typically has a solid appearance on ultrasound but may be cystic or have a mixed echogenic pattern.

❏❏ **A term male infant is noted to have multiple genitourinary anomalies at birth consistent with the classic bladder exstrophy / epispadias complex. How must the exstrophic bladder be maintained prior to surgical intervention?**

The mucosa of the bladder must be protected while the candidacy for surgery is discussed. Noncontact care may consist of placing the child in an incubator without a diaper and with saline mist to keep the mucosa moist. Alternatively, the bladder mucosa may be protected by a plastic wrap to prevent the mucosa from sticking to clothing or to the diaper. Broad spectrum antibiotics may be started to sterilize the bladder wall prior to surgical intervention.

❏❏ **A 39-week-old term infant has a firm right scrotal mass at birth. The mass is painless and does not transillumate. The overlying skin is erythematous and indurated. What is the most likely diagnosis?**

The most common cause of a scrotal mass at birth is testicular torsion. The differential diagnosis for the described presentation includes incarcerated inguinal hernia, scrotal hematoma, tumor and more rarely, ectopic spleen or adrenal tissue.

❏❏ **How is neonatal testicular torsion anatomically different from testicular torsion in adolescents?**

Neonatal testicular torsion is extra-vaginal since the tunica vaginalis is not adherent to the surrounding dartos fascia of the scrotal wall until 4 to 8 weeks of age. Torsion in the neonate, therefore, involves the testis, spermatic cord and overlying tunica vaginalis. Testicular torsion in the adolescent, meanwhile, is intravaginal as the tunica vaginalis is fixed to the dartos fascia.

❏❏ **An infant with a firm scrotal mass at birth is diagnosed with testicular torsion. The infant is hemodynamically stable and the contralateral testis is normal. Is surgical exploration and detorsion with orchiopexy necessary?**

It is well known that successful testicular salvage in the event of neonatal testicular torsion is exceedingly rare. Exploration with an intent of salvage alone is not justified. The role of scrotal exploration with contralateral testicular fixation due to the potential for asynchronous torsion until the tunica vaginalis adheres to the scrotal wall remains controversial. Clearly, however, if bilateral torsion is suspected, then exploration despite the low incidence of salvage is necessitated.

❏❏ **A male infant delivered at an estimated 34-weeks gestational age without prenatal care demonstrates failure to thrive and neonatal ascites. The infant is noted to have a diminished, dribbling urinary stream. What is the most likely diagnosis?**

The most common cause of bladder outlet obstruction in the male newborn is posterior urethral valves. An abdominal mass, failure to thrive and neonatal ascites are among the most common presenting symptoms. Clearly the widespread use of prenatal ultrasound has directed early investigation in patients with posterior urethral valves.

❑❑ **Prenatal sonography at 22-weeks reveals bilateral hydroureteronephrosis with a distended bladder consistent with posterior urethral valves. Attempts at placement of a vesicoamniotic shunt are unsuccessful. Labor is induced at 32-weeks. What is the initial radiological workup at birth?**

Recognition of prenatal hydronephrosis suggests the need for repeat sonography at birth to establish a baseline view of the renal collecting systems. A voiding cystourethrogram should also be performed and often demonstrates a thick trabeculated bladder with a distended posterior urethra.

❑❑ **A 35-week gestational age male infant with apparent posterior urethral valves (PUV) on voiding cystourethrogram (VCUG) has tense abdominal distension with a fluid wave and a urine output of 0.2 ml/kg/hr despite aggressive fluid resuscitation. What is the most likely diagnosis?**

Neonatal urinary ascites occurs in 7% of male infants with PUV. The diagnosis is based on clinical and radiological evidence and can be confirmed by a diagnostic tap of the ascites. When bladder outlet obstruction is suspected, catheter drainage is initiated followed by drainage of ascites only if respiratory compromise is suspected.

❑❑ **A 32-week gestational age infant is delivered after induction of labor for oligohydramnios and hydronephrosis. A cystic mass is noted on the ventral surface of the penoscrotal junction. What finding is expected on the voiding cystourethrogram (VCUG)?**

A cystic mass at the penoscrotal junction especially with dribbling urinary stream is likely the rare finding of anterior urethral valves. VCUG will likely show a large ventral diverticulum due to a crescentic cusp on the ventral aspect of the urethra. Vesicoureteral reflux may also be seen with this condition.

❑❑ **A term male infant is brought to the emergency room with fever, irritability and weight loss. The infant is uncircumcised. Until what age is the infant more at risk for urinary tract infection (UTI) than circumcised male infants?**

Regardless of phimosis, the presence of foreskin predisposes an infant to UTI until 3 to 6-months of age versus age matched circumcised infants. Colonization of the newborn prepuce diminishes as a risk factor beyond 6-months of age.

❑❑ **An uncircumcised male infant is referred for a clean-catch urine culture revealing 50,000/ml staphylococcous epidermidis. Is a voiding cystourethrogram (VCUG) indicated?**

Further evaluation in this child should not commence until a repeat culture is obtained using urine specimen collected in another manner. While plastic bag collected urine cultures are useful if negative, a confirmation must be sought with a catheterized specimen or suprapubic aspirate. If, however, a single organism with a colony count greater than 100,000/ml in a symptomatic infant is obtained, then a UTI should be treated even in a plastic bag obtained urine specimen.

❑❑ **On initial examination, a term infant has left-sided cryptorchidism and a mid-shaft hypospadias. What is the incidence of intersex disorder in this patient with these findings?**

Phenotypic males with cryptorchidism and hypospadias are estimated to have a 20% to 30% incidence of intersex disorders. Similarly, male phenotype with bilateral impalpable testes and perineal hypospadias alone should initiate an investigation of intersexuality.

❑❑ **What familial risk factors increase risk of intersex states in infants?**

Most intersex disorders result from autosomal recessive inheritance and inquiry as to siblings with abnormal genitalia, infant death or abnormal events at puberty is necessary. Maternal ingestion of androgenic medication (Danozol), progestational agents or drug abuse should also be carefully and investigated.

❑❑ **A term infant with severe hypospadias and unilateral cryptorchidism is suspected to have an intersex disorder. What is the most common intersex disorder with this presentation?**

The most common type of intersex state in patients with severe hypospadias, a testis on one side, and nonpalpable undescended testis is mixed gonadal dysgenesis. This patient likely has a testis on one side and streak gonad on the contralateral side.

❑❑ **Physical exam of a 37-week-old infant shows a hypertrophied clitoris and partially fused, rugated labioscrotal folds. The karyotype is 46 XX. What is the diagnosis and the most likely cause?**

The infant is likely a female pseudohermaphrodite. This group constitutes 60% -70% of all intersex cases in the neonatal period. Congenital adrenal hyperplasia is the etiology in the majority of female pseudohermaphrodites due to the increased ACTH secretion secondary to defective production of cortisol.

❑❑ **An infant is suspected of having congenital adrenal hyperplasia (CAH). What life-threatening condition must be considered, and how is it diagnosed?**

The only life-threatening cause of ambiguous genitalia is the salt-wasting form of CAH. Infants with the most severe form of CAH, 3ß-ol-dehydrogenase deficiency, rarely survive. Infants with the more common 21-hydroxylase deficiency at the zona glomerulosa and fasciculata show a deficient production of mineralocorticoids and the subsequent salt-wasting condition. A salt-wasting crisis typically manifests one week following birth. Following medical stabilization of the patient in an intensive care setting, a plasma 17-hydroxyprogesterone level should be checked and a 24-hour urine collection to measure 17-ketosteroids and pregnanetriol should be initiated.

❑❑ **A 2-week-old infant is brought to the emergency room with profound hypotension and hyperkalemia. Genital examination demonstrates virilization. What treatment should be administered?**

The salt-wasting form of congenital adrenal hyperplasia should be suspected and must be aggressively treated initially with a bolus infusion of 20 ml/kg normal saline. Cortisol replacement is started with a hydrocortisone sodium succinate bolus at 50 mg/m^2 followed by an infusion of 50 to 100 mg/m^2 added to intravenous fluids. For this critically ill infant, deoxycorticosterone (DOCA) at 1-mg to 2-mg should be injected intramuscularly every 12 to 14 hours.

❑❑ **A one-week-old female infant is evaluated in the emergency room for failure to thrive. Physical exam reveals hypertension and virilization of the genitalia with hypertrophy of the clitoris. An arterial blood gas sample is consistent with metabolic acidosis and the potassium level is 6.5 mg / dl. What is the most likely diagnosis?**

Congenital adrenal hyperplasia (CAH) with an enzymatic block at the level of 11ß-hydroxylase is most consistent with this presentation and constitutes 5% of cases of CAH. A deficiency at this enzymatic level results in accumulation of 17-hydroxyprogesterone and androgens as well as the potent mineralocorticoid deoxycorticosterone. Hyperkalemic acidosis, hypervolemia with hypertension are presenting features.

❑❑ **A term-female infant is oliguric at 48-hours of age. Physical exam reveals a palpable, distended bladder and an erythematous interlabial mass. Renal sonography reveals hydronephrosis of the left upper pole. What is the most likely diagnosis?**

The most common cause of urethral obstruction in the female infant is an obstructing ureterocele. In addition, 80% of ureteroceles are associated with the upper pole ureter of a minimally functioning duplicated system. The sonographic findings are consistent with a ureterocele arising from a duplicated collecting system.

❑❑ **Antenatal sonography of a 25-week gestational age female fetus reveals right-sided hydronephrosis and an intravesical cystic dilatation consistent with a ureterocele. Follow-up postnatal sonography, however demonstrates persistent hydronephrosis but no obvious ureterocele. What are likely technical errors during sonography that may confound the diagnosis?**

There are common errors in sonographic technique that may render the diagnosis of ureteroceles difficult. If the bladder is overdistended, then the ureterocele may become effaced and be invisible on ultrasound and even on voiding cystourethrogram. Additionally, if the injected contrast is too concentrated, the ureterocele may become obscured on radiologic imaging. If the bladder is completely empty at time of sonography, on the other hand, a large ureterocele may mimic the wall of the bladder and distinction between the bladder wall and ureterocele may be difficult.

❑❑ **A neonate is noted to have deficiency of abdominal wall musculature, diffuse dilatation of the urinary tract and hydronephrosis. The patient is without cardiopulmonary complications and clinically stable. Does this patient require acute urological intervention to address the upper tract dilatation?**

Rarely does a case of Group 2 prune-belly syndrome described above require urgent urological intervention. Ultrasonography and serial electrolytes are used to assess parenchymal reserve and extent of uropathy. A diuretic renal scan should be performed. Patients presenting with Group 1 characteristics, on the other hand, including oligohydramnios, pulmonary hypoplasia, cardiac anomalies, urachal abnormalities or pneumothorax require intervention for the cardiopulmonary abnormalities prior to other aspects of care.

❑❑ **The neonate with prune-belly syndrome described in the previous question may be expected to have up to an 85% rate of vesicoureteral reflux. Should a voiding cystourethrogram (VCUG) be immediately performed to determine the grade of reflux and subsequent treatment?**

Instrumentation of a neonate with prune-belly syndrome is associated with a high-risk of infection and should be performed only with antibiotic prophylaxis.

ENURESIS

Sang Won Han, M.D. and Koon Ho Rha, M.D.

❑❑ **A normal seven-year-old boy suddenly develops daytime urinary frequency every 20 minutes without incontinence. His symptom is limited to daytime only, and no enuresis was reported. Medicosurgical history, physical exam, urinalysis, and brief ultrasound of the kidneys and bladder are normal. What is the most appropriate management option?**

The daytime urinary frequency syndrome is a benign condition, which occurs, in otherwise normal children who have no associated daytime incontinence or nighttime symptoms. The etiology is generally unknown and a conservative approach is not unreasonable. Symptoms usually resolve in two to four months and are characteristically unaffected by anticholinergic drugs.

❑❑ **An otherwise normal six-year-old boy wets his bed two or three times a week at night. He has no urinary symptoms during the daytime. What is the most most likely cause of his nocturnal enuresis?**

Nocturnal enuresis is usually due to maturational delay. Additional support for the concept of maturational lag comes from observation of a generalized but not pathologic immaturity in many younger enuretics, who may show a tendency towards passivity, late walking, and other minor evidences of developmental delay. Anatomic abnormalities such as ureteocele may be responsible for both diurnal and nocturnal wetting.

❑❑ **A seven-year-old boy has been taking imipramine for 3 months due to enuresis. What is the most potent pharmacologic effect of imipramine on the lower urinary tract?**

Three major actions of imipramine in the urinary tract are antimuscarinic action, direct inhibition of bladder smooth muscle and analgesic effect. It also causes CNS sedation and blockade of norepinephrine re-uptake. However the most important action in the bladder is the direct relaxant effect.

❑❑ **The only diagnosis that can be excluded in a four-year-old boy with incontinence based on history alone is what?**

Primary enuresis. The diagnosis of enuresis can be made after five years of age.

❑❑ **A six-year-old girl has been suffering from marked urinary frequency and urgency for two weeks. Physical exam is normal, and her urinalysis and culture are normal. The next step should be?**

Observation. In case of a pediatric benign condition, evaluation should be minimal if no significant complication is eminent. In most cases the spontaneous improvement is a rule.

❑❑ **The mother of 5-year-old boy who still wets his bed at night was concerned about the chance of recovery at the age of 15. What is the percentage of recovery you can tell to this mother?**

99%.

❑❑ **The parents of a six-year-old girl who still wets her bed at night tell the pediatrician that her older brother was also an enuretic. What percentatge of children at age 5 are enuretic?**

Approximately 15 per cent of normal children still wet at night at age 5-years. Enuresis is defined as an involuntary discharge of urine. The term is often used alone, imprecisely, to describe wetting that occurs only at night during sleep. It is more accurate, however, to refer to nighttime wetting as nocturnal enuresis and to distinguish it from daytime wetting, or diurnal enuresis. The age at which enuresis becomes inappropriate depends on the statistics of developing urinary control, the pattern of wetting, and the sex of the child. Nocturnal enuresis occurring after the age of 5 or by the time the child enters grade school is generally considered a cause for concern. With a spontaneous resolution rate of about 15 per cent per year, 99 per cent of children are dry by the age of 15 years.

❑❑ Parents of an infant boy are curious about enuresis, since both of the parents were enuretic themselves. They wish to find out what the first event is in the development of bowel and bladder control?

In terms of continence, children develop nocturnal bowel continence before daytime bowel or bladder continence. The enuretic seldom exhibits an abnormality in bowel function or bladder function during the day, and control of the bladder function by night is the last event to occur. The usual sequence of development is: 1) nocturnal bowel continence, 2) daytime bowel continence, 3) daytime bladder continence and finally, after several months, nocturnal control of bladder function. This sequence of achieving urinary control can be deterred by external factors.

❑❑ A pediatrician consulted urology for a urodynamic evaluation of a six-year-old boy. Would you expect to see pelvic floor muscle activity during spontaneous detrussor contractions?

No. Studies have reported uninhibited contractions in more than 50 per cent of these patients and sleep cystometrograrns recorded from enuretics show spontaneous bladder contractions that are more frequent and of greater amplitude than those of non-enuretics. However, if concomitant electromyography is performed, it is found that during spontaneous bladder contractions, pelvic floor muscle activity is quiet. Additionally, a functional reduction in bladder capacity is the most important urodynamic finding in enuretics, however, under anesthesia, these children prove to have a normal bladder capacity.

❑❑ An otherwise normal six-year-old boy wets his bed two or three times a week at night. What may be some of the contributing factor in his condition?

Enuresis is caused by nonorganic disturbances effecting normal development, such as social factors and stress, which can modify the urinary control. An increased prevalence of enuresis has been found in children from deprived environments and in talking, and retardation in skeletal maturation, which may reflect delayed maturation of regulatory central nervous system functions. It is proposed that enuresis is a sleep disorder but recent studies indicate that enuretic sleep patterns are not appreciably different form the sleep patterns of normal children, and that most enuretics do not wet as a consequence of sleeping too deeply.

❑❑ Enuretic children are known to have normal bladder capacity under anesthesia, but exhibit decreased functional capacity. What is the predicted average bladder capacity in a eight-year-old boy?

The predicted bladder capacity in children i.e. average capacity (ml)=[age (years) + 2] x 30 up until 10 years of age. Thus, if a child is 8 years old: (8+2) x 30 or 300 ml.

❑❑ A six-year-old boy with enuresis, frequency and urgency, uninhibited detrussor contractions and decreased functional capacity had been taking various remedies for his enuresis. After a thorough evaluation of his condition, the physician recommended anticholinergics. Which of his conditions is anticholinergic therapy proven most effective?

Anticholinergic medication in this setting will have greatest impact on uninhibited bladder contractions.

❑❑ A six-year-old boy had been taking various remedies for his enuresis. He has evidence of bladder hyperactivity, frequency and urgency, detrussor instability, day and night incontinence as well as pure nocturnal enuresis. Which of his conditions has anticholinergic therapy been proven most ineffective?

Pure nocturnal enuresis with normal cystogram. Anticholinergic drug therapy has been effective for enuresis in just 5% to 40% of patients. However, since anticholinergics eliminate uninhibited bladder contractions and increase bladder capacity, this therapy may be effective for enuretic patients with symptoms of bladder hyperactivity, such as urgency, frequency, and day and night incontinence, and highly effective in patients with proven uninhibited bladder contraction.

☐☐ **T/F: A daughter of diplomat who just returned from Sweden told her doctor that she had been satisfied with desmopressin (DDAVP) in the treatment of her enuresis. You can assure her that DDAVP has proven effectiveness in her condition.**

True. European clinical studies have proven the effectiveness of DDAVP in the treatment of enuresis.

☐☐ **T /F: A seven-year-old daughter of diplomat who just returned from Sweden told her doctor that she had been satisfied with desmopressin (DDAVP) in the treatment of her enuresis. DDAVP can be administered as a nasal spray or in oral form.**

True. Effective routes of administration of DDAVP include both intranasal as well as oral administration. Additionally, simply limiting fluids to reduce urine output is not generally effective. However, the importance of antidiuretic hormone (ADH) levels is now elucidated. Measurements of urinary and serum ADH demonstrate an absence or reversal of the normal circadian rhythm in enuretics who have lower than normal excretion desmopressin (DDAVP), a synthetic analog of ADH, which has become available. It is given both orally and nasally, and has an effect lasting 7 to 10 hours. DDAVP has been shown to be more effective than placebo in treating enuresis, with response rates up to 60%, especially in older children. Limitations are the relative expensive cost and recurrence upon discontinuation.

☐☐ **An eight-year-old boy had been taking imipramine before camping for 2 years and is very satisfied. Would you expect imipramine to have an antidepressant effect at anti-enuretic doses?**

No. Imipramine taken at anti-enuretic doses will have impact on REM sleep, light NREM sleep, anticholinergic as well as sympathetic input to the bladder but will not have any antidepressant action.

☐☐ **An eight-year-old boy had been taking imipramine before going camping for 2 years and is very satisfied. What are the different actions of the medication that you can tell the patient and his family about?**

This medication is known to have weak anticholinergic activity, direct antispasmodic activity, alpha sympathetic inhibitory action and inhibition of norepinephrine reuptake. The medication will not cause a decrease in bladder capacity. Imipramine, a tricyclic antidepressants, is the most widely used anti-enuretic agent. Enuresis can be cured in more than 50 per cent of children and will be improved in another 15 to 20 per cent, however up to 60 per cent of patients will relapse upon discontinuation. Its peripheral effects increase bladder capacity by (1) weak anticholinergic activity (ineffective in abolishing uninhibited detrusor contractions); (2) direct antispasmodic activity (inapparent at clinically effective antienuretic doses) (3) complex effect on sympathetic input to the bladder (prevents norepinephrine action on alpha receptors and enhances its effect on beta receptors by inhibiting norepinephrine reuptake). Imipramine effects on the central nervous system include its antidepressant activity and its action on sleep. Imipramine significantly alters sleep patterns by decreasing the time spent in REM sleep and increasing the time spent in light NREM sleep. It is unlikely that the effect of imipramine against enuresis is related to antidepressant activity because such an effect requires much higher dosage and its onset is delayed.

☐☐ **A mother of an enuretic child is curious about the various methods of treatment available today. Currently, what is the most effective treatment for enuresis?**

Management of enuresis has been divided into pharmacologic therapy and behavior modification. Modification of behavior has been quite successful but only for the very motivated parents and child. Bladder training, was developed to increase functional bladder capacity, but has not seen much success. Another method of alternative behavior modification is responsibility reinforcement, such as reward and motivation. This also requires active child participation to succeed.

It has been reported that the most effective therapy of treating enuresis is conditioning therapy, as in the bell alarm method. Superior results have been reported with this method compared to other forms of behavior therapy, as well as pharmacologic therapy with imipramine and DDAVP.

☐☐ **A 20-year-old army recruit was referred to an army hospital after his confession of enuresis. He had not been free of bed wetting throughout his life. What advise can you give him regarding diet to help minimize his problem?**

Enuresis is found in more than 1 per cent of the population, often with overt abnormalities on urodynamic studies such as uninhibited bladder activity. The extent of the investigation is usually more thorough than those carried out in younger enuretics. Cessation of compounds that might increase nocturnal urine output, such as caffeine, should be strongly advised before recommending other forms of treatment.

❑❑ **A 6-year-old girl is being evaluated for both nocturnal and diurnal enuresis. Work-up with history and physical examination, neurologic examination, urinalysis, and urine culture are normal. What is the next appropriate step?**

Most children with enuresis do not have a definite lesion. A careful history, physical examination, and urinalysis with culture are needed for all children with bed wetting and are usually sufficient. Radiographic studies such as IVP or VCUG are not normally recommended. In patients with diurnal enuresis, normal history and physical examination, no evidence of neuropathy and a negative urine, the urinary tract anatomy should be screened. This can be accomplished noninvasively and satisfactorily with an ultrasound examination of the kidneys, ureters, and bladder before and after voiding.

INTERSEX

James Mandell, M.D.

❏❏ **What structure undergoes condensation and shortening to promote descent of the testis?**

The gubernaculum which anchors the testis to the genital region condenses to allow descent.

❏❏ **What cell type is responsible for producing mullerian inhibiting substance (MIS)?**

The fetal sertoli cells produce MIS.

❏❏ **What enzyme converts testosterone into dihydrotestosterone?**

The conversion is mediated by 5-alpha reductase.

❏❏ **Mullerian inhibiting substance prevents the development of which female reproductive structures?**

MIS prevents the development of the oviduct, uterus, cervix and upper third of the vagina.

❏❏ **What physical findings are most suggestive of congenital adrenal hyperplasia?**

The findings include an apparent hypospadias (enlarged clitoris with fused labio-scrotal folds and single urogenital opening), hyperpigmented genital skin and non-palpable gonads.

❏❏ **What laboratory tests are most often used to confirm the presence of congenital adrenal hyperplasia?**

The most efficient tests include karyotype and plasma 17-hydroxyprogesterone.

❏❏ **What imaging studies are the most helpful in identifying infants with congenital adrenal hyperplasia?**

Use of the pelvic ultrasound (to look for the presence of a uterus) and a flouroscopic genitogram to look for a vaginal connection to a urogenital sinus are often helpful.

❏❏ **Which of the intersex conditions is inherited in a fairly consistent pattern?**

Congenital adrenal hyperplasia is associated with an enzymatic deficiency at the 21 or 11- beta hydroxylase position, and is commonly inherited in an autosomal recessive manner.

❏❏ **What is the typical appearance of a patient with complete testicular feminization syndrome?**

These patients appear as normal phenotypic females with normal development of secondary sexual characteristics. On examination, these patients prove to have a short blind ending vagina with no internal mullerian duct structures. Since MIS is present during embryogenesis the mullerian duct strucutures do not develop. Development of the external male external genitalia, dependent upon dihydrotestosterone, is also absent due to the lack of the androgen receptor.

❏❏ **What is the most common demonstrable defect seen in patients with complete testicular feminization syndrome?**

The most common finding is absence of high-affinity binding of dihydrotestosterone.

❑❑ **What is the genetic focus for determination of male gonadal development?**

The genetic focus is the testis determining factor on the short arm of the Y chromosome.

❑❑ **At what stage in fetal development can one see a differentiation between male and female phenotypes?**

Between the sixth to eighth week of gestation, the indifferent gonad differentiates into male or female characteristics.

❑❑ **What are the clinical presentations that most often lead to the diagnosis of complete testicular feminization?**

Patients with this disorder most commonly present as females with bilateral inguinal hernias or with ammenorhea at puberty.

❑❑ **What is the anatomic anlage of the male internal genital structures and what causes their differentiation?**

The wollfian duct system develops into the vas deferens and epididymus under the influence of testosterone.

❑❑ **What is the most common genotype in patients with true hermaphoditism?**

The most common karyotypic finding is 46 XX.

❑❑ **What is the most common cause of intersex in children in this country?**

The most common finding is congenital adrenal hyperplasia in genetic females.

❑❑ **What is the most common biochemical defect found in patients with congenital adrenal hyperplasia?**

An enzymatic defect at the 21-hydroxylase position in the adrenal conversion of cholesterol to cortisone is the most common finding.

❑❑ **What are the most common gonadal malignancies associated with a dysgenetic gonad and the presence of a Y chromosome?**

The most common malignancies are gonadoblastomas and dysgerminomas.

❑❑ **What is the most common karyotypic finding in Klinefelter's syndrome?**

The most common finding is an additional X chromosome (47XXY or 46XX,XXY).

❑❑ **What is the histopathologic finding in patients with pure gonadal dysgenesis?**

Bilateral streak gonads and underdeveloped mullerian structures are found.

NEUROGENIC VOIDING DYSFUNCTION

George Young, M.D.

❏❏ Describe the effects on voiding following a cerebrovascular accident?

The effects on micturition are divided into acute and long term. The initial period of shock may be associated with urinary retention secondary to detrusor areflexia. The most common long-term sequelae is detrusor hyperreflexia. Sensation and compliance are generally intact.

❏❏ What effect does Alzheimer's disease have on voiding?

Dementia involves the loss of grey and white matter from the frontal lobes. Incontinence may ensue and may be secondary to detrusor hyperreflexia with voluntary sphincter activity or may be due to loss of awareness to void.

❏❏ Does outlet obstruction exist in patients with Parkinson's disease?

Voiding dysfunction exists in 35 % to 70 % of patients with Parkinson's disease. The most common symptoms are urgency, frequency, nocturia and urge incontinence. The most common finding on urodynamics is detrusor hyperreflexia with smooth sphincter synergy. In contradistinction to patients post CVA, those patients with Parkinson's generally do not have outlet obstruction and subsequently respond poorly to prostatectomy. This may be due to poorly sustained bladder contractions and poor sphincter relaxation.

❏❏ What is Shy-Drager Syndrome?

This disorder results from cell loss and gliosis in the cerebellum, substantia nigra, intermediolateral columns of the spinal cord and Onuf's nucleus. Clinically, patients demonstrate orthostatic hypotension, anhydrosis and certain degrees of Parkinsonian symptoms plus autonomic dysfunction. Diagnostically, these individuals are identified by the uncommon findings of an open bladder neck (in contrast to Parkinson's patients) and striated sphincter denervation on EMG.

❏❏ How does Multiple Sclerosis affect voiding?

MS is a demyelinating disease that most commonly involves the posterior and lateral columns of the cervical spinal cord. Fifty percent to 90% of these patients have voiding dysfunction at some point. The most common findings is detrusor hyperreflexia. Thirty percent to 65% of these patients have striated sphincter dyssynergia.

❏❏ The sacral spinal cord begins at what level and ends at which spinal cord level?

It is important to distinguish between spinal column segment (bone level) and the corresponding cord level. The sacral spinal cord begins at the column level of T12-Ll. It terminates as the cauda equina at spinal column level L2.

❏❏ What is the voiding pattern observed in a complete cord injury above the sacral reflex?

Most commonly, these lesions result in detrusor hyperreflexia, absent sensation below the level of the lesion, smooth sphincter synergy and striated sphincter dyssynergia. Lesions above the sympathetic outflow tract T7 or T8 (spinal column level of T6) may also result in smooth sphincter dyssynergia.

❏❏ **A diver suffers from a complete spinal cord injury at the level of T8, what pattern of voiding would be expected immediately following the accident?**

The immediate result is a period of spinal shock. There is generally bladder areflexia and acontractility. Some EMG activity may be present at the external sphincter but there is no voluntary control. Urinary retention is the most common finding initially; and is typically managed with a Foley catheter. The areflexic period generally lasts 6 to 12 weeks but may persist up to one to two years.

❏❏ **While performing cystoscopy on a patient with a high cervical cord injury he develops hypertension, flushing, sweating and bradycardia. What is the problem, and what should be done?**

This is a classic description of autonomic hyperreflexia. It arises from massive autonomic discharge in patients with cord injuries above the sympathetic outflow tract (T6 to T8). Prevention is based on use of spinal anesthesia and the use of oral Nifedipine (10 mg) 30 minutes prior to the procedure. Initial management of symptoms is withdrawl of the stimulus and alpha blockade.

❏❏ **Two days following a lumbar laminectomy, a 61-year-old male is in urinary retention. What is the treatment?**

Disc disease is commonly associated with voiding dysfunction. The most common finding is that of detrusor areflexia. Generally, patients present with symptoms of poor emptying. Interestingly, laminectomy may not improve the bladder dysfunction. Treatment in this male would consist of catheter placement and urodynamic studies.

❏❏ **What is diabetic cystopathy?**

This is a term that describes the effects of diabetes on the urinary bladder. The most recent evidence points to both a sensory and motor dysfunction. Urodynamically, these bladders demonstrate impaired sensation, increased capacity, decreased contractility and impaired flow patterns. Pressure / Flow studies can differentiate poor bladder emptying from outlet obstruction. Timed voiding plays a pivotal role in therapy.

❏❏ **What are the pathways and influences involved in normal micturition?**

Voluntary control is exerted by the cerebral cortex by release of tonic inhibitory signals to the Pontine Micturition Center (PMC). The PMC initiates voiding by stimulation of parasympathetics at S2-S4 causing detrusor contraction and inhibition of sympathetic fibers T11-L2 and somatic fibers of the pudendal nerve causing relaxation of the bladder neck and proximal urethra and the external sphincter, respectively.

❏❏ **What are some of the causes of urinary retention in females?**

Etiologies of retention in women include; multiple sclerosis, spina bifida occulta, viral sacromyeloradiculitis, lumbar disc protrusion-cauda equina syndrome, bladder neck obstruction, pseudomyotonia and reflex sympathetic dystrophy.

❏❏ **What are the urodynamic parameters used to diagnose bladder neck obstruction in women?**

While validated nomograms do not exist the following findings are highly suggestive of obstruction: sustained detrusor contraction of normal or high pressure, poor flow of urine, lack of bladder neck funneling on fluoroscopy. All of these findings must be accompanied by a synergic external urethral sphincter or bladder neck obstruction to exist.

❏❏ **How do Kegel exercises reduce incontinence?**

These exercises not only produce a direct physical obstruction to urinary leakage but they also can help abolish uninhibited detrusor contractions. This is accomplished by stimulation of afferent sacral nerves at low frequencies (below the pain threshold of C fibers). This causes inhibition of efferent pelvic nerve firing thereby reducing detrusor activity.

❏❏ **What is the failure rate of pelvic floor biofeedback?**

Biofeedback works by bringing to conscious control that which was previously unconscious. The most important factor in the success of therapy is a well-motivated patient. In fact, attrition rates remain as high as one-third even in well-established centers.

❑❑ **The first recordable event of the micturition reflex is?**

Cessation of sphincter EMG activity.

❑❑ **What is the distinction between the smooth and the striated urinary sphincters?**

The smooth sphincter refers to a physiologic rather than an anatomic sphincter. It is located at the smooth musculature of the bladder neck and the proximal urethra. Control is involuntary. In contrast, the striated sphincter is anatomic and includes the skeletal muscle surrounding the membranous urethra in men and the middle segment of the urethra in females. This sphincter also includes the striated muscle surrounding the urethra in both men and women. The outer portion of this sphincter is under voluntary control.

❑❑ **According to Wein, what are the three factors necessary for (1) normal bladder and urine storage to occur, and (2) normal bladder emptying to occur?**

The factors necessary for storage of urine are:

1. Accommodation of urine at low pressure with appropriate sensation.
2. A closed outlet at rest and one that remains so with increases of intra-abdominal pressure.
3. No involuntary bladder contractions.

Requirements for normal emptying are:

1. A contraction of adequate magnitude and duration.
2. Lowering of outlet resistance when this contraction occurs.
3. No anatomic outlet obstruction.

❑❑ **What is the Q-tip test?**

This test is designed to uncover urethral hypermobility A Q-tip is inserted to the level of the bladder neck. At this point the resting angle from the horizontal is determined. After the patient strains, the degree of rotation is assessed. Hypermobility is defined as greater than 30 degrees from the horizontal on either resting or straining.

❑❑ **In patients with neurogenic voiding dysfunction, what urodynamic finding has the highest correlation with the development of upper tract damage?**

Detrusor-sphincter dyssynergia correlates highest with upper tract damage.

❑❑ **In patients with bladder outlet obstruction, what is the opening pressure on pressure-flow studies?**

These patients have opening pressures greater than 80 cm H_2O.

❑❑ **What cord segment is evaluated with the bulbocavemous reflex?**

This test evaluates the integrity of the S2-S4 segments.

❑❑ **A Valsalva leak point pressure less than what is diagnostic of intrinsic sphincter deficiency?**

A pressure less than 60 cm H_2O is evidence for intrinsic sphincter deficiency.

❑❑ **Why is pharmacotherapy using acetylcholine like drugs not clinically useful in facilitating bladder emptying?**

These drugs are rapidly hydrolyzed by cholinesterases thereby limiting their efficacy.

❐❐ **What factors may contribute to urinary incontinence following radical prostatectomy?**

Any one of the following or combination may contribute to incontinence:

1. residual outlet obstruction.
2. detrusor instability.
3. sphincteric incompetence.
4. pre-existing neurologic disease.

❐❐ **Briefly summarize the parasympathetic innervation of the bladder?**

Parasympathetic efferents from the pelvic nerves S2-S4. The ganglion is located near the organ and the neurotransmitter is acetylcholine. The receptors are muscarinic (M2 / M3) and stimulation results in bladder contraction.

❐❐ **What is the role of sympathetic innervation of the bladder and outlet?**

Together they promote bladder storage via the hypogastric nerve (T10-L2). Alpha (bladder base and prostate) and beta (bladder body) receptors exist on the bladder and alpha-receptors are on the prostatic capsule. Beta activation results in inhibition of muscle contraction. Alpha activation results in increased outlet resistance.

❐❐ **What are the general factors which contribute to urinary incontinence in women?**

Predisposing factors such as anatomy and collagen status. Inciting factors such as childbirth and previous surgery. Promoting factors such as infection and obesity. Decompensating factors such as aging.

❐❐ **When evaluating incontinence in geriatric patients what does the pneumonic DIAPPERS refer to?**

Delirum, Infection, Atrophic vaginitis, Psychological problems, Pharmaceuticals, Excess urine output, Restricted mobility, Stool impaction.

❐❐ **What broad categories of medications may be associated with urinary incontinence?**

ACE inhibitors, alcohol, alpha-adrenergic agonists and antagonists, calcium channel blockers, diuretics, medications that affect incontinence, narcotics, sedatives and hypnotics and Vincristine.

❐❐ **What is the most common type of urinary incontinence in the elderly?**

Urge incontinence is the most common cause of urinary incontinence in the elderly. Many conditions that are prevalent in this population predispose them to this type of incontinence including: cerebrovascular accidents, Parkinson's disease, spinal cord injury, multiple sclerosis and benign prostatic hyperplasia.

❐❐ **Is urinary incontinence a normal consequence of aging?**

While age-related changes are present in the elderly and predispose them to incontinence, this should not be considered a normal part of aging and a thorough evaluation is indicated.

❐❐ **What are the indications for urodynamics testing in the incontinent patient?**

Any patient who reports a history of a failed incontinence procedure or previous radical pelvic surgery, patients with mixed symptoms (including both stress and urge), history of a neurologic disorder and most importantly any patient in whom stress incontinence is not demonstrated on physical exam.

URODYNAMICS

Gamal M. Ghoniem, M.D.

❑❑ **T/F: A high post-void residual urine volume correlates with both the symptoms and urodynamic findings associated with bladder outlet obstruction.**

False. A high post-void residual volume does not necessarily mean bladder outlet obstruction. This condition can be present in association with any physical bladder outlet obstruction or it can be present in association with a poorly contracting bladder. Conversely, this condition may not be present in patients with severe bladder outlet obstruction if they have enough detrusor function to overcome the outlet obstruction. Elevated post-void residual volumes when present do not necessarily lead to infection.

❑❑ **A 40-year-old female had a uroflow with Qmax of 50 ml/sec, a mean of 25 ml/sec, and a configuration that looks like a bread loaf standing on end. The most likely single diagnosis is:**

Sphincteric incontinence with low outlet resistance.

❑❑ **What are the two events most likely to produce a similar electromyographic pattern?**

Striated sphincter dyssynergia and Valsalva voiding both produce similar EMG patterns of increased activity. Patients with these conditions void in the absence of coordination between the detrussor muscle and the sphincteric unit.

❑❑ **During the act of volitional voiding what would you expect a normal EMG pattern to look like?**

During the act of normal volitional voiding the EMG should be silent.

❑❑ **At initiation of normal voiding, which event happens first?**

The initial measurable event upon voiding is decreased EMG activity. This precedes an increase in detrusor pressure and a decrease in maximum urethral pressure.

❑❑ **What is the relationship between pressure and flow during normal micturition in men and women?**

Normal urinary flow in young healthy males should be 15-25 mL / second and the associated detrussor pressure should be less than 40 cm H_2O. Women typically void with similar or slightly higher peak flow rates but the associated detrusor pressures are lower and usually approximate 30 cm H_2O. Interestingly, identical results on repeated measurements are difficult to obtain with repeated pressure flow studies in the same healthy individual.

❑❑ **What does an intermittent flow pattern in an individual with normal deep tendon and bulbocavemosus reflexes and normal perineal sensation most likely indicate?**

Intermittent flow in an otherwise normal individual is most suggestive of abdominal straining. The neurologically intact patient cannot have detrusor hyperreflexia or detrusor sphincter dyssynergia.

❑❑ **A patient with incontinence shows evidence of low compliance by urodynamics. The Valsalva leak point pressure is 20 – 30 cm H_2O. What would you tell the patient her risk of upper tract deterioration is?**

Valsalva leak point pressures less than 40 cm H_2O will actually protect the upper tracts from pressure induced hydronephrosis and subsequent deterioration in renal function. The lower the leak pressure, the less likely upper tract deterioration will happen, when bladder compliance is low.

❑❑ **In phase 2 (the tonus limb) of the cystometrogram, bladder compliance is most dependent upon which factor?**

Viscoelastic properties of the detrusor. Other neural factors like cerebral inhibition of reflex bladder activity and intact thoracolumbar spinal cord are more active in the final phase.

❑❑ **What is the most important parameter in uroflowmetry with volumes between 150 and 350 ml: maximum flow rate or average flow rate?**

Maximum flow rate is most indicative of normal detrussor function.

❑❑ **A patient, with no evidence of neurologic disease, has evidence of involuntary detrusor contractions during the filling phase of a CMG. What is your diagnosis? Detrusor instability or poor compliance?**

Detrusor instability. In the presence of neurological disease, identical findings on a CMG would lead to the diagnosis of detrusor hyperreflexia.

❑❑ **Can detrusor hyperreflexia and overactive detrusor function be used as interchangeable terms?**

No. Detrusor hypeneflexia is always due to neurologic disorder.

❑❑ **What is the Valsalva's leak point pressure?**

The Valsalva leak point pressure is the pressure at which passive urethral resistance is overcome by increasing abdominal pressure and urine leaks through an otherwise closed sphincter. This is not a measure of detrusor function and the result can be affected by the presence of a large cystocele.

❑❑ **How is detrusor pressure (P det) calculated ?**

Pves-Pabd (vesical pressure-abdominal pressure). The detrusor pressure is important in recognizing pressure increases due to abdominal and not true vesical pressure, e.g., straining.

❑❑ **What does high bladder compliance relate to?**

Bladder accommodation. High compliance does not relate to high leak pressure.

❑❑ **What does the static infusion urethral pressure profile most accurately predict?**

Intrinsic sphincter deficiency. It does not predict striated sphincter dyssynergia or urethral obstruction.

❑❑ **What is the most common urodynamic findings seen in patients with CVA?**

Detrusor hyperreflexia, normal compliance, smooth sphincter synergia, and striated sphincter synergia.

❑❑ **T/F: In patients with cerebral infarction, the upper tracts are at minimal risk of deterioration.**

True. Immediately following the injury, these patients often manifest detrusor areflexia. As they convalesce, patients with cerebral lesions, (CVA, subdural hematoma, closed head injuries, brain tumors, etc...) most commonly develop detrusor hyperreflexia. They can have uninhibited motor neurogenic bladders with detrusor hyperreflexia. The bladder activity in these patients is characterized as complete coordinated incontinence. These patients void at normal pressures, but in an uninhibited manner with coordination between the detrusor muscle and sphincter mechanism. In these cases there is no detrusor sphincter dyssynergia, and high pressure voiding is not a common finding.

❑❑ **When do you most likely see pseudodyssynergia ?**

In a patient with a cerebrovascular accident. In these patients the sensation is intact.

❑❑ **A 72-year-old male develops urgency, frequency, and urge incontinence following a CVA. Prior to his CVA, he complained of a decreasing stream and hesitancy. His postvoid residual is 130 ml. What is the most likely cause of his high residual?**

Benign prostatic hyperplasia with bladder outlet obstruction would be the most likely explanation for his elevated post-void residual volume. CVA causes detrusor hyperreflexia.

❑❑ **Are suprapontine lesions (stroke, dementia, etc.) usually associated with detrusor sphincter dyssynergia?**

No. They are usually associated with detrusor hyperreflexia or detrusor areflexia, phasic detrusor instability, or detrusor overactivity

❑❑ **A 21-year-old male patient with cerebral palsy and severe mental retardation has day and night incontinence. What is the most practical and informative urodynamic evaluation?**

A post-void residual plus renal ultrasound. In this situation, with an uncooperative patient, videourodynamic studies, pressure-flow studies, or even simple cystometry are not likely to impact your management.

❑❑ **What are the urodynamic findings in a complete spinal cord transection at cord level T10 after spinal shock has disappeared?**

Detrusor hyperreflexia, striated sphincter dyssynergia, and smooth sphincter synergia.

❑❑ **What are the urodynamic findings in patients with voiding dysfunction secondary to ShyDrager syndrome ?**

An open bladder neck at rest, decreased detrusor compliance, striated sphincter denervation.

❑❑ **Are uninhibited detrusor contractions diagnosed by filling CMG always due to bladder outlet obstruction?**

No. They can be caused by neurologic diseases that affect upper motor neuron function.

❑❑ **What are the urodynamic findings generally associated with autonomic hyperreflexia?**

Detrusor hyperreflexia, striated sphincter dyssynergia, and smooth sphinter dyssynergia. Lesions above T6 are usually associated with smooth sphincter dyssynergia.

❑❑ **Which condition is detrusor striated sphincter dyssynergia most frequently associated with?**

Suprasacral spinal cord injury. It is absent in Parkinson's disease, stroke, myelomeningocele, and radical pelvic surgery.

❑❑ **What is the most common urodynamic abnormality in patients with voiding dysfunction secondary to multiple sclerosis?**

Detrusor hyperreflexia. The second most common dysfunction is striated sphincter dyssynergia.

❑❑ **At approximately which spinal cord column level does the sacral spinal cord begin and end?**

T12-L2.

❑❑ **Two weeks after an abdominoperineal resection, a 70-year-old male with minimal voiding symptoms prior to his surgery has a post-void residual of 400 ml. What are the most likely urodynamic abnormalities and what is the preferred management strategy?**

Detrusor areflexia and low compliance will result from pelvic nerve injury, and the best management would be CIC with or without anticholinergics.

❏❏ **What is the most common cause for upper urinary tract deterioration in the SCI patient?**

Striated sphincter dyssynergia. This results in elevated detrusor pressures, high residual urine, hydronephrosis with secondary urinary infections, and renal failure.

❏❏ **What is the best treatment for a T-10 paraplegic with Type I striated sphincter dyssynergia, Grade 1 reflux, a postvoid residual of 250 cc, no hydronephrosis, normal compliance, and unsustained detrusor contractions?**

Intermittent catheterization. The description fits a safe reservoir; only CIC is indicated.

❏❏ **A C 5-6 SCI female patient has low bladder compliance, an incompetent bladder neck, urethral erosion, and Grade 1 hydronephrosis. What would be the best treatment?**

A bladder neck closure or obstructive sling with ileovesicostomy.

❏❏ **A C 5-6 male SCI patient has no change in postvoid residual urine following external sphincterotomy. What is the most likely reason?**

Impaired bladder contractility. Less common conditions like inadequate sphincterotomy, smooth muscle dyssynergia, and urethral stricture can cause large residuals.

❏❏ **During cystoscopy, a C7 quadriplegic patient complains of sweating and headache. His blood pressure has rapidly risen to 210/120. What is the best initial management?**

Empty the bladder. In this emergency situation, the offending cause, i.e., distention, should be treated immediately, and usually this is enough to control the autonomic hyperreflexia. Other measures, like oral nifedipine or even phentolamine intravenously, are not effective enough in controlling this serious situation. Unattended serious complications like stroke can happen.

❏❏ **A C5 quadriplegic on external condom catheter drainage has recurrent episodes of autonomic dysreflexia. Urodynamic evaluation shows high-pressure detrusor contractions and prolonged external sphincter dyssynergia. What is the best option for management?**

A bladder augmentation with subsequent clean intermittent catheterization will minimize the furture morbidity in this individual.

❏❏ **What is the main indication for pressure-flow studies?**

To help distinguish detrusor hypocontractility from urethral obstruction low-flow conditions, with or without large residual urine, which can result from any of these conditions.

❏❏ **What percent of men with symptoms of prostatism are found to have urodynamically proven outlet obstruction?**

30%

❏❏ **What study yields a definitive diagnosis of bladder outlet obstruction?**

A pressure/flow study is the gold-standard for the diagnosis of bladder outlet obstruction.

❏❏ **What is the clinical presentation of tethered cord syndrome?**

Patients typically present in infancy with detrussor areflexia and urinary retention.

❏❏ **What are the characteristics of diabetic cystopathy?**

An increased bladder capacity, impaired detrusor contractility, and decreased bladder sensation, with diminished urinary stream.

□□ What are the factors that lead to a favorable outcome following prostatectomy in patients with Parkinson's disease?

Normal intravesical voiding pressures with decreased flow rate, urethral sphincter contractions which can voluntarily interrupt the urinary stream, adequate voluntary detrusor contractions, and perceived urgency. On the contrary, decreased detrusor contractility is not favorable.

□□ What are the strong indications for a urodynamic evaluation?

Spina bifida, sacral agenesis, high imperforate anus, and monitoring of a patient with spinal cord injury are all indications for a urodynamic evaluation.

□□ What is the estimated bladder capacity of a healthy two-year-old male?

120 ml. A simple formula to use is: age in years + 2 = capacity in ounces.

□□ What is the initial management of the newborn with myelodysplasia?

The initial management should include: serum electrolytes, BUN, serum creatinine, measurement of residual urine, renal sonogram and VCUG. The urodynamic studies the day prior to spinal closure are not indicated.

□□ When should urodynamic studies be performed for myelomeningocele patients?

Urodynamics are helpful in the newborn period as a baseline study. This is important in order to assess the relative risk of the upper tracts based upon the bladder dynamics and to monitor any changes during the course of the disease.

□□ Why has vesicostomy been demonstrated to be effective in initial management in infants born with posterior urethral valves?

A vesicostomy is a simple and safe procedure in infancy, bringing the dome of the bladder to the skin. This results in upper tract decompression in 90 percent of the cases. Reflux is not a problem, since voiding pressures are eliminated. The risks of urethral injury are avoided, since valve ablation may be delayed. In addition, vesicostomy dosen't cause a permanent reduction in bladder capacity.

□□ A 3-year-old boy received a vesicostomy at 4-months of age secondary to posterior urethral valves. He now presents with progressive hydronephrosis and a serum creatinine of 2.5 mg/dL. A CMG revealed low bladder compliance. What is the next best step in management?

A high urinary diversion would be appropriate. Other management strategies are usually not effective, e.g., augmentation cystoplasty and vesicostomy closure or CIC.

□□ To further characterize the cause of a 350 cc residual urine in a 60-year-old, non insulin dependent diabetic, what is the most informative study?

A simultaneous detrusor pressure/flow study.

□□ A 50-year-old female with urgency and frequency following a suspension procedure voids with a detrusor pressure of 50 cm H_2O at a peak flow of 12 ml/sec. The most likely diagnosis is:

Urethral obstruction. Irritative bladder symptoms with high voiding pressures are indicative of outlet obstruction after a suspension procedure.

□□ A 53-year-old female underwent needle suspension one year ago. She complains of continuous urinary incontinence in upright positions. Seventeen years ago she underwent abdominal hysterectomy and retropubic suspension. Videofluorourodynamics show an open bladder neck with minimal hypermobility, no involuntary contractions, and good bladder capacity, with low Valsalva's Leak Pressure. What is the best operative option?

A pubovaginal sling procedure. The patient has intrinsic sphincter deficiency (ISD) and would not benefit from repeat suspension.

❑❑ **A 55-year-old man has had a detubularized right colon orthotopic continent diversion. He has done well for one year, but now complains of increasing incontinence. Pouch urodynamics revealed several pressure spikes. What is the mechanism most likely responsible for his incontinence?**

A return of coordinated bowel contractions.

❑❑ **Why is nocturnal enuresis common with orthotopic diversions?**

Because of loss of the spinal reflex arc recruiting external sphincter contraction.

❑❑ **How can you best describe cecal contractions?**

Intermittent high-pressure contractions. They are usually massive contractions and not peristaltic.

LOWER URINARY TRACT OBSTRUCTION

Steven C. Stewart, M.D. and Gregory Stewart, M.D.

☐☐ **Increased urinary pressure behind a tight urethral stricture can have what effect on the proximal epithelium and spongiosum?**

The epithelium may become thickened proximally or may appear normal. Regardless of epithelial changes, spongiofibrosis may develop for a considerable distance both proximally and distally. Surgical repair may fail if this underlying fibrosis is not recognized.

☐☐ **T/F: Congenital urethral strictures are a common etiology of stricture disease.**

False. Congenital urethral strictures are rare and are probably overestimated. Histopathologically they differ from acquired strictures in that their walls consist of smooth muscle rather than scar tissue.

☐☐ **T/F: Urethral stricture development secondary to gonorrhea tends to result in discreet lesions within the bulbar urethra.**

False, while infectious strictures tend to develop within the bulbar urethra, they also tend to involve considerable length of the urethra and underlying spongiosum.

☐☐ **Urethral stricture following cardiothoracic surgery with bypass may occur in up to 22% of cases. Which portion of the urethra is most at risk for stricture development?**

Pendulous urethra. Etiology may be related to local tissue ischemia / hypoxia during the bypass portion of the operation.

☐☐ **Prior to repair of a completely obliterative urethral stricture optimal radiographic evaluation includes which studies.**

In addition to a retrograde urethrogram, a voiding cystourethrogram is essential to identify the proximal extent of the stricture.

☐☐ **T/F: Substitution urethroplasty tends to fail earlier than anastamotic repair.**

False, anastomotic repair tends to fail within the first year, while substitution urethroplasty has been shown to fail at a rate of 4% per annum with a 60% successful outcome rate after 10 years.

☐☐ **When treating a urethral stricture with progressive weekly dilations, what is the largest caliber dilator that should be used?**

Current recommendations are to not exceed 24 French dilator.

☐☐ **When treating a urethral stricture with visual urethrotomy, the 12 o'clock incision was made too deep. What specific complication can occur?**

Peyronie's like reaction resulting in ventral chordee.

☐☐ **What is the most common problem reported following stenting of a urethral stricture?**

Recurrent stricture at the distal or proximal end of the stent.

❑❑ **Why is anastomotic urethroplasty generally inappropriate for treating pendulous urethral strictures?**

The resulting urethral shortening is sufficient to cause ventral chordee.

❑❑ **What is the disadvantage of using scrotal skin for urethral reconstruction?**

A high incidence of dermatitis can lead to restenosis.

❑❑ **Which type of bulbar urethral stricture lends itself best to anastomotic urethroplasty?**

Short strictures usually <1 cm in length and due to trauma.

❑❑ **If delayed surgical repair of pelvic urethral distraction injury is selected, how long should one delay the repair?**

3-months is generally consider to be a sufficient period of time to allow for resolution of tissue edema, periurethral hematoma and "stabilization" of the injury. Longer delays do not result in shortening of the distraction injury.

❑❑ **T/F: Nongonococcal urethritis has been shown to be related to urethral stricture?**

False.

❑❑ **Retrograde urethrography may exacerbate a urethral stricture by what mechanism?**

Excessive pressure may cause extravasation; inappropriate contrast selection not suitable for IV injection may compound the problem.

❑❑ **T/F: Given that surgical management of urethral strictures carries a success rate of greater than 90% in many cases, non-operative stricture management is no longer appropriate in these cases?**

False, some patients prefer to live with periodic dilations rather than undergo surgery.

❑❑ **What are the two specific contraindications to using an indwelling urethral stent?**

Patients who have undergone prior substitution urethral reconstruction, particularly with skin; and patients with deep spongiofibrosis.

❑❑ **When performing substitution urethroplasty over fibrosed spongiosum, which is considered superior, graft or flap substitution?**

Flap substitution. In cases where the underlying blood supply is in question, a flap, which carries its own blood supply, has a more predictable outcome.

❑❑ **Meatal strictures associated with balanitis xerotica obliterans are best managed with what approach?**

A formal meatal reconstruction is usually necessary as dilation in this condition rarely results in a long-term response.

❑❑ **With regard to repeat direct visual internal urethrotomy, how does the success rate compare with the first procedure?**

Subsequent procedures do not result in an increase in the success rate of an internal urethrotomy. Success rates are generally hard to define, but curative success rates have been reported between 20% to 35%.

PROSTATIC HYPERPLASIA

W. Bruce Shingleton, M.D.

❑❑ **The development of the transition zone of the prostate begins at what week of embryologic development?**

This occurs at week 16 of development of the fetus.

❑❑ **What effect does finasteride have on serum testosterone levels?**

There is no change in serum testosterone levels.

❑❑ **What percent of patients with BPH will have symptom improvement or stabilization without treatment?**

Up to 50% of patients with BPH will have symptom stabilization or improvement regardless of whether treatment is started.

❑❑ **What percent of the ejaculate arises from the prostate gland?**

Prostatic secretions constitute 15% of the total ejaculate volume.

❑❑ **What is the average weight of the prostate in an adult male age 40?**

At this age, the mean weight of the prostate is approximately 20 grams.

❑❑ **The prostate is in contact with how many and what fascial layers?**

The 3 fascial layers which abut the prostate include Denonvilliers posteriorly, the endopelvic fascia cranially, and the lateral pelvic fascia.

❑❑ **What artery provides the major source of blood for the prostate?**

The prostatovesicular artery arising from the inferior vesical artery is the main source of arterial blood to the prostate.

❑❑ **The plexus of Santorini drains into what major veins?**

This venous complex drains into the hypogastric veins.

❑❑ **The urethra divides the prostate into what areas?**

The urethra demarcates the prostate into the fibromuscular (ventral) and glandular (dorsal) areas.

❑❑ **The transition zone constitutes what percentage of the prostate?**

The transition zone comprises 4-5% of the glandular prostate.

❑❑ **What is the largest zone of the prostate?**

Typically the peripheral zone is the largest zone accounting for approxiamtely 75% of the prostate gland.

❑❑ **The fibromuscular stroma is composed of mainly what type of tissue?**

Smooth muscle fibers are the main component of the fibromuscular stroma.

❑❑ What cell types are present in the acinar epithelium?

There are two cell types, glandular cells and basal cells.

❑❑ BPH is the most common cause of what urologic symptom?

Gross painless hematuria.   BPH is commonly associated with gross painless hematuria in men older than 60 years. When present one must perform a complete evaluation to rule out neoplasm as an etiology.

❑❑ Finasteride has what effect on prostatic tissue levels of 5 alpha - DHT?

Finasteride decreases 5 alpha – DHT prostatic tissue levels.

❑❑ Finasteride produces what side effects in regard to sexual function?

The side effects include decreased libido, decreased ejaculatory volume and erectile dysfunction.

❑❑ The majority of alpha-1 adrenoceptors are located where in the GU tract?

The alpha-1 receptors are located mainly in the bladder neck and prostate.

❑❑ Post-obstructive diuresis is thought to be due to what factor?

The obstruction results in altered function of the collecting duct cells manifested as a loss of renal concentrating ability with resultant diuresis. The ability to acidify the urine is also often impaired with an obstructive process. The ensuing post-obstructive diuresis will resolve once the collecting ducts have regained their ability to conserve a fluid load and the renal medullary interstitium has regained is osmotic gradient.

❑❑ What is the reported incidence of urethral stricture after TURP?

Urethral strictures have a reported incidence of 2.7% to 20% following TURP.

❑❑ During a transurethral resection of the prostate (TURP) a large venous sinus is opened. What are the next steps to be performed?

Lower the height of the irrigation fluid to decrease further fluid absorption. Diligent efforts to endoscopically gain control of the bleeding should be undertaken, but can be difficult. Therefore, it may be necessary to quickly finish the resection and place a Foley catheter with appropriate traction, which will usually tamponade the bleeding. Serum electrolyte studies are appropriate to monitor for TUR syndrome (dilutional hyponatremia), and intravenous Lasix should be administered to help minimize the dilutional hyponatremia that can be associated with the unroofing of a large venous sinus.

❑❑ T/F: Transurethral incision of the prostate (TUIP) is useful regardless of the size of the prostate?

False. Success with this technique is typically limited to a prostate 30 grams or less in size.

❑❑ What alternative minimally invasive treatment modalities are available for use in anticoagulated patients?

Laser prostatectomy and transurethral electrovaporization (TUVP) have been successfully used in anticoagulated patients for the treatment of BPH.

❑❑ Define the temperature range for hyperthermia and thermotherapy of the prostate?

Temperatures > 44.5^0 C constitute thermotherapy and temperatures < 44^0 C are termed hyperthermia.

❏❏ **The outer zone of the prostate is of what embryologic origin?**

The endoderm gives rise to the outer (peripheral) zone of the prostate.

❏❏ **What percent of men develop symptoms secondary to BPH?**

Fifty percent of men with BPH will have symptoms as they age.

❏❏ **How many isoenzymes exist for 5-alpha reductase?**

There are two isoenzymes, Type I and Type II with Type II being the major isoenzyme in the prostate.

❏❏ **What two growth factors are important in the development of BPH?**

Transforming growth factor alpha and epidermal growth factors have been identified as the major growth factors in the development of BPH.

❏❏ **Does androgen ablation have any effect on the cell population of the prostate?**

Epithelial cells are mainly affected by a decrease in androgens and show varying degrees of atrophy as compared to stromal cells.

❏❏ **What alpha-receptor subtype is most numerous in the prostate?**

Alpha 1A is the most prevalent alpha-receptor subtype in the prostate.

❏❏ **What is the relationship between symptoms score and degree of obstruction as determined by pressure flow study?**

Various studies have shown no correlation between symptom score and pressure study regarding degree of obstruction.

❏❏ **T/F: Finasteride administration results in castrate levels of DHT?**

False. Conversion of testosterone to DHT by Type II 5-alpha reductase (which is not blocked by finasteride) occurs in the skin and liver.

❏❏ **What is one disadvantage of Nd:YAG laser prostatectomy versus TURP?**

There is no tissue specimen available for histologic examination in patients treated by laser.

❏❏ **Does treating BPH with hyperthermia cause a temporary rise in serum PSA?**

In a review of clinical trials of hyperthermia treatment, post-treatment PSA was not significantly elevated following hyperthermia treatment for BPH.

❏❏ **T/F: Electrovaporization of the prostate (TVP) requires a shorter operative time than TURP?**

True. During TVP, only a small segment of the prostate is treated at a given interval versus a larger surface area covered by each pass of the loop of the resectoscope resulting in longer operative time for TURP.

❏❏ **What is the danger of using distilled water during transurethral surgery?**

The development of intravascular hemolysis will occur with the use of distilled water.

❏❏ **What is the danger of increasing the height of irrigation fluid during transurethral surgery?**

Fluid absorption during TURP has been estimated at 20 ccs per minute of resection time. The height of the irrigant may cause increased fluid absorption across open venous sinuses.

❏❏ **Prostatic secretions include:**

A high level of zinc is present in prostatic secretions.

❏❏ **What is the anatomic female equivalent to the prostate gland?**

The Skene glands in the female urethra are the homologue to the male prostate.

❏❏ **What typical female malignant neoplasm can arise in the prostate?**

Endometrial carcinoma can occur at the prostatic utricle.

❏❏ **What is the site of origin for endometrial carcinoma of the prostate?**

The utricle is the site of endometrial carcinoma in men.

❏❏ **The treatment of TUR syndrome includes:**

Symptomatic dilutional hyponatremia must be managed aggressively. Calculation of the total body sodium deficit using the following formula: (0.6 x weight in Kilos) x (desired serum Na^+ – the measured serum Na^+) = total body Na^+ deficit. This value divided by 513 milliosmoles/L gives you the liters of 3% saline that must be administered to correct the total body sodium deficit. One-half the total body deficit should be corrected in the first 2 hours and the remainder over the next 6 hours. Failure to correct the Na^+ deficit can have lethal results.

❏❏ **What drugs penetrate into the prostatic fluid?**

Trimethoprim-sulfamethoxazole and fluoroquinolones are the only drugs that achieve therapeutic levels in the prostatic parenchyma.

❏❏ **Where are Cowper's glands located?**

They are located within the urogenital diaphragm.

❏❏ **The blood supply to the prostate arises from how many groups of arteries?**

Two, a urethral and capsular group.

❏❏ **Lymphatic drainage of the prostatic urethra is to what lymph nodes?**

The obturator and external iliac lymph nodes are the main lymphatic drainage group.

❏❏ **T/F: Saline is safe to use for irrigation during transurethral surgery?**

False. Saline irrigation results in dissipation of electric current and renders the resectoscope useless.

❏❏ **Bacterial prostatitis is caused by what gram-positive organism?**

The gram-positive organism is enterococcus.

❏❏ **Where are prostatic calculi located within the prostate?**

The calculi are located between the prostatic adenoma and the surgical capsule.

❏❏ **Where in the prostatic cell is testosterone converted to 5-alpha dihydrotestosterone?**

This conversion occurs in cytoplasm.

FEMALE INCONTINENCE

Dominick J. Carbone, Jr., M.D. and Shlomo Raz, M.D.

❑❑ Define female urinary incontinence.

Female incontinence denotes the involuntary loss of urine per urethra. This is often socially embarrassing and impacts negatively on a patient's quality of life. It is important to identify the fluid lost as urine and not fluid from another source, peritoneal or uterine. Also, one must be sure that the urine is coming per urethra and not from a urinary fistula.

❑❑ Describe bladder abnormalities associated with urinary incontinence.

Detrusor overactivity: The bladder responds to filling with involuntary detrusor contractions leading to urinary incontinence. These may or may not result from a neurologic condition.

Sensory urgency: The bladder responds to early filling with a sensation of a strong need to void. This usually does not result in urinary incontinence, but severely impacts on a patient's quality of life.

Incomplete bladder emptying: The bladder does generate an adequate contractile force to empty and always contains an "excess" volume of urine. This may result in overflow incontinence.

Low bladder compliance: Compliance is defined as the change in volume over the change in pressure as measured during a cystometrogram. The result is expressed in millimeters per centimeter of water. A value above 20 ml/cm H_2O is considered normal. Compliance is dependent upon the viscoelastic properties of the detrusor. A variety of factors may affect the "normal" function of the viscoelastic properties of the bladder.

❑❑ Describe outlet abnormalities associated with urinary incontinence.

Urethral hypermobility: The pelvic floor fails to support the vesical neck and proximal urethra. This results in either the vesical neck and proximal urethra being situated *below* the inferior margin of the symphysis pubis at rest, or they descend from a position situated *above* the inferior margin of the symphysis pubis during stress.

Intrinsic sphincter deficiency: The internal urethral sphincter fails to maintain continence even at low detrussor pressures (0 cm H_2O to 60 cm H_2O) with resultant leakage of urine per urethra.

❑❑ Describe the classification of outlet abnormalities associated with urinary incontinence.

Type 0:   The vesical neck and proximal urethra are *closed* at rest and situated *above* the inferior margin of the symphysis pubis. During stress, the vesical neck and proximal urethra open and descend, however, no leak occurs. This is probably due to momentary voluntary contraction of the external urethral sphincter during the examination.

Type 1:   The vesical neck and proximal urethra are *closed* at rest and situated *above* the inferior margin of the symphysis pubis. During stress, the vesical neck and proximal urethra open and descend less than 2 cm with associated leakage of urine. Cystocele is minimal or absent.

Type 2A: The vesical neck and proximal urethra are *closed* at rest and situated *above* the inferior margin of the symphysis pubis. During stress, the vesical neck and proximal urethra open and descend greater than 2 cm with associated leakage of urine. A significant cystourethrocele is typically present.

Type 2B: The vesical neck and proximal urethra are *closed* at rest and situated *below* the inferior margin of the symphysis pubis. During stress, the vesical neck and proximal urethra open with or without further descent and leakage of urine occurs.

Type 3:   The vesical neck and proximal urethra are *open* at rest regardless of position. The urethral sphincter fails with leakage of urine either due to gravity or minimal stress.

❒❒ **Describe the symptoms associated with urinary incontinence.**

Urge incontinence: Involuntary loss of urine associated with a sudden strong desire to void.

Stress incontinence: Involuntary loss of urine during coughing, sneezing or increases in intrabominal pressure.

Positional incontinence: Involuntary loss of urine with any change in position not associated with increases in intraabdominal pressure.

Unconscious incontinence: Involuntary loss of urine without the awareness of urgency or stress.

Continuous leakage: Continuous involuntary loss of urine.

Nocturnal enuresis: Involuntary loss of urine that occurs only during sleep.

Post-void dribble: Involuntary loss of urine after voiding.

Overflow incontinence: Loss of urine accompanied by urinary retention.

❒❒ **Can stress incontinence induce urge incontinence?**

Yes. Urgency may result from compensatory responses initiated in the incontinent patient. For example, once the initial symptom of stress incontinence is noticed, the patient may urinate frequently to keep the bladder empty thus reducing the chance of stress-related incontinent episodes. As the bladder accommodates to these lower volumes, decreased bladder capacity and/or compliance may ensue. Subsequently, when the bladder distends beyond its reduced functional capacity, the patient experiences sensory urgency, frequency and urinary incontinence. Alternatively, urgency may be a product of urine passage into the proximal urethra with stress leakage. Correction of the stress incontinence may eliminate the urgency.

❒❒ **Distinguish detrusor instability vs. detrusor hyperreflexia.**

Both are conditions of detrusor overactivity. Detrusor instability describes involuntary bladder contractions *without* a neurologic etiology. Detrusor hyperreflexia describes involuntary bladder contractions *with* a neurologic etiology.

❒❒ **Is urge incontinence the same as detrusor overactivity?**

Yes. Urge incontinence implies involuntary bladder contractions. These may not be identifiable on urodynamics given that patients can suppress involuntary contractions.

❒❒ **List the components of normal urinary continence in response to increases abdominal stress.**

Normal continence in the female is a product of several forces working together. These forces include the proper *anatomic location* of the sphincteric unit, the critical functional and anatomic *urethral length*, the *mucosal coaptation* of the urethral surface and the increased urethral pressure generated by *reflex pelvic contractions* at the time of stress. Failure of one of the components of this delicate balance will not invariably produce stress incontinence because of the compensatory effect of the other forces

❒❒ **List the structures that provide normal pelvic support.**

The fascia of the pelvic floor may be collectively referred to as the *levator fascia*. Although the fascia works in an integrated fashion to provide pelvic support, certain areas of the fascia have been separately described because of their importance in supporting individual female pelvic structures.

The *pubourethral ligaments* connect the midportion of the urethra with the inner surface of the inferior pubis. Laterally this midportion of the urethra is supported by segments of the levator fascia just below their attachments to the pubis. Collectively, these may be referred to as the *midurethral complex*.

The *urethropelvic ligaments* (periurethral fascia) connect the proximal urethra and bladder neck laterally to the tendinous arch of the obturator muscle.

The *vesicopelvic ligaments* (pubocervical fascia) connect the bladder base laterally to the tendinous arch of the obturator muscle.

The *cardinal-sacrouterine ligaments* connect the uterine cervix and isthmus to the sacral vertebrae.

The *broad ligaments* connect the uterine body to the pelvic sidewall.

❏❏ Describe the urethral "washer effect".

The female urethra consists of a 4-cm tube of inner epithelium and outer muscularis. The infolded epithelium is enclosed by a rich vascular sponge, which in turn is surrounded by a fibromuscular and smooth muscle coat. This submucosa, consisting of loosely woven connective tissue scattered throughout with smooth muscle bundles and an elaborate vascular plexus, provides a compressive "washer effect" vital to the mechanism of continence. The effectiveness of this washer is estrogen dependent.

❏❏ Distinguish between abdominal, valsalva, bladder and detrusor leak point pressures.

Adbominal/Valsalva LPP: At a bladder volume of 150 – 200 cc, patients voluntarily increase abdominal pressures by incremental straining (valsalva). The abdominal pressure at which leakage occurs defines the abdominal or valsalva LPP. In the normal patient, urine loss should never occur during abdominal straining even at high pressures.

Detrusor/Bladder LPP: The pressure in the bladder during voluntary voiding when urine exits from the urethra defines the detrusor or bladder LPP. In the normal patient, urine exits the urethra at relatively low bladder pressures during voiding. A bladder LPP greater than 40 cmH$_2$0 puts the upper tracts at risk.

❏❏ What is the role of the history?

Because urinary symptoms may be similar despite disparate etiologies, the history is often nondiagnostic when considering female urinary incontinence. There is a 30% error in diagnosing stress urinary incontinence if only the history is used. Evaluation of the incontinent female must include a history, physical examination, and adjuvant testing. However, because more than one symptom is often present, it is essential to determine the relative severity of each complaint. It is important to focus on the *chief presenting symptom* in deciding the next diagnostic or therapeutic step.

❏❏ Describe several adjuvant office tests in assessing female urinary incontinence.

Q-tip test: Assesses mobility of the urethra. With stress, the tail of the applicator will transcribe an arc of 0 – 30 degrees in most women. Movement of greater than 35 degrees suggests urethral hypermobility.

Stress testing: Assesses urethral leak with stress. With the bladder full, the patient is asked to cough or strain. The patient with stress incontinence will immediately lose urine as a brief, small squirt associated with the stress. The position is variable. Eighty percent of patients will leak in the lithotomy position, an additional 10% of patients will leak at an incline of 45 degrees, while the final 10% of patients will only leak in the standing position.

Marshall-Bonney test: Assesses urethral continence with repositioning of the proximal urethra and vesicle neck. Without compressing the urethra, using either two fingers (Bonney) or ringed forceps (Marshall) the urethra is elevated behind the pubic bone and the patient strains. Continence, a positive test, suggests that surgical correction of the urethral hypermobility will eradicate the incontinence. False-positive results occur because obstruction of the urethra can occur during the maneuver.

Speculum examination: Assesses concomitant pelvic floor defects. Urethral hypermobility may be measured with a Q-tip, but a speculum is necessary to evaluate the anterior vaginal wall, the vaginal apex, an enterocele, a rectocele, the anal sphincter and the perineal body.

❏❏ What are the indications for urodynamic testing?

When results of simpler diagnostic tests have been inconclusive.

When empirical treatments have proved unsuccessful.

When the patient complains of incontinence but it cannot be demonstrated clinically.

In symptomatic patients that have previously undergone corrective surgery.

In patients with a history of prior radical pelvic surgery.

In patients with known or suspected neurologic disorders.

☐☐ What are the indications for cystoscopy?

In all patients with urgency as a complaint, bladder pathology such as bladder stone, bladder cancer and carcinoma-in-situ must be ruled out. All patients with hematuria should undergo cytologic examination, cystoscopy and upper tract evaluation. Patients with pure stress urinary incontinence may undergo preoperative cystoscopy to evaluate for incidental coexisting disease.

☐☐ Describe several radiographic evaluations useful in assessing female urinary incontinence.

Cystogram with voiding films (VCUG): Often obtained videourodynamics, these tests are useful in comparing resting and straining films. AP films can reveal the presence or absence of a cystocele. Lateral films are helpful in identifying urethral position at rest and hypermobility with straining. Urinary leak may be observed on the lateral straining films.

Ultrasound: Useful in identifying urethral mobility and prolapse, ultrasound can be performed transabdominally, transrectally, or transvaginally. The quality of the examination is highly dependent upon the skills of the ultrasonographer.

MRI: Usually reserved for cases of more severe prolapse, the MRI is very helpful in identifying cystocele, uterine prolapse and rectocele. It is also useful in revealing any concomitant pelvic pathology when hysterectomy is being considered as part of pelvic repair. Use of the HASTE sequence MRI is particularly helpful in identifying urologic pathology.

☐☐ What is the role of Kegel exercises and estrogens in female urinary incontinence?

Kegel exercises: If performed properly and diligently, Kegel exercises can strengthen the levator musculature which can lead to an increase in urethral pressure, better urethral reflex response to stresses, reduction of cystocele, and improved cough-urethra pressure transmission in stress urinary incontinence. These exercises are also useful for urge incontinence. By increasing pudendal activity to the sphincter muscles this may in turn stimulate a reflexive inhibitory input to the detrusor, thereby suppressing involuntary bladder contractions.

Estrogens: Lack of estrogen causes the urethral mucosa and underlying blood vessels to atrophy, leading to a decreased compressive washer effect. In women who are estrogen deficient, estrogen causes hypertrophy and thickening of the urethral mucosa and engorgement of the blood vessels beneath.

☐☐ Identify several behavioral modifications for a woman with urge incontinence.

Timed voiding: Instruct the patient void on a timed schedule. The specific interval should be based on voiding before the development of urgency. Increase the interval after several weeks without urgency. Prompt voiding: Instruct the patient not to delay voiding. Additionally, the patient must concentrate on completely relaxing and emptying the bladder during the void.

Fluid restriction: Limit the fluid intake for patients that are drinking excessively. Avoid caffeine containing beverages and fluid consumption after dinner.

☐☐ Distinguish between the pharmacologic treatments for a woman with urge incontinence.

Anticholinergics: Antagonize the muscarinic receptors of the bladder resulting in increased total bladder capacity, decreased amplitude of bladder contraction, and increased bladder volume before first bladder contraction. (e.g. – Propantheline bromide, Hyocyamine)

Antispasmodics: Primarily cause relaxation of detrusor smooth muscle in addition to anticholinergic effects and local anesthetic effects. (e.g. – Oxybutin chloride, Dicyclomine hydrochloride, Flavoxate hydrochloride, Tolterodine)

Tricyclic antidepressants: Unique in the ability to increase urethral outlet resistance due to adrenergic stimulation on the smooth muscle of the bladder neck and proximal urethra in addition to anticholinergic effects and a sedative action that may be related to antihistaminic properties (e.g. – Imipramine hydrochloride, Amitriptyline hydrochloride)

Calcium-channel blockers: Uncommon as first-line agents, calcium channel blockers inhibit the inflow of calcium after membrane depolarization and have the potential of relaxing the smooth muscle of the bladder (e.g. – Nifedipine)

❏❏ **What is the role of surgery for urge incontinence?**

Bladder augmentation allows for increased total bladder capacity and physical interruption of the overactive detrusor muscle. It is used as a last resort after exhausting all possible pharmacologic interventions for urge incontinence. Today, additional options before surgical intervention include the use of electrical stimulation to inhibit involuntary bladder contractions or laparoscopic myomectomy (autoaugmentation). Bladder augmentation is not effective in the elderly population.

❏❏ **What is the role for needle suspension for stress urinary incontinence?**

Needle suspension prevents urethral descent with stress. It has been effective in the treatment of urethral hypermobility but does not affect incontinence due to intrinsic sphincter deficiency.

❏❏ **What is the role for periurethral collagen injection for stress urinary incontinence?**

Collagen is used as a bulking agent. It is effective in the treatment of intrinsic sphincter deficiency, but does not affect incontinence due to urethral hypermobility.

❏❏ **What is the role for suburethral sling for stress urinary incontinence?**

Suburethral (pubovaginal) sling procedures effectively prevent urethral descent with stress and improve the urethral washer effect. Therefore, slings are equally effective for urethral hypermobility and intrinsic sphincter deficiency. However, there are increased postoperative risks of retention with detrussor instability.

❏❏ **An elderly woman presents with urinary urgency and frequency. Ultrasound evaluation determines her post-void residual to be 350 cc. What is the diagnosis?**

This patient has detrusor hyperactivity with impaired contractility (DHIC). DHIC represents the coexistence of detrusor overactivity and bladder weakness rather than a distinct entity and is common in the elderly patient. Treatment is difficult since pharmacologic treatment of the detrusor overactivity often exacerbates the retention. This requires clean intermittent catheterization which is often difficult in the elderly population.

❏❏ **A 46-year-old woman, gravida 4, para 4, presents with urgency, frequency and urinary incontinence. Physical examination is normal, Marshall test is negative and urodynamic evaluation reveals a normally compliant bladder without involuntary bladder contractions. What is the diagnosis?**

This patient has classic urge incontinence. It is important to focus on the chief presenting symptom in evaluating a patient with urinary incontinence. Despite the obstetrical history and the lack of involuntary bladder contractions, the diagnosis remains urge incontinence.

❏❏ **A woman presents with complaints of urgency and precipitous voiding shortly following a cough or sneeze. What is the diagnosis?**

This patient has stress-induced urge incontinence. Stress incontinence is the involuntary loss of urine during coughing, sneezing or increases in intraabdominal pressure. The described patient loses urine after the intraabdominal pressure has returned to normal and continues to empty her bladder precipitously. This suggests an involuntary bladder contraction occurring due to the stress stimulus.

❏❏ **A woman presents with urodynamically demonstrated stress incontinence with urinary urgency. What is the treatment of choice?**

Treatment of the stress incontinence. Urgency may result from compensatory responses initiated by the incontinent patient. Alternatively, urgency may be a product of urine passage into the proximal urethra with stress leakage. In 65% of patients with mixed stress and urge incontinence, correction of the stress incontinence will resolve the urgency.

❑❑ **A woman presents with urinary incontinence immediately following only repair of a large cystocele. What is the diagnosis?**

Stress urinary incontinence. The full bladder contributes to normal continence by creating a valvular effect through limited posterior rotation of the bladder base against a well-supported urethra during stress. Cystoceles exacerbate this valvular effect and may mask underlying urethral dysfunction. Correction of a large cystocele in this setting leads to incontinence due to either urethral hypermobility or intrinsic sphincter deficiency.

❑❑ **Immediately following a needle bladder neck suspension, a woman complains of persistent stress urinary incontinence. What is the diagnosis?**

Intrinsic sphincter deficiency. Needle suspension corrects urethral hypermobility but is ineffective against intrinsic sphincter deficiency. Periurethral collagen injection corrects intrinsic sphincter deficiency but is ineffective against urethral hypermobility. Suburethral sling procedures correct both deficiencies.

UPPER URINARY TRACT OBSTRUCTION

Uday Kumar, MS, F.R.C.S. and David M. Albala, M.D.

❑❑ **In evaluating upper tract obstruction, which is the radiopharmaceutical of choice?**

99mTc-mercaptoacetyltriglycine (MAG3). It is more efficiently excreted by the kidney than DTPA, delivers a lower dose of radiation to the kidney than OIH and provides better visualization of the anatomy of obstruction than other agents.

❑❑ **What is the basis of the Whitaker test?**

It provides urodynamic evidence of mechanical obstruction of the upper tract at a given flow rate. As it is an invasive test, it is only used in cases with extreme dilatation of the upper tract or when renal function is too poor for adequate diuretic response.

❑❑ **What are the phases in pressure changes in the ureter after unilateral occlusion of the ureter?**

Following unilateral occlusion, there is a rise in both ureteric pressure and renal blood flow for 1-1.5 hours. Then in phase 2, there is a continued rise in ureteric pressure while renal blood flow declines (5 hours). In the final phase both renal blood flow and ureteric pressure fall.

❑❑ **What are the causes of postobstructive diuresis?**

Postobstructive diuresis occurs after relief of bilateral ureteric obstruction or obstruction of a solitary kidney. It may be classified as physiologic, when caused by retained urea, sodium and water, or pathologic when caused by impaired concentrating ability or sodium absorption.

❑❑ **What is the embryological basis of retrocaval ureter?**

The persistence of the posterior cardinal vein as the major portion of the inferior vena cava causes medial migration of and compression of the right ureter.

❑❑ **What are the types of retrocaval ureter?**

There are two types. Type I or the "low loop type", is the most common and the dilated proximal portion assumes a reverse J. Type II or the "high loop" is rarer. In this case the ureter goes behind the vena cava at the level of or just above the UPJ.

❑❑ **How common is hydronephrosis in pregnancy?**

Unilateral or bilateral hydronephrosis occurs by the third trimester of pregnancy in 90% -95% of asymptomatic patients. In more than 80% of patients, right-sided hydronephrosis predominates.

❑❑ **T/F: In the treatment of ureteric obstruction due to endometriosis, hormonal therapy is the treatment of choice?**

False. Surgery is more likely to be successful. The choice of surgery depends on the extent of ureteric involvement and the patient's desire to have more children. Ureterolysis with unilateral or bilateral oophorectomy and hysterectomy may be required. In severe cases, nephrectomy may be needed.

❑❑ **How common is ureteral injury following hysterectomy?**

In routine hysterectomy, the incidence varies from 0.5% to 3% and is bilateral in one of every six cases. After radical hysterectomy, the incidence varies from 10% - 15%.

□□ How is ureteral involvement in Crohn's disease treated?

Rarely is ureterolysis required for ureteral involvement in Crohn's. Medical or surgical therapy for Crohn's disease is usually effective in resolving ureteral involvement. It may also be indicated in some cases with severe retroperitoneal fibrosis with encasement of the ureter.

□□ What are the causes of retroperitoneal fibrosis (RPF)?

Two thirds of cases are idiopathic. Other causes include prolonged use of methysergide and other ergot derivatives. RPF can occur secondary to other disease processes of the retroperitoneum like hemorrhage, urinary extravasation, trauma, peri-aneurysmal inflammation, radiation therapy, surgery, inflammatory bowel disease, collagen disease and fat necrosis.

□□ What are the symptoms of retroperitoneal fibrosis?

In about 90% of cases, there is a characteristic pain with a girdle type distribution. The pain is dull and non-colicky. Later it becomes severe and unrelenting. The pain may be relieved by aspirin and not by narcotics. Rarely there may be features of compression of the great vessels. Uremia is a late feature.

□□ What are the features of retroperitoneal fibrosis on intravenous urography?

There is medial deviation of the ureters on IVU. Though this finding is present in up to 20% of normal studies, in RPF the displacement extends higher than the normal variant. There is usually associated obstruction and hydronephrosis. CT or MRI is most useful in establishing a diagnosis.

□□ How is retroperitoneal fibrosis treated?

Any suspected medication like methysergide is withheld. If the patient is uremic, renal drainage should be established with ureteral stenting or nephrostomy tube placement. Steroid therapy may be useful in some but bilateral ureterolysis is required in most cases.

□□ What is pelvic lipomatosis?

Pelvic lipomatosis a proliferative disease of unknown etiology involving the mature fatty tissues of the pelvic retroperitoneum. It occurs exclusively in men in the third to sixth decade of life and is more common in African American men. This benign condition may lead to compression of the pelvic viscera including the ureters.

□□ What conditions may be associated with pelvic lipomatosis?

It may be associated with cystitis cystica, cystitis glandularis, adenocarcinoma of bladder, chronic UTI, hypertension, superficial thrombophlebitis, VU reflux, RPF, non-tropical chyluria and Proteus syndrome.

□□ How is pelvic lipomatosis diagnosed?

Plain KUB x-ray may show the radiolucent area in the bony pelvis. On IVP, the bladder base is noted to be elevated and the bladder itself takes on a pear-shape. CT is useful to confirm the diagnosis.

□□ How common is bilaterality in UPJ obstruction?

Bilateral UPJ obstruction is seen in 10-40% of cases.

□□ T/F: UPJ obstruction occurs more commonly in males and on the left side?

True. The ratio of male to female is more prominent in infancy (2: 1). Left-sided lesions are more common. In infancy about two thirds of UPJ obstructions are on the left.

⬚⬚ How common is the finding of an aberrant lower polar vessel in UPJ obstruction?

The incidence varies from 15% - 52%. Though some cases are no doubt caused by the aberrant vessel, especially in adults, in most cases it is felt to be a concomitant finding rather than the cause.

⬚⬚ Vesicoureteric reflux and UPJ obstruction are found together in what proportion of cases?

In about 10% (minor degree of reflux has been quoted in up to 40%). Severe cases of VU reflux can cause marked tortuosity of the ureter and secondarily give rise to UPJ obstruction.

⬚⬚ What are the congenital anomalies associated with UPJ obstruction?

UPJ obstruction in contralateral kidney (10% - 40%), renal dysplasia and multicystic disease of contralateral kidney, unilateral renal agenesis, duplicated collecting system, VU reflux and the VATER complex.

⬚⬚ What is the investigation of choice for UPJ obstruction?

A diuretic renogram is the best non-invasive method to determine if a dilated upper tract is obstructed or not.

⬚⬚ What test is useful to determine whether a hydronephrotic kidney is salvageable or not?

A quantitative renal scan using technetium-99-DMSA is useful to determine whether a patient will benefit from pyeloplasty or not. If a kidney contributes less than 10% of the overall renal function, it should probably be removed.

⬚⬚ How is resistive index (on ultrasound examination) defined?

(peak systolic velocity - lowest diastolic velocity) / peak systolic velocity.

⬚⬚ What is the basis for the use of resistive index (RI) in the diagnosis of obstructive uropathy?

A decrease in renal blood flow and an increase in renovascular resistance are hallmarks of obstructive uropathy. There is a more marked reduction in diastolic blood flow than systolic causing a rise in RI.

⬚⬚ What conditions other than obstructive uropathy can cause RI to be elevated?

Values above the normally accepted 0.70 may be found in children especially infants, in medical renal diseases, dehydration, hypotension and a low heart rate.

⬚⬚ What are the determinants of the curve obtained during diuretic renography?

The curve depends on the tracer used, the patient's hydration status, the dose and timing of the administration of the diuretic and the overall renal function. The shape, size and distensibility of the renal pelvis, its outlet resistance, gravity and bladder filling, also influence the curve.

⬚⬚ What are the patterns of curves described on the diuretic renogram?

Type I (normal), Type II (obstructed), Type IIIa (dilated unobstructed) and Type IIIb (equivocal).

⬚⬚ Can urinary biochemical markers be used in the diagnosis of upper tract obstruction?

N-B-Acetyl glucosaminidase (NAG), B-2-microglobulin and transforming growth factors (TGF-P) have been found to be elevated in the urine of patients with renal obstruction. The utility of these markers is yet to be determined.

⬚⬚ What are the ultrasound findings of UPJ obstruction in the neonate?

The pelvis is seen as a large medial sonolucent structure, surrounded by smaller, rounded sonolucent structures representing the dilated calyces. Sometimes, the infundibular communications between the dilated calyces and the renal pelvis may be seen.

☐☐ T/F: It is difficult to distinguish antenatally between severe hydronephrosis and multicystic dysplastic kidneys (MDK)?

True. The ultrasound findings of MDK are lack of reniform shape of the kidney, multiple cysts of varying size and no evidence of collecting system. In severe hydronephrosis the distinction may be difficult.

☐☐ What are the indications for intervention in UPJ obstruction?

The presence of symptoms from obstruction, impairment of renal function or development of infection or stones. Patients with solitary kidneys and bilateral UPJ obstruction should have intervention. The timing of repair in infants is controversial, as it is difficult to determine which kidneys are at risk.

☐☐ A dismembered pyeloplasty is not suitable for which cases?

When the UPJ obstruction is associated with lengthy or multiple proximal ureteral strictures or when the renal pelvis is small, intrarenal and relatively inaccessible.

☐☐ When is preoperative drainage of a kidney with UPJ obstruction indicated?

When there is infection associated with obstruction, uremia due to obstruction in a solitary kidney or bilateral disease and rarely in the patient with severe unrelenting pain.

☐☐ How is UPJ obstruction treated in the adult?

Until recently, open surgery (i.e. pyeloplasty) was the only option. Minimally invasive alternatives now available include, endopyelotomy (antegrade or retrograde), cautery wire balloon incision (Acucise device) and laparoscopic pyeloplasty.

☐☐ When an endopyelotomy is performed, where is the incision made?

If a direct endoscopic incision is performed, a direct lateral cut is the safest. This appears to have the least likelihood of encountering a crossing vessel. In one study, a posterior-crossing vessel was found in 6.2% of cases, whereas no vessels were found crossing the UPJ laterally.

☐☐ What factors predict a poor outcome after endopyelotomy?

Poor renal function, massive hydronephrosis and the presence of a crossing vessel result in a reduced success rates.

☐☐ What are the possible complications of endopyelotomy?

Hemorrhage is the most commonly encountered problem. Rarely ureteral avulsion, ureteral necrosis, arteriovenous fistula formation, hematoma, urinoma and urinary infection have been reported.

☐☐ When hydronephrosis is noted in a horseshoe kidney what is the likely cause?

The obstruction is usually due to a UPJ obstruction and not due to pressure on the ureter from the isthmus.

☐☐ What are the basic techniques used in open pyeloplasty?

There are two fundamental techniques. A pelvic flap is used in Culp and DeWeerd, Scardino and Prince and Foley Y-plasty operations. An Anderson-Hynes pyeloplasty is the dismembered type.

☐☐ Which part of the nephron is most resistant to damage from hydronephrosis?

The glomerulus. Glomerular changes are not evident until 28 days of obstruction. In contrast, distal tubular and proximal tubular atrophy is seen at 7 and 14 days, respectively.

❑❑ How does urine exit the kidney in complete obstruction?

In acute obstruction with high pressures, like ureteral calculi, urine exits through a rupture in the fornices. In low-pressure obstruction, urine exits via lymphatic channels and in chronic hydronephrosis, it is mostly into the renal venous channels.

❑❑ What is the incidence of UPJ obstruction?

Urinary dilatation is detected in utero in one in 100 pregnancies; of these, significant uropathy is seen in one in 500. UPJ obstruction is responsible for 40% of these, placing the incidence of UPJ obstruction at 1: 1250 births.

❑❑ What is the crescent sign on the excretory urogram in a patient with UPJ obstruction?

The calyceal crescents represent transversely oriented collecting ducts and signify recoverable renal function.

❑❑ What are the causes of PUJ obstruction?

A. Intrinsic:
1. congenital - adynamic muscular segment
2. ureteral mucosal folds
3. high insertion of ureter into renal pelvis

B. Extrinsic:
1. Aberrant lower pole vessel
2. Retroperitoneal fibrosis
3. Retroperitoneal tumors

C. Secondary:
1. Renal calculi
2. Fibroepithelial polyps
3. Tumors
4. Failed pyeloplasty

❑❑ Which is the most common cause of UPJ obstruction?

Intrinsic causes are the most common, with an adynamic muscular segment (congenital) occurring frequently.

❑❑ Where is the most common site for ureteral strictures to occur?

Ureteral strictures occur most commonly at the ureteropelvic junction. The second most common area of stenosis is at the ureterovesical junction.

INTESTINAL SEGMENTS IN UROLOGY

Bolent Akduman, M.D. and Laurence Klotz, M.D.

◻◻ **What is the advantage of stomach over other intestinal segments for urinary diversion?**

Stomach is less permeable to urinary solutes, it acidifies the urine, it has a net excretion of chloride and protons rather than a net absorption of them, and it produces less mucus.

◻◻ **T/F: The jejunum is a good option as an intestinal segment for urinary intestinal diversion.**

False. The jejunum is usually not employed for reconstruction of the urinary system because its use often results in severe electrolyte imbalance.

◻◻ **T/F: The incidence of postoperative bowel obstruction in patients who have segments isolated from the colon is less than that occurring with ileum.**

True. Postoperative bowel obstruction occurs in about 10% of patients who have bowel segments isolated from the ileum for urinary tract reconstruction compared to 4% of patients who have bowel segments isolated from colon.

◻◻ **What are the most common aerobic organisms in the bowel?**

Escherichia coli and Streptococcus faecalis.

◻◻ **What are the most common anaerobic organisms in the bowel?**

Bacteroides species and Clostridium species.

◻◻ **T/F: A mechanical bowel preparation reduces the concentration of bacteria as well as the total number.**

False. The mechanical preparation reduces the amount of feces, whereas the antibiotic preparation reduces the bacterial concentration.

◻◻ **What are the common adverse effects of antibiotic bowel preparation?**

Diarrhea. Pseudomembranous enterocolitis, monilial overgrowth resulting in stomatitis, malabsorption of protein, carbohydrate, and fat are the other disadvantages.

◻◻ **What is the etiologic agent of pseudomembranous enterocolitis?**

Clostridium difficile. C difficile elaborates cytotoxin A and cytotoxin B which cause diarrhea and enterocolitis.

◻◻ **Which factors contribute to a potential anastomotic breakdown?**

Poor blood supply, local sepsis, drains placed in contact with an anastomosis, and performance of an anastomosis on previously irradiated bowel. Poor blood supply and local sepsis cause ischemia whereas drains placed on the anastomosis increase the likelihood of an anastomotic leak.

◻◻ **What are the complications of intestinal anastomoses?**

Stenosis, obstruction, pseudo-obstructions (Ogilvie's syndrome) (acute colonic pseudo-obstruction characterized by massive colonic dilatation in the absence of mechanical cause), intestinal leak, hemorrhage, fistulas, wound infections, pelvic abscesses, sepsis. 1% of these complications require operations.

☐☐ **What are the common causes of the bowel obstruction following construction of intestinal anastomoses?**

Adhesions, and recurrent cancer.

☐☐ **What are the consequences of persistent infection in intestinal segments?**

Strictures and renal deterioration. Persistent infection of the intestine exposed to urine may result in stricture, bacterial seeding of the upper tracts, and renal deterioration.

☐☐ **In a patient with a continent diversion, you diagnose elongation of the intestinal segment. What is the next step?**

Catheterize the pouch. The elevated intraluminal pressure may result in deterioration of renal function and a volvulus of the segment.

☐☐ **Which type of abdominal stoma is preferable when a collection device is worn?**

Protruding stoma. It has a lower incidence of stomal stenosis and fewer peristomal skin problems.

☐☐ **What is the potential complication of the abdominal stoma placed lateral to the rectus sheath?**

Parastomal hernia. Ideally, the stoma should be placed through the belly of the rectus muscle.

☐☐ **Which stomas are associated with an increased likelihood of parastomal hernias?**

The incidence of parastomal hernias for end stomas is 1%-4%, compared to 4%-20% for loop stomas.

☐☐ **What are the options if an ileal conduit won't reach the skin?**

a)   Turnbull stoma (ie, loop ileostomy).
b)   Excise mesentery from the terminal part of loop.
c)   Mobilize the base of mesentery.
d)   Redo the loop.

☐☐ **T/F: The pressure within the renal pelvis in refluxing conduit diversions is elevated above normal.**

False. Peristaltic ureteral contractions dampen pressure transmission from intestine to renal pelvis, as a result it is not elevated above normal.

☐☐ **Which of the small bowel anti-refluxing procedures has the lowest incidence of stricture as an ureterointestinal anastomosis?**

LeDuc procedure (mucosal trench). It has also the highest success rate in preventing reflux.

☐☐ **How long are patients at risk for ureterointestinal strictures?**

Late strictures (>10 years) are not uncommon. They are at risk for ureterointestinal strictures for the life of anastomosis.

☐☐ **Is ureteral stenosis in a patient with a ureterointestinal anastomosis more common on one side than the other? Why?**

Ureterointestinal anastamotic strictures occur more commonly with the left ureter. Blood supply to the ureter may be compromised where the ureter crosses over the aorta beneath the inferior mesenteric artery.

Additionally, aggressive stripping of adventitia and angulation of the ureter at the inferior mesenteric artery can result in ischemia and subsequent stricture formation.

□□ A patient is considered for a continent diversion. His serum creatinine exceeds 2.0 mg/dl. How should he be evaluated to determine whether he is a candidate?

Criteria for candidacy for a continent diversion include the ability to achieve a urine pH of 5.8 or less following an ammonium chloride load test, a urine osmolality $\geq$ 600 mOsm/kg in response to water deprivation, a glomerular filtration rate > 35 ml/minute, and no more than minimal proteinuria.

□□ List the contraindications to an ileal conduit.

Short bowel syndrome, inflammatory small bowel disease, and previous extensive radiation to ileum.

□□ What is the optimal site for a stoma in jejunal conduit?

Left upper quadrant. The portion of jejunum to be utilized should be as distal as possible.

□□ Which is the most common electrolyte abnormality in patients who have an ileal conduit?

Hyperchloremic metabolic acidosis. It is seen as a late complication in 13 % of patients.

□□ Which kind of electrolyte abnormalities are seen in patients with a jejunal conduit?

Hyponatremic, hypochloremic, hyperkalemic metabolic acidosis. Sodium chloride replacement and thiazides are the treatment of choice.

□□ Which part of colon is the most appropriate segment for a conduit in patients requirng an intestinal pyelostomy?

Transverse colon. It is an excellent segment when an intestinal pyelostomy needs to be performed.

□□ Which part of colon is the most appropriate segment to use as a colon conduit in patients who have received extensive pelvic irradiation.

Transverse colon. This segment of bowel typically lies outside the treated field in patients undergoing pelvic irradiation. The isolated segment will be well supplied by the middle colic artery.

□□ Which part of colon is the most appropriate segment as a colon conduit in patients undergoing a pelvic exenteration?

Sigmoid colon. No bowel anastomosis needs to be made.

□□ What is the contraindication to the use of sigmoid colon in addition to disease of the segment and extensive pelvic irradiation.

If the internal iliac arteries have been ligated and the rectum has been left in situ, use of the sigmoid colon is contraindicated. It may result in sloughing of rectum or its mucosa.

□□ What are the contraindications to the use of colonic segments?

Inflammatory large bowel disease and severe chronic diarrhea.

□□ What are the main advantages of an ileocecal conduit.

Long segments of ileum are available when long segments of ureter need to be replaced. It also provides colon for the stoma, and finally, a non-refluxing anastamosis can be performed.

□□ Which electrolyte abnormalities are seen when the stomach is used for urinary diversion?

Hypochloremic, hypokalemic metabolic alkalosis. This is a more significant problem if the patient has concomitant azotemia.

❏❏ **What is the medical treatment for hypochloremic hypokalemic metabolic alkalosis?**

Proton pump blockers (Omeprazole) and acidification with dilute hydrochloric acid (0.1N HCL, arginine hydrochloride and oral NH_4Cl.

❏❏ **What is the likely diagnosis of a patient with jejunal conduit who has lethargy, nausea, vomiting, dehydration, muscular weakness, and an elevated temperature?**

Metabolic disturbance. Hyponatremia, hypochloremia, hyperkalemia, azotemia, and acidosis are seen in patients with jejunal conduits.

❏❏ **How effective is IV hyperalimentation for the treatment of the metabolic disturbances in a patient with a jejunal conduit?**

Administering hyperalimentation solutions may exacerbate the syndrome.

❏❏ **What are the symptoms of the electrolyte abnormality that occurs with ileal and colonic diversions.**

Easy fatigability, anorexia, weight loss, polydipsia, and lethargy. Exacerbation of diarrhea is often seen in patients with a ureterosigmoidostomy.

❏❏ **What is the treatment of persistent hyperchloremic metabolic acidosis in patients with ileal conduits if an excessive sodium load is undesirable?**

Chlorpromazine and nicotinic acid. Both result in inhibition of cyclic AMP which impedes chloride ion transport, so HCO_3 levels increase.

❏❏ **Which kind of urinary diversion has the highest possibility of hypokalemia?**

Ureterosigmoidostomies. Ileal segments reabsorb some of the potassium when exposed to high concentrations of potassium in the urine whereas colon do not.

❏❏ **What is the mechanism of hyperchloremic acidosis in patients with ileal diversions?**

Ionized transport of ammonium is responsible for hyperchloremic acidosis in patients with ileal diversions. When ammonium substitutes for sodium in the Na/H antiport, NH_4 is coupled with the exchange of bicarbonate for chloride. So, NH_4 is absorbed across the lumen into the blood in exchange for H_2CO_3. In addition, potassium channels in bowel lumen may contribute to ammonium entry to the blood.

❏❏ **What are the mechanisms causing potassium depletion in patients with urinary diversion?**

It is due to renal potassium wasting, osmotic diuresis, and gut loss through intestinal secretion.

❏❏ **What is a consequence of the treatment of metabolic acidosis by $NaHCO_3$ alone.**

Severe hypokalemia. The treatment must involve both correction of the acidosis with bicarbonate and replacement of potassium.

❏❏ **T/F: Serum concentrations of urea and creatinine are less accurate measures of renal function after enteric diversion.**

True. Urea and creatinine are reabsorbed by both the ileum and the colon.

❏❏ **What are the most likely causes of altered sensorium in a patient with urinary diversion.**

Magnesium deficiency, drug intoxication, hyperammonemia, or diabetic hyperglycemia (this is not a consequence of the intestinal diversion).

❏❏ What is the treatment of ammoniagenic coma?

Draining the urinary intestinal diversion to prevent urine exposure to the intestine for extended periods of time, administration of neomycin to reduce the ammonia load from enteric tract, limitation of protein consumption should be done to limit the patient's nitrogen load. In severe cases, arginine glutamate, 50 gms. in 1000 ml of 5 % dextrose in water intravenously to complex the ammonia in the gut and to prevent its absorption. Additionally, lactulose may be given orally or per rectum.

❏❏ Which classes of drugs can be problematic in patients with urinary intestinal diversion regarding drug toxicity?

Drugs which are absorbed by the gastrointestinal tract and excreted unchanged by the kidney. This includes phenytoin, certain antibiotics, and methotrexate.

❏❏ In which type of urinary diversion is altered sensorium most commonly found?

Ureterosigmoidostomy. It has been reported for those with ileal conduits as well.

❏❏ What is the most common cause of osteomalacia in patients with urinary diversion?

Acidosis. Other causes are vitamin D resistance and excessive calcium loss by the kidney.

❏❏ A patient with urinary diversion has hip pain, lethargy, and proximal myopathy. What is your diagnosis?

Osteomalacia.

❏❏ What are the abnormalities in serum chemistry in a patient who develops osteomalacia?

The calcium is either low or normal, the alkaline phosphatase is elevated and the phosphate is low or normal.

❏❏ In a patient with osteomalacia, you corrected acidosis, and provided dietary calcium. What is the next step?

1-alpha-hydroxycholecalciferol should be administered. This is a vitamin D metabolite that is more potent than vitamin D_2.

❏❏ Which patients with asymptomatic bacteriuria and an intestinal diversion should be treated?

Only patients with predominant cultures of Proteus or Pseudomonas should be treated. Other bacteria should not be treated.

❏❏ What is the most common cause of stone formation in conduits and pouches?

Foreign body such as staples or nonabsorbable sutures. Persistent infection, hypercalciuria are the other factors.

❏❏ Loss of which bowel segment may cause vitamin B_{12} and bile salt malabsorption?

Terminal ileum.

❏❏ What is the effect of vitamin B_{12} deficiency?

Vitamin B_{12} deficiency results in anemia, neurological degeneration.

❏❏ Loss of which segment of bowel is associated with folic acid malabsorption?

Jejunum. In addition, malabsorption of fat and calcium may be seen.

❑❑ **What is the most common histologic type of cancer seen in association with urinary intestinal diversion?**

Adenocarcinoma.

❑❑ **A 27-year-old male with spina-bifida undergoes and ileal conduit undiversion. How should the defunctionalized segment be managed?**

Excision of the segment is appropriate. If left in situ, it has malignant potential.

❑❑ **Which segments of the small intestine are most likely to have been radiated in a patient receiving pelvic radiation?**

The last two inches of the terminal ileum and 5 feet of small bowel beginning approximately 6 feet from the ligament of Treitz are the two portions of the small bowel that may lie within the confines of the pelvis and as such may be exposed to pelvic irradiation and pelvic disease. In a postradiated patient, one should try to avoid using these two segments of the small intestine in any reconstructive procedure.

❑❑ **Where are the three vulnerable points involving the vascular supply to the colon located?**

Sudeck's critical point located between the junction of the sigmoid and superior hemorrhoidal arteries, the midpoints between the middle colic and right colic arteries and between the middle colic and left colic arteries are tenuous anastomotic areas. If the colon were transected in these regions, the anastomosis might be at risk because of compromised blood supply.

❑❑ **T/F: Hypergastrinemia may occur following gastric pouch orthotopic bladder formation.**

True. Hydrochloric acid produced by the parietal cells in the body of the stomach has a negative feedback on antral gastrin secretion. When the body of the stomach is removed this negative feedback mechanism may be impaired.

❑❑ **What is the lipid profile of a patient in whom 60 to 100 cm. ileum are removed from the fecal stream?**

Serum cholesterol decreases while triglycerides increase.

❑❑ **What are the major consequences of lipid malabsorption seen in patients with ileal resection?**

The deficiency of fat soluble vitamins (A, D, E, K), and an increase in incidence of gallstones and renal stones.

❑❑ **What length of time is required for the depletion of vitamin B_{12} stores in the complete absence of absorption in a patient who has an extensive terminal ileum resection?**

3 to 4 years. Partial malabsorption may take up to 30 years to become clinically manifest.

❑❑ **What are typical neurological manifestations of vitamin B_{12} deficiency?**

Peripheral neuropathy, optic atrophy, subacute combined degeneration of the spinal cord and dementia.

❑❑ **In which part of the intestinal segments used for urinary diversion does the least net water movement occur?**

Stomach. It is followed by colon, ileum, and jejunum, respectively.

❑❑ **What is the most accurate means of determining renal function in patients with urinary diversion?**

Measurement of renal function with serial serum determination of 51Cr-EDTA after bolus injection is the most accurate method of determining renal function. This agent crosses the intestinal mucosa in negligible quantities.

❏❏ **A patient with invasive TCC of the bladder wishes to have an orthotopic neobladder. What are the absolute contra-indications to a neobladder?**

The only absolute contraindication is the presence of TCC at the urethral resection margin. Prostatic urethral TCC is associated with an increased risk of urethral recurrence, but if the resection margin is negative a neobladder is still an option in these patients.

❏❏ **A patient is diagnosed with a recurrent invasive lesion in the urethra following radical cystectomy and neobladder construction. What is your treatment?**

Urethrectomy. Convert to a continent diversion if possible, or remove the reservoir and convert to a conduit.

❏❏ **Which kind of neobladder is the most amenable for conversion of a patient to a conduit?**

Studer neobladder. It has 15 to 20 cm isoperistaltic proximal ileal limb.

❏❏ **What should the upper level of sustained bladder pressure be in a patient with a continent neobladder?**

40 cm H_2O. Sustained pressures over 40 cm H_2O put the upper tract at risk.

❏❏ **What is the most common complaint of a patient with an orthotopic diversion?**

Nocturnal enuresis. The loss of native bladder and its reflexes, and the production of an increased urine volume are responsible for this complaint.

URINARY DIVERSION AND UNDIVERSION

Christopher L. Coogan, M.D. and Thomas G. Matkov, M.D.

❑❑ **What is the electrolyte abnormality most commonly seen when stomach is used in the urinary tract?**

Hypochloremic metabolic alkalosis. This is secondary to the HCl secretion by the stomach segment, involving the H^+/K^+ ATPase secretory mechanism of the gastric mucosa.

❑❑ **What is the electrolyte abnormality most commonly seen when jejunum is used in the urinary tract?**

Hyponatremic, hypochloremic, hyperkalemic metabolic acidosis. This has been termed the "jejunal conduit syndrome". This syndrome can be quite debilitating, resulting in nausea, anorexia, lethargy, fever and even death. The more proximal the segment used, the more likely the syndrome is to develop, secondary to the increased surface area available, due to increased villi and microvilli. The jejunum should be used only when there are no other acceptable segments available for use.

❑❑ **What is the electrolyte abnormality most commonly seen when ileum or colon is used in the urinary tract?**

Hyperchloremic metabolic acidosis. This is caused by the substitution of ammonium for sodium in the Na/H transport. Therefore ammonium chloride is absorbed into the bloodstream in exchange for carbonic acid (CO_2 and H_2O).

❑❑ **What is the cause of the altered sensorium occasionally associated with intestinal conduits?**

Magnesium deficiency, drug intoxication, or abnormalities of ammonia metabolism. This should be treated with drainage of the urinary intestinal diversion (foley or rectal tube) and treating the underlying condition.

❑❑ **T/F: Continent urinary diversions are generally associated with fewer metabolic abnormalities.**

False. Given the longer dwell time of urine in contact with the intestinal segment used, both neobladders and continent urinary diversions are associated with a higher risk of electrolyte and metabolic abnormalities.

❑❑ **What is the most common stomal complication following urinary diversion?**

Stomal stenosis. The incidence is reported to be 20 - 25% for ileal conduits and 10 - 20% for colon conduits. Other complications include bleeding, bowel necrosis, dermatitis, parastomal hernias, and stomal prolapse.

❑❑ **Which segment of bowel is most suitable for non-refluxing uretero-intestinal anastomoses?**

Colon. Numerous anastomoses (Leadbetter and Clarke, Goodwin, Strickler, and Pagano) employ the seromuscular strength of the tenia to create a backing for the submucosal tunnel needed for the anti-reflux procedure.

❑❑ **Briefly describe the Bricker uretero-intestinal anastomosis.**

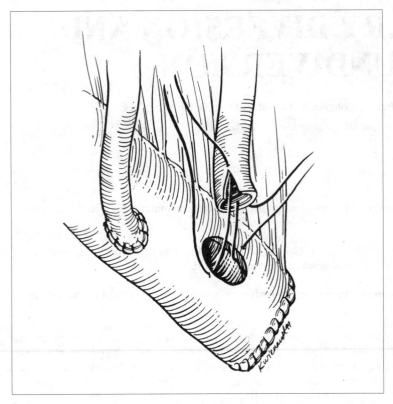

Fig.1

The Bricker anastomosis is a refluxing end-to-side anastomosis. It involves spatulating the distal end of the ureter, and stitching the full thickness of the bowel to the full thickness of the ureter. This anastomosis boasts both technical ease as well as a low complication rate. (Fig. 1)

❑❑ **Briefly describe the Wallace uretero-intestinal anastomosis.**

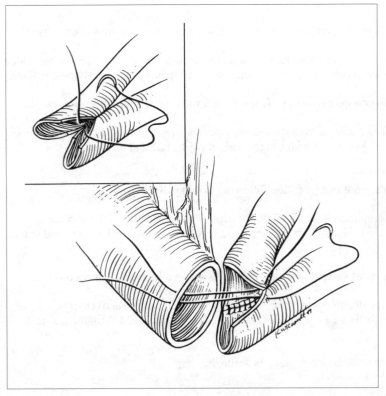

Fig.2

The Wallace anastomosis is a refluxing end-to-end anastomosis. Different techniques are described, but the concept is that the ureteral ends are spatulated and sewn together into a common opening. This "common ureter" is then anastomosed to the end of the intestinal segment used. It has a lower stricture rate due to the wide anastomosis, but is not recommended for patients with extensive carcinoma-in-situ or a high likelihood of recurrence in the ureter. Recurrence in the distal aspect of one ureter could block the egress of both ureters, causing bilateral obstruction. (Fig. 2)

❏❏ **What is the generally accepted cut-off value of serum creatinine at which continent diversions and orthotopic neobladders are no longer considered?**

2.0 mg/dl. Due to the extended dwell time of urine in contact with the intestinal segments used, continent diversions and orthotopic neobladders should be considered only for those patients with good renal function.

❏❏ **What long-term effects can urinary intestinal diversion have on the bony skeleton?**

Osteomalacia. Osteomalacia (or renal rickets) has been reported most commonly with ureterosigmoidostomy, but also with colon and ileal conduits, and ileal ureters. It is thought to be secondary to acidosis, vitamin D resistance, and excessive calcium loss by the kidney.

❏❏ **T/F: Approximately 75% of urine specimens from ileal conduits are infected.**

True. Intestine, in contrast to urothelium, generally lives symbiotically with bacterial flora. Most patients have no sequelae from their chronic bacteriuria, and are not treated unless they develop symptoms.

❏❏ **What is the urinary diversion procedure that puts the patient at the highest risk for development of carcinoma of the intestinal segment?**

Ureterosigmoidostomy. Following ureterosigmoidostomy, as many as 40% of patients will develop tumors at the ureterosigmoid anastamosis given sufficient time. About half of the tumors are adenocarcinoma and the rest are benign polyps. The mean latency period between ureterosigmoidostomy and the diagnosis of tumor is 26 years.

❏❏ **If performing undiversion following ureterosigmoidostomy, what must be done to minimize the risk of tumorigenesis?**

The distal ureteral stumps must be removed from contact with the colonic epithelium. Adenocarcinoma has been reported to occur when the ureterointestinal anastomoses were left in situ, even when the diversion is defunctionalized.

❏❏ **Briefly describe the Mitrofanoff procedure.**

The Mitrofanoff procedure is the creation of a continent, catheterizable urinary diversion. It is usually performed with the appendix, which is anastomosed to the conduit (or bladder) in a tunneled fashion (similar to a ureteroneocystostomy). The other end of the appendix is brought out to the anterior abdominal wall, and is utilized for clean intermittent catheterization.

❏❏ **In patients who have received extensive pelvic radiation, which intestinal segment is preferred for creation of a conduit?**

The transverse colon. Given its position within the abdominal cavity, it is the most likely to have remained unaffected by previous pelvic radiation.

❏❏ **What is the blood supply of the appendix?**

The appendiceal artery, a branch usually off of the ileocolic artery, which arises from the superior mesenteric artery.

❏❏ **What is the source of continence for orthotopic neobladders?**

In both the male and female, the preserved striated external sphincter is the source of continence. Daytime continence rates of greater than 95% can be expected if this mechanism is surgically spared.

❑❑ What are the two phenomena thought to be responsible for nocturnal enuresis following orthotopic neobladder procedures?

First, the spinal reflex arc that recruits external sphincter contraction is gone, as the native bladder (and therefore the afferent nerves) has been removed. The other hypothesis is that there is a significant re-absorption and re-circulation of urinary constituents and metabolites that stimulate increased urinary volume, resulting in nocturnal enuresis.

❑❑ Briefly describe the ureterointestinal anastomosis described by Studer and colleagues.

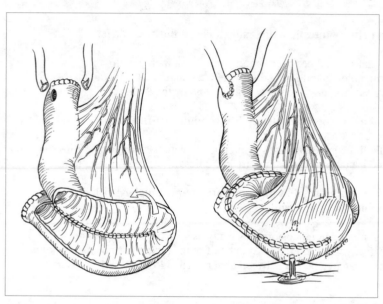

Fig.3

The Studer ileal neobladder incorporates a novel approach to prevent reflux. The proximal limb of small bowel is left intact for a length of 20-25 cm., and the neobladder is constructed from the distal 35-40 cm. of ileum. The ureters are then anastomosed to the intact proximal limb in a standard (Bricker) ureterointestinal refluxing anastomosis. This proximal limb of ileum retains its peristaltic integrity, effectively dampening back-pressure on the upper urinary tract. (Fig. 3)

❑❑ What tumor location in women is a contraindication to orthotopic neobladder formation after radical cystectomy?

Bladder neck involvement. Patients with bladder neck involvement often have involvement of the anterior vaginal wall, and orthotopic neobladder formation could compromise the margins of resection.

❑❑ What tumor location in men is a contraindication to orthotopic neobladder formation after radical cystectomy?

The prostatic urethral stroma. It is recommended that all men being considered for an orthotopic neobladder undergo formal transurethral resection of the prostatic urethra, and are candidates only if the prostatic stroma is free of disease.

❑❑ What are the four basic methods of achieving continence in a urinary diversion?

The Mitrofanoff principle, the ileocecal valve, the nipple valve, and the hydraulic valve.

❑❑ What is the continence mechanism in an Indiana pouch?

The buttressed ileocecal valve. Neourethral pressure profiles show that the continence zone is confined only to the area of the ileocecal valve, rendering imbricating sutures necessary only for this area.

□□ Describe the Benchekroun hydraulic ileal valve.

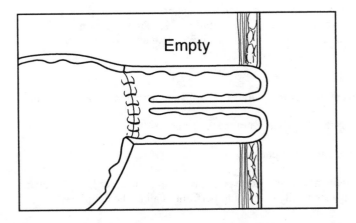

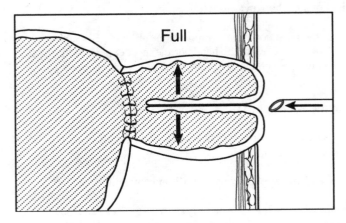

Fig.4

12-14 cm. of ileum is selected, and reverse intussusception is performed, such that serosa covers the entire segment and mucosa apposes mucosa. The ends are then sutured in position, allowing space between sutures to allow the mucosal surface to fill with urine as pouch pressures increase. The blunt serosal end is secured to the abdominal wall, and catheterization is done so that the catheter passes through a serosally lined channel into the conduit. When pressures rise in the conduit, urine flows into the mucosal space of the valve, coapting the serosal surface, ensuring continence. (Fig. 4)

□□ What is the most common complication of the Benchekroun hydraulic ileal valve?

Stomal stenosis. Stomal stenosis requiring surgical revision has been reported in up to 73% of patients undergoing this procedure. Devagination of the valve is another complication, with a reported incidence of up to 36%.

□□ What is the "pipe stem" deformity of the ileal conduit, and what is the cause?

The "pipe stem" deformity of an ileal conduit is the radiographic appearance on loopogram of strictured areas along the course of the loop. This results in a thin, non-compliant loop with decreased peristalsis and propulsion of urine with subsequent deterioration of the upper urinary tracts. The cause is vascular insufficiency. Treatment usually requires replacement of the entire loop.

□□ What is the incidence of stones in patients with ileal conduits?

Approximately 20%. The etiology of stone formation is multifactorial. Staples and non-absorbable sutures may act as a nidus for stone formation. There is an increased incidence of bacteruria following intestinal diversion, which may also cause stone formation.

❏❏ T/F: Patients with continent diversions are at increased risk of reservoir stones.

True. This is secondary to the increased urinary excretion of calcium, magnesium and phosphate in continent diversions as compared to ileal conduits. Also, patients with long segments of ileum used for reconstruction (continent diversions and orthotopic neobladders) may have secondary hyperoxaluria.

❏❏ What is "pouchitis"?

Pouchitis is a condition described in continent urinary diversions that is manifested by pain in the region of the pouch and increased pouch contractility. This may result in temporary failure of the continence mechanism. Antibiotic treatment usually results in resolution of these symptoms.

❏❏ What is the continence mechanism of the Kock pouch?

The surgical principle used in achieving continence by the Kock pouch is the intussuscepted nipple valve. This surgical procedure is felt to be the most technically difficult to perform of all of the continence mechanisms.

❏❏ What are the most common complications of the Kock pouch?

Nipple failure resulting in loss of continence is the most common complication following Kock pouch formation. This can be expected in 10 to 15% of cases even in the hands of the most experienced surgeon. Another complication of the Kock pouch that is unique is the higher incidence of stones, secondary to the use of staples on the intussuscepted nipple valve.

❏❏ What is the continence mechanism of the Penn pouch?

The Mitrofanoff principle. The Penn pouch was the first conduit to utilize the Mitrofanoff principle, using the appendix tunneled into the tenia of the ascending colon.

❏❏ What is a potential drawback to the use of the appendix as a continence mechanism?

The appendix has a small luminal diameter, allowing catheterization only with a 12 or 14 Fr catheter. Since intestinal reservoirs produce large amounts of mucus, this often makes irrigation and emptying difficult. Also, the appendix may be surgically absent or of insufficient length for use.

❏❏ What are the contraindications to ureterosigmoidostomy?

Hydronephrosis, pelvic radiation, neurogenic bladder, renal or hepatic dysfunction. Dilated upper tracts are more subject to reflux and obstruction, which can be deleterious to renal function. Previous pelvic radiation will likely involve both the sigmoid and the pelvic ureters. Patients with neurogenic bladder usually have associated functional bowel abnormalities as well. Renal insufficiency is a contraindication to any continent diversion. Patients with hepatic dysfunction should not undergo ureterosigmoidostomy because of the risk of ammonia intoxication.

❏❏ What is essential in the pre-operative evaluation of patients selected for rectal bladder urinary diversion or ureterosigmoidostomy?

Anal sphincter integrity testing. Patients should be required to retain an enema solution of liquid and solid material in an upright and ambulatory position without soilage for a specified amount of time.

❏❏ T/F: Renal insufficiency is a contraindication to urinary undiversion.

False. Many candidates for undiversion will likely have renal insufficiency, either secondary to their underlying pathology or the diversion itself. If transplantation becomes necessary in these patients, it is better done into a functioning lower urinary tract than a urinary diversion.

❏❏ With what intestinal segment is the "hematuria-dysuria" syndrome associated?

Stomach. Following gastrocystoplasty, the urine is markedly acidic, which can lead to bladder pain, dysuria, and hematuria in approximately 30% of patients.

❏❏ **What is the gastrointestinal consequence of the loss of the ileocecal valve?**

In the short-term, this results in frequent bowel movements and diarrhea. Most patients recover bowel regularity following intestinal adaptation or pharmacologic therapy, but some patients have steatorrhea or diarrhea refractory to medical management following loss of the ileocecal valve.

❏❏ **T/F: Refluxing ureterointestinal anastomoses have a higher incidence of renal deterioration than non-refluxing anastomoses following conduit formation in patients with normal ureters.**

False. In patients with normal peristaltic contractions of the ureter, there does not seem to be detrimental pressure transmission to the renal pelvis in patients with refluxing anastomoses. Additionally, the presence of non-refluxing anastomoses does not prevent bacterial colonization of the renal pelvis.

❏❏ **What are the contraindications to ileal conduit formation?**

The contraindications to ileal conduits are short bowel syndrome, inflammatory disease of the small intestine, and previous radiation to the pelvis.

❏❏ **What is the most common composition of stones formed in urinary diversions?**

The stones are usually of mixed composition, and may be made up of struvite, calcium oxalate, calcium phosphate, and uric acid. Foreign materials may act as a nidus for stone formation within the diversion.

MALE INFERTILITY

Mark R. Licht, M.D.

☐☐ **The pituitary hormones FSH and LH act on which cells in the testicle and what are the mediators of feedback inhibition from these cells to the pituitary gland?**

FSH acts on the Sertoli cell and inhibin is the mediator of feedback inhibition, while LH acts on the Leydig cell and testosterone is the mediator.

☐☐ **Which cells in the testicle create the blood-testis barrier excluding sperm from recognition by which body system?**

Tight junctional complexes between adjacent Sertoli cells create the blood-testis barrier making the seminiferous tubule an immunologically privileged site.

☐☐ **A germ cell undergoes how many meiotic divisions before producing a mature sperm?**

Germ cells undergo multiple mitotic divisions to produce many primary spermatocytes which then undergo 2 meiotic divisions to first produce secondary spermatocytes and then spermatids.

☐☐ **Aside from sperm transportation, what is the most important function of the epididymis?**

Sperm maturation occurs along the length of the epididymis resulting in sperm which are capable of fertilizing eggs.

☐☐ **Prostate specific antigen (PSA) plays what role in male fertility?**

The protein secreted by prostate epithelium serves as a protease enzyme involved in semen liquefaction.

☐☐ **Which substance produced in the seminal vesicle is the major energy source for sperm metabolism?**

Fructose.

☐☐ **What is the role of the acrosome and where is it located?**

The acrosome forms a cap on the sperm head and contains the enzymes necessary for drilling into the zona pellucida of the egg.

☐☐ **Do the testicle, epididymis, and vas deferens share the same embryological origin?**

No. The testicle develops from coelomic epithelium of the genital ridge and underlying mesenchyme. Primordial germ cells migrate to this area. The epididymis and vas deferens, however, develop from the Wolffian (mesonephric) duct.

☐☐ **A patient develops retrograde ejaculation after RPLND for testis cancer. Which nerves were likely injured and which class of medications may be used to treat the problem?**

Thoracolumbar sympathetic nerves control closure of the bladder neck during seminal emission via norepinephrine. Alpha-adrenergic agonist drugs have been used to stimulate closure of the bladder neck.

☐☐ **A patient presents with azoospermia, low ejaculatory volume and a semen pH of 5. Post-ejaculation urine is negative for sperm. What is the next test that should be performed and what is the most likely diagnosis?**

Transrectal ultrasound of the prostate should be performed to rule out ejaculatory duct obstruction.

❐❐ **Men with non-obstructive azoospermia can have DNA microdeletions in which genes on which chromosome?**

The AZF (AZoospermia Factor) genes present on the Y chromosome.

❐❐ **Men with congenital absence of the vas deferens (CAVD) can have mutations in which gene?**

The cystic fibrosis gene on chromosome 7.

❐❐ **A patient is found to have unilateral congenital absence of the vas deferens. The presence of which organ needs to be confirmed?**

The ipsolateral kidney may be absent due to lack of development of the mesonephric duct.

❐❐ **A patient with primary infertility is found to have a normal sperm count, but zero motility. Viability staining shows that the sperm are alive. Semen culture and antisperm antibody testing is negative. Which syndrome must be suspected?**

Immotile cilia syndrome. If the patient also has chronic sinusitis, bronchiectasis, and situs inversus then he has Kartagener's syndrome.

❐❐ **A patient with Klinefelter's syndrome has a small number of sperm in his ejaculate. What would his karyotype most likely reveal?**

46, XY/ 47, XXY mosaic.

❐❐ **What is the normal adult testicular size?**

It is 20 cc or greater in volume and at least 4 cm in length.

❐❐ **A patient is undergoing a vasectomy reversal. Fluid expressed from the proximal end of the vas is thick and pasty and no sperm are seen on microscopy. What is the next step the surgeon should undertake?**

Explore the epididymis to rule out an epididymal obstruction.

❐❐ **An azoospermic patient with unilateral congenital absence of the vas and anormal testicle has an atrophic opposite testis with a normal vas deferens. What surgical procedure may restore sperm to the ejaculate?**

A crossover vasoepididymostomy.

❐❐ **A patient seen for infertility complains of a new onset right varicocele. What pathological entity should be suspected?**

An imaging study should be performed to rule out a right-sided retroperitoneal mass.

❐❐ **In performing a sub-inguinal varicocelectomy, the testicular artery is inadvertently ligated and divided. By what blood supply might the testicle still survive?**

The deferential artery and the cremasteric artery also supply blood flow to the testicle.

❐❐ **An azoospermic patient who previously underwent surgery for a pituitary tumor is found to have undetectable levels of FSH and LH. What form of therapy may restore spermatogenesis?**

Treatment with intramuscular HCG and HMG can replace absent FSH and LH and turn on sperm production in the testicle.

❐❐ **What morphologic semen characteristics comprise the stress pattern often seen in patients with a varicocele?**

Increased numbers of sperm with tapered heads, immature germ cells, and amorphous sperm cells.

❐❐ **The laboratory reports an increased number of round cells on semen analysis. What can these cells represent?**

Round cells are either prematurely released immature germ cells or white blood cells representing inflammation or infection. Immunohistochemical staining and the Endtz test can distinguish between the two.

❐❐ **A patient with azoospermia is found on transrectal ultrasound of the prostate to have a midline cystic structure causing dilation of the ejaculatory ducts and seminal vesicles. What is the origin of this structure and what procedure may restore sperm in the ejaculate?**

The cyst is likely a Mullerian duct remnant and transurethral resection of the ejaculatory ducts (TURED) may unroof the obstructing cyst and allow sperm to be present in the semen.

❐❐ **A patient with azoospermia has extremely small testicular size (6 cc volume) and an FSH of 26. The most likely diagnosis is?**

Primary testicular failure or hypergonadotropic hypogonadism.

❐❐ **A patient with neuropathy secondary to diabetes mellitus develops anejaculation. If he fails alpha sympathomimetic oral therapy, the next treatment option to obtain sperm would be?**

Either microsurgical vasal or epididymal sperm aspiration to obtain sperm for use with IVF.

❐❐ **What percentage of patients undergoing varicocelectomy for infertility can expect to have improvement in semen parameters and which parameters are most often improved?**

Approximately 70% of patients will have improvement in semen parameters after varicocelectomy. Motility is most often improved followed by count and then morphology.

❐❐ **A patient with a history of unilateral testicular torsion presents with primary infertility. A semen analysis reveals a normal volume and count, but significantly low motility as well as sperm agglutination. There is no evidence of infection. What condition should be tested for and by which means?**

In a patient with torsion, cryptorchidism, infection, obstruction or trauma and the above noted semen parameters antisperm antibodies should be suspected. The direct immunobead assay is used to test for antisperm antibodies.

❐❐ **A patient presents with primary infertility. On exam he has normal male secondary sex characteristics and slightly decreased testicular size. Semen analysis reveals normal volume and pH, but azoospermia. FSH is slightly elevated, LH and testosterone are normal. What is the most likely histologic finding on testis biopsy?**

Germ cell aplasia or Sertoli-only syndrome in which the seminiferous tubules are lined by Sertoli cells and no germ cells are present.

❐❐ **A patient with azoospermia and bilateral varicoceles underwent a testicular biopsy that revealed late maturation arrest. What treatment option may result in the appearance of sperm in the ejaculate?**

Bilateral varicocelectomy has been reported to reverse late maturation arrest in some cases resulting in completion of spermatogenesis.

❐❐ **A couple presents with primary infertility. The male partner has normal semen parameters. The female partner's evaluation is also negative. A post-coital test on 2 occasions, however, reveals** no sperm in the cervical mucus. What assisted reproductive procedure may increase this couple's chance of conceiving?

Intrauterine insemination (IUI) is a useful form of treatment for bypassing cervical female factor infertility.

❏❏ **A patient with primary infertility and oligoasthenoteratospermia has low-normal levels of FSH, LH and testosterone. What form of empirical medical therapy may help improve his semen parameters?**

Clomiphene citrate (Clomid) has been used in these cases. While most patients will experience an increase in FSH, LH and testosterone, only a small subset of patients will obtain an improvement in semen parameters.

❏❏ **A patient with azoospermia is found to have very low levels of FSH, LH and testosterone. He also reports anosmia. What is the diagnosis?**

This patient with hypogonadotropic hypogonadism has Kallmann's syndrome.

❏❏ **A patient with primary infertility reports having had the mumps at age 6. Is this a clinically significant factor in his infertility?**

No. Prepubertal mumps does not appear to affect the testicle while postpubertal mumps orchitis can result in significant testicular damage and atrophy.

❏❏ **A body builder who abuses anabolic steroids presents with azoospermia. What is the mechanism for this failure of sperm production and is it reversible?**

Exogenous androgenic steroids suppress gonadotropin secretion and interfere with spermatogenesis. This form of hypogonadism is usually reversible after discontinuation of steroid use, but in some cases it is permanent.

❏❏ **A paraplegic with a cervical spinal cord injury has anejaculation. What is the preferred treatment option for sperm acquisition?**

Vibratory stimulation applied to the frenulum of the penis can result in antegrade ejaculation via the ejaculation reflex arc. If this fails, electroejaculation or microsurgical vasal or epididymal sperm aspiration can be used to obtain sperm.

❏❏ **A patient who has undergone a vasectomy wishes to have a reversal. On examination he has bilateral sperm granulomas and the sites of the vasectomy are high in the straight segments of the scrotal vas deferens. Are these findings more indicative of the need for vasovasostomy or vasoepididymostomy at the time of surgical exploration?**

Vasovasostomy. Sperm granuloma and longer vasal length proximal to the site of obstruction are associated with a lower incidence of secondary epididymal obstruction.

❏❏ **What are considered to be the normal values for count, motility and morphology on a semen analysis?**

A count of greater than 50 million, motility of greater or equal to 50%, and 50% or more normal forms by WHO criteria define baseline criteria for fertility.

❏❏ **A patient with primary infertility is found to have severe oligospermia with only 100 motile sperm in his ejaculation on repeat evaluations. Evaluation reveals no correctable or treatable conditions and empirical medical therapy fails to improve his count. What option is available for this patient to conceive his own biological child?**

Small numbers of sperm can be used to fertilize ova in an IVF cycle employing intracytoplasmic sperm injection (ICSI) where individual sperm are directly injected into an individual ovum.

❏❏ **A couple has one 4-year-old child and are now having difficulty conceiving again. The male partner has oligoasthenospermia and normal hormonal testing. What abnormality can be expected on physical exam?**

A varicocele is found in as many as 80% of men with secondary infertility. A varicocele has been shown to cause progressive worsening of semen parameters.

❏❏ **A patient is found to have a normal count and zero motility. Which 2 lab tests can help distinguish between immotile sperm and dead ones?**

The hypo-osmotic swelling test and viability staining can be used. Living sperm experience bulging of the plasma membrane and curling of the tails from fluid absorption under hypo-osmotic conditions. Both tests reflect the integrity of the plasma membrane in living versus dead sperm.

❏❏ **What percentage of couples are infertile and how often is a male factor present?**

15% of couples are infertile and in 50% of the cases, a male factor is present.

❏❏ **What percentage of men with unilateral and bilateral cryptorchidism will have oligospermia on semen analysis?**

30% of men with unilateral and 50% of men with bilateral cryptorchidism will have oligospermia on semen analysis.

❏❏ **A tall, thin patient presents for infertility evaluation. He is found to have gynecomastia. What will his testicular exam reveal? What will his semen analysis show? What is the underlying cause for his condition?**

This patient with Klinefelter's syndrome will have small, firm testes and azoospermia on semen analysis. His karyotype of 47 XXY results from non-dysjunction of the meiotic chromosomes of the gametes of either parent.

❏❏ **What commonly inhaled illegal substance is associated with infertility and by what mechanism?**

Marijuana can lead to a decrease in sperm concentration and motility and abnormal morphology as well as decreased serum testosterone levels and gynecomastia. The drug alters the hypothalamic-pituitarygonadal axis.

❏❏ **A patient receives 4 courses of cisplatin-based chemotherapy for testicular cancer. Immediately after treatment he is azoospermic. What are the chances that spermatogenesis will return and how long can it take?**

This patient has an 80% chance of complete return of baseline sperm production. It may take up to one year after treatment for sperm production to begin and several years to reach steady-state levels.

❏❏ **How long does the process of spermatogenesis take? How long does it take for a sperm to appear in the ejaculation?**

It takes 74 days for a mature sperm to develop from a primitive germ cell, or spermatogonia. Including ductal transit time, the time from spermatogenesis to ejaculation is approximately 3-months.

❏❏ **A 13-year-old boy is found to a have a grade 2 left sided varicocele on a school sports physical exam. His testicles are of equal, normal size and consistency. GNRH stimulation test reveals a normal LH and FSH response. Would you recommend elective varicocelectomy at this time?**

15% of all males have a varicocele and only a small percentage of these men will have difficulties with fertility. With no evidence of decreased testicular volume and no exaggerated FSH release in response to GNRH, elective surgery would not be indicated at this time.

❑❑ **A patient with primary infertility is found to have increased numbers of WBC's in the semen. What are the possible causes? What needs to be tested for? Can seminal WBC's have an adverse affect on sperm function?**

Pyospermia may be due to either genital tract infection or an inflammatory immunologic response. Cultures to rule out urinary and genital tract infection should be performed. The etiology is sometimes never uncovered and pyospermia can resolve without specific treatment. Seminal WBC's can produce reactive oxygen species (ROS) which adversely affect sperm function.

❑❑ **How does testicular radiation exposure lead to infertility? How long after radiation therapy can it take for spermatogenesis to return? How long should a patient wait before trying to conceive after gonadal exposure to radiation?**

Ionizing radiation is lethal to sperm by increasing free radical formation. It also alters sperm head morphology and damages sperm chromatin structure. It can take up to 5 years for spermatogenesis to return. Direct effects on DNA can result in numerical and structural chromosomal abnormalities, therefore, conception should be avoided for 2 years.

SEXUAL FUNCTION AND DYSFUNCTION

Mark R. Licht, M.D.

❏❏ **According to the Massachusetts Male Aging Study, what percentage of men age 60 complained of complete or moderate erectile dysfunction (ED)?**

40%

❏❏ **What is Buck's fascia and what structures does it surround?**

It is the deep layer of the penile fascia that covers both the corpora cavernosa and corpus spongiosum in separate fascial compartments. The dorsal artery, deep dorsal vein, and dorsal nerve lie beneath Buck's fascia.

❏❏ **A patient experiences cylinder autoinflation of his three-piece inflatable penile prosthesis. What is the cause and how can this be prevented?**

Autoinflation occurs when pressure around the reservoir is high enough to force fluid back through the pump into the cylinders at a time when inflation is not desired. This is due to either insufficient space created for the reservoir at implantation or formation of a tight capsule due to device inflation during early healing. Active deflation of the device may increase the reservoir volume or else surgical exploration and incision of the capsule is necessary.

❏❏ **Are the two corpora cavernosa completely separate structures?**

No. The intercavernous septum is incomplete distally. Openings provide communication between the corpora. Hence, intracavernosal pharmacological injection to treat ED need only be injected into one corpora.

❏❏ **The arterial supply to the penis arises from which blood vessel?**

The internal pudendal artery branches after passing through Alcock's canal. The penile artery then divides into the dorsal artery of the penis, the deep cavernous artery and the bulbourethral artery.

❏❏ **Which part of the autonomic nervous system provides excitatory input to the penis?**

The parasympathetic nervous system with its preganglionic neurons originating in sacral spinal cord segments S 2 - 4.

❏❏ **What is penile prosthesis SST deformity and how is it corrected?**

Downward bowing of the glans after penile prosthesis implantation is called the SST deformity named after the airplane's nose. It is the result of either distal corporal underdilation or cylinder undersizing at the time of implantation or post-operative anatomical changes, which have left the glans unsupported. Surgical correction includes redilating the corpora and resizing the device. Occasionally, glans fixation is required to add stability.

❏❏ **What structures comprise the penile corporal veno-occlusive mechanism?**

The tunica albuginea compresses the exiting emissary veins and subtunical venules as the penis engorges with blood. This venoocclusion limits blood flow out of the penis and allows for rigidity.

◻◻ **What is the most common organism identified as the cause of periprosthetic infection? Which patients are at higher risk for infection?**

Staphylococcus epidermidis is the organism most often cultured from infected prostheses. Patients with poorly controlled diabetes, immunocompromised patients and spinal cord injury patients are at higher risk for infection. Increased risk of infection is also associated with subsequent implant operations and surgical revisions.

◻◻ **What is the anatomical relationship of the cavernous nerves which innervate the penis to the prostate?**

The cavernous nerves which are branches of the pelvic plexus travel posterolateral to the apex of the prostate at the 5 o'clock and 7 o'clock positions.

◻◻ **What is the role of cavernosography in the evaluation of erectile dysfunction?**

In a patient in whom venous leak is clinically suspected and then documented by dynamic infusion cavernosometry, contrast injection into the corpora demonstrates the sites of abnormal leaking veins for surgical repair.

◻◻ **A patient with sickle-cell anemia presents to the ER with a 4-hour history of painful priaprism. What is the underlying mechanism? What is the initial form of management?**

Sludging of sickled red blood cells in the corpora leads to prolonged erection. Initial conservative management with hydration, alkalinization, analgesia and transfusion is often successful. If not, then corporal aspiration and injection of an alpha adrenergic agent should be employed.

◻◻ **What is the principle neurotransmitter responsible for parasympathetic-mediated penile smooth muscle relaxation?**

Nitric oxide.

◻◻ **During dynamic infusion cavernosometry, the flow rate of saline required to maintain a normal intracavernosal pressure is 20 ml/min. What is this representative of?**

Venous leak. A maintenance flow rate of 6 ml/min or less represents normal veno-occlusive function if maximal smooth muscle relaxation has been achieved.

◻◻ **A 35-year-old male with ED due to a pelvic fracture and a 65-year-old male with ED secondary to long-standing hypercholesterolemia and hypertension undergo pelvic angiography. What are the expected findings?**

The younger man would likely have a focal stenosis of the penile or cavernosal artery, while the older man would most likely have diffuse stenotic plaques.

◻◻ **A patient is seen for a complaint of decreased libido and ED. Physical examination is normal. What is an appropriate initial endocrine evaluation?**

A morning free and total testosterone level is a good initial screening test. If abnormal, it should be repeated along with prolactin, LH, and FSH levels.

◻◻ **If a patient has documented primary hypogonadism with normal serum prolactin levels, what options exist for testosterone supplementation?**

Currently, testosterone can be safely administered by either depot IM injection or by transdermal patch. Oral testosterone is also available in a form which bypasses the liver and the first pass effect. A topical gel is nearing FDA approval.

◻◻ **What class of antihypertensive medication is most often associated with ED?**

Beta blockers.

❑❑ What group of antidepressant medications has been used successfully to treat premature ejaculation? What is the mechanism of action?

The selective serotonin re-uptake inhibitors have been used to treat premature ejaculation as they have been found to prolong the latency phase of the ejaculatory reflex.

❑❑ A patient with idiopathic low-flow priapism fails to respond to repeated corporal aspiration, irrigation and injection of an alpha adrenergic agonist. What is the next appropriate form of treatment?

Patients who fail conservative therapy need surgical intervention to allow for penile detumescence and attempt to save potency. First a distal cavernosal-spongiosum shunt (El Ghorab) should be attempted. If not successful, a proximal shunt created by anastamosing the spongiosum of the urethra to the corpus cavernosum (Quackles) should be tried.

❑❑ What role does penile Doppler ultrasound play in the diagnosis of ED?

Measurement of the peak systolic velocity (PSV) and end diastolic velocity (EDV) in the cavernosal arteries after smooth muscle relaxation brought about by the administration of a vasodilating agent serves as a screening tool for vasculogenic ED. A PSV less than 35 cm/sec is indicative of arterial disease while a EDV greater than 5 cm/sec predicts patients who may have venous leak.

❑❑ Which areas in the brain control erection and ejaculation?

The medial preoptic area and the paraventricular nucleus of the hypothalamus has been identified as the supraspinal center for erection and ejaculation.

❑❑ Which drugs are most commonly used alone or in combination for intracavernosal pharmacological injection therapy?

The vasodilating agents prostaglandin El, phentolamine and papavarine.

❑❑ What is the neuronal mediator of penile detumescence?

Contraction of the cavernous smooth muscle in response to sympathetic nervous input leads to penile detumescence.

❑❑ Which artery is most commonly used to bypass obstruction in a penile artery during revascularization surgery?

The inferior epigastric artery is the most commonly used source of new arterial inflow.

❑❑ What surgical treatment options exist for a patient with symptomatic Peyronie's disease?

Patients with a stable plaque and difficulty or inability to penetrate due to penile angulation are surgical candidates. Surgical options include plaque incision / excision with grafting, penile placation procedure, or implant of a penile prosthesis.

❑❑ A patient reports priapism after blunt perineal trauma. What is the likely mechanism? How is this best managed?

This patient most likely has high-flow priapism caused by a cavernosal artery to cavernosal tissue fistula. This can be diagnosed by penile color Doppler ultrasound. As high-flow priapism does not represent an emergency conservative management with either observation or compression can be attempted. Definitive therapy, however, often requires cavernosal arterial embolization or ligation. Impotence is a possibility after this form of therapy.

❑❑ **During distal dilation of the corpora for placement of an inflatable penile prosthesis, a tear is made in the urethra with the dilator at the level of the urethral meatus. What is the best form of management?**

A cylinder should not be placed in the corpora on the side of the injury. No direct attempt should be made to close the urethral tear. After it has healed over a catheter, a cylinder can be placed on that side 4-6 weeks later.

❑❑ **A patient with a 3-piece inflatable penile prosthesis is explored for suspected periprosthetic infection. At surgery, gross pus is found around the cylinders. What is the best form of management?**

All components of the device should be removed and drains should be placed in all of the component sites. The wound can be closed primarily. Postoperatively, the drains should be irrigated with antibiotic solution for 3-5 days and are then removed. Prosthesis reimplantation can be attempted in 4 to 6 months.

❑❑ **Which patients are candidates for penile venous ligation surgery? How successful is this surgery?**

Patients with a history of ED and documented venous leak by pharmacological cavernosometry and cavernosography and no evidence of arterial insufficiency are candidates for venous ligation surgery. The short-term surgical success rate is approximately 60%.

❑❑ **What is nocturnal penile tumescence (NPT)? When does it occur? How is the rigidity of these erections measured?**

NPT is the normal cycle of night-time erections which occur in healthy males of all ages. These erections occur during REM sleep. Rigidity can be measured either by a technician with axial buckling pressure in a sleep laboratory or by radial compression from the loops of a home monitor device.

❑❑ **What are some of the causes of false positive and false negative NPT results?**

False positive NPT results are defined as normal testing but true underlying organic ED. This is seen with neurogenic ED (i.e. MS) and with pelvic steal syndrome (penile blood shunted to the gluteus muscles with pelvic thrusting). False negative results are defined as inadequate NPT, but no organic ED. This is seen in elderly patients, patients with major depression and sleep disorders as well as those with anxiety (first night effect). Also certain medications can alter the sleep cycle and NPT. Nocturnal erections are testosterone dependent so patients with hypogonadism may not have NPT, but may have normal erotic erections.

❑❑ **What is the mechanism of action of Sildenafil citrate (Viagra)?**

It is a selective phosphodiesterase (PDE) 5 inhibitor. It inhibits the breakdown of nitric oxide-induced elevation in CGMP thereby potentiating smooth muscle relaxation in the penis.

❑❑ **What are the most common side effects of Viagra? In which groups of patients is the drug contraindicated?**

The most common side effects are headache, dyspepsia, and facial flushing. Rarely, patients experience a blue color tint to their vision. The drug is contraindicated in patients who are using nitrates and those with severe heart disease who should not engage in any exertional activity such as sexual intercourse.

❑❑ **What is the mechanism of action of Yohimbine and what side effects are associated with the drug? Does it have any proven utility in treating ED?**

Yohimbine is an alpha-2 adrenoreceptor antagonist with central and peripheral actions. Side effects include headache, anxiety, palpitations, nausea, and blood pressure elevation. No placebo-controlled study has shown a statistically significant advantage to Yohimbine in the treatment of ED.

❑❑ **What is MUSE? How is it administered? What are it's most significant side effects?**

MUSE is prostaglandin E1 in a semi-solid pellet form for intra-urethral injection. An applicator is placed into the distal urethra and the pellet is dislodged. The pellet then dissolves and is absorbed into the corpus spongiosum. Venous channels then transfer the drug to the corpus cavernosum. Hypotension and syncope have been reported in up to 4% of patients.

☐☐ **What are the possible risks of androgen supplementation in men with ED and low-normal testosterone levels?**

Testosterone supplementation can increase the symptoms of BPH, have a stimulatory effect on prostate cancer, increase LDL and decrease HDL cholesterol. Additionally, it can increase sodium retention, and increase hematocrit.

☐☐ **What are the reported side effects of intracavernosal injection therapy for ED?**

Bleeding, pain, and infection are minor side effects which can be obviated with instruction of good injection technique. Priapism and corporal fibrosis are more serious complications.

☐☐ **What are the reported side effects of vacuum erection device use?**

Pain is the most common side effect followed by penile bruising and numbness. The ejaculate is often trapped in the urethra by the constriction band and the base of the penis proximal to the band pivots during intercourse.

☐☐ **What conservative non-surgical options exist for the treatment of Peyronie's disease?**

Oral therapy using vitamin E and Potaba has been used extensively. Intra-lesional injection of the calcium channel blocker verapamil has been reported as has the use of low dose radiation to the plaque.

☐☐ **What is the pathophysiology of ED in diabetic patients?**

Neuropathy and vascular small vessel disease are commonly known factors. Diabetes is also associated with decreased levels of circulating testosterone as well as damage to endothelial and smooth muscle function in the penis.

☐☐ **Spinal cord injury patients can have either reflex erections from tactile stimulation or psychogenic erections. What cord level of injury separates the two groups?**

Patients with injuries above T10-12 often have reflex erections and rarely have psychogenic erections, while patients with a level of injury below T12 often experience psychogenic erections and do not get reflex erections.

☐☐ **What is the physical sequence of events of ejaculation? Which portion of the nervous system controls ejaculation?**

Ejaculation is entirely under sympathetic nervous control. First the bladder neck closes. Then the contents of the vasa and the prostate are expelled into the prostatic urethra. Subsequently, the contents of the seminal vesicles are expelled into the prostatic urethra followed by rhythmic contraction of the bulbospongiosus muscle, which propels the ejaculate out of the urethra.

☐☐ **Which commonly used drugs have been associated with impairment in ejaculation and orgasm?**

Alcohol, amitriptyline, haloperidol, prazosin, thiazides, and imipramine are all associated with impairment in ejaculation and orgasm.

☐☐ **What is the mechanism of hyperprolactinemic hypogonadism? How is it treated?**

Hyperprolactinemia leads to disruption of the normal pulsatile secretion of GNRH by the hypothalamus thereby leading to decreased LH and FSH secretion by the pituitary gland. Dopamine agonists such as bromocriptine are used to treat hyperprolactinemia.

❏❏ **A man hears a "pop" as his penis buckles during intercourse. This is followed by pain and swelling. What has occurred? How is it treated?**

The patient has sustained a penile fracture due to rupture of the tunica albuginea of the corpus cavernosum fallowed by blood extravasation and subcutaneous hematoma formation. If the tear and hematoma is small,the patient can be managed conservatively with ice and compresses. If, however, the tunical tear is large and there is a large or expanding hematoma surgical exploration and repair of the tunical tear is indicated.

❏❏ **A patient with clinical evidence of a penile fracture and a ventral hematoma also has gross hematuria. What concurrent injury should be suspected? How is it diagnosed and treated?**

This patient has sustained an injury to the corpus spongiosum as well as a cavernosal tear. He should have a retrograde urethrogram to diagnose the site and extent of the urethral inujury. Surgical exploration should follow and both the cavernosal and spongiosal injuries repaired. Conservative management for these injuries is not recommended as it risks a high incidence of urethral stricture formation.

❏❏ **After placement of a three-piece inflatable penile prosthesis a patinet has bloody urine. What has likely occurred? How is this complication best avoided?**

The patient has most likely sustained a bladder injury during reservoir placement. This type of injury is prevented by draining the bladder completely with a catheter prior to the retropubic dissection.

ADULT URINARY TRACT INFECTIONS

David M. Albala, M.D. and Uday Kumar, MS FRCS

❑❑ **How common are urinary tract infections in young women?**

UTIs occur in about 1% of schoolgirls (aged 5-14 years). This proportion rises to 4% by young adulthood.

❑❑ **Should patients with asymptomatic bacteriuria be treated?**

Pregnant women, children under 4 years of age, severe diabetics and patients with Proteus infections should be treated regardless of symptoms.

❑❑ **Which bacteria are urea-splitting?**

Majority are Proteus and Providentia species. Pseudomonas, Klebsiella, Staph. epidermidis, and mycoplasma are also capable of producing urease. E.coli is not a ureasplitting organism.

❑❑ **What is emphysematous pyelonephritis?**

It is a rare complication of pyelonephritis that can occur in diabetics. Non-resolving pyelonephritis despite therapy and the triad of fever, vomiting and flank pain should be investigated. Presence of intra-parenchymal gas on plain KUB or CT is diagnostic.

❑❑ **What is significant bacteriuria?**

The number of bacteria that exceeds the number usually caused by contamination. $\geq 10^2$ cfu / ml of a known pathogen in a patient with dysuria would be significant. Previously $\geq 10^2$ had been the cut off limit. However, 20-40% of women with symptomatic UTIs had colony counts between 10^4-10^5.

❑❑ **What are bacterial pili?**

Bacteria have surface structures called adhesins that aid their binding to mucosal surfaces. The most important adhesins are long filamentous appendages called pili or fimbriae.

❑❑ **What is phase variation?**

Changes in environmental growth conditions of bacteria can cause them to rapidly shift between piliated and nonpiliated phases.

❑❑ **What patient genetic factors affect susceptibility to UTIS?**

Variation in bacterial adherence to vaginal, urethral and buccal cell surfaces is genetically determined. Women with non-secretor blood group phenotypes are more prone to UTIS.

❑❑ **How common are E. coli infections?**

In the community setting, E. coll account for 85% of the UTIS. In the hospital setting, this proportion reduces to 50%.

❑❑ **What tests are used to localize UTI to the upper or lower tract?**

Fairley bladder washout and Stamey ureteral catheterisation tests.

⬜⬜ How accurate are clinical signs in localising UTI to the upper or lower tract?

<50%. Fever and loin pain with significant bacteriuria, traditionally taught to be diagnostic of pyelonephritis may occur with cystitis alone. Conversely, in patients with only bladder symptoms, upper tract is often involved.

⬜⬜ What is the recommended duration of therapy for uncomplicated UTIS?

In a patient with a structurally normal urinary tract, a single dose or 3 day course of antimicrobial treatment is adequate. Success rates are lower with single dose therapy compared to multi-day regimens. In men all UTIs should be presumed complicated and treated 7 days or more and an underlying cause sought.

⬜⬜ Is antibiotic prophylaxis necessary for TUPP?

No, if the pre-op urine shows no growth ($< 10^2$ cfu / ml) prophylaxis is not necessary. In patients with significant growth, urethral catheters, risk of endocarditis or whose bacterial status is unknown, prophylaxis is warranted. Risk of bacteremia is 50% if antimicrobials are not given when UTI is present.

⬜⬜ What antibiotics are suitable as prophylaxis for transrectal biopsy of the prostate?

Metronidazole with ampicillin or trimethoprim-sulphamethoxazole is often used. A fluoroquinolone is a suitable alternative.

⬜⬜ When are imaging studies needed in UTI?

Infections in males, febrile infections, failure to respond to appropriate therapy, bacterial persistence and suspected urinary obstruction warrants imaging studies.

⬜⬜ What are the common causes of unresolved bacteriuria during therapy?

A. Bacterial resistance to drug (resistance may develop during course of therapy)
B. Mixed bacterial growth with varying drug susceptibilities
C. Rapid reinfection with new organism
D. Renal insufficiency
E. Papillary necrosis
F. Staghorn calculus
G. Self-inflicted infections or deception taking medications
H. Urinary obstruction

⬜⬜ What is bacterial persistence?

Despite clearance of bacteriuria with appropriate antimicrobial treatment, the same organism can reappear in the urinary tract from a site within the urinary tract that was excluded from the high concentrations of the antimicrobial agent e.g. struvite stone.

⬜⬜ Which antibiotics are suitable for long-term low-dose prophylaxis?

Nitrofurantoin, TMP-SMX, TMP, Cephalexin. A low dose of the antibiotic is given, typically at bedtime for 6-12 months.

⬜⬜ Are there alternatives to long-term low-dose prophylaxis?

Intermittent self-start therapy or post-intercourse therapy may be used instead.

⬜⬜ What does urinary microscopy show in patients with acute pyelonephritis?

Numerous white cells and bacteria. VvBCs exhibit Brownian motion of cytoplasm (glitter cells). Granular and leucocyte casts. Bacteria may be seen in casts.

❏❏ **T/F: Nitrofurantoin and TMP-SMX are ineffective against Pseudomonas species.**

True. TMP alone or with SMX is effective against most uropathogens except enterococci and Pseudomonas sp. Nitrofurantoin is ineffective against Proteus and Pseudomonas sp.

❏❏ **Why does Infection with Proteus cause more concern than E. coli?**

Patients who have protracted infection with Proteus risk formation of struvite calculi due to the alkalinization caused by the urea-splitting bacteria. This leads to precipitation of Ca, Mg, NH4 and P04 salts. E. coli does not produce urease.

❏❏ **T/F: Prophylactic antibiotics should be given to catheterized patients to reduce risk of UTI.**

False. This does not reduce risk of infections. In fact, they give rise to infection with organisms resistant to several antibiotics.

❏❏ **What are the radiological features of xanthogranulomatous pyelonephritis?**

Usually unilateral. IVU shows renal calculi in 38-70%, non-ftinctioning kidney in 27 - 80%, renal mass in 62% and calyceal deformity in 46%. On CT scan, large renal mass with renal pelvis tightly surrounding a central calcification is seen.

❏❏ **What are the diagnostic features of malacoplakia on histology?**

Large histiocytes called von Hausemann cells and small basophilic calculospherules called Michaelis-Guttmann bodies which may be intra or extracytoplasmic.

❏❏ **Why should a hydatid cyst not be aspirated?**

The contents of a hydatid cyst are highly antigenic and may cause anaphylaxis if it ruptures and spills during aspiration.

❏❏ **What is the initiator of gram-negative septic shock?**

Endotoxin, a lipopolysaccharide component of bacterial cell wall activates the macrophages and humoral pathways in septic shock. Most of the toxicity of endotoxin is contributed by Lipid A, which is bound to the core oligosaccharide.

❏❏ **Why do post-menopausal women have UTIs more frequently?**

Lack of estrogen causes changes in vaginal pH and microflora including loss of lactobacilli and colonization with E.coli. In addition, some women may have residual urine after voiding.

❏❏ **When is screening for bacteriuria worthwhile?**

The first trimester of pregnancy. There appears to be little advantage in screening healthy women.

❏❏ **T/F: In women with bacteriuria, acute pyelonephritis occurs more commonly in pregnant women than in non-pregnant women.**

True. Non pregnant women with screening bacteriuria (SCBU) rarely develop pyelonephritis in contrast to 28% of pregnant women with SCBU.

❏❏ **Which antimicrobials are suitable for use in pregnancy?**

Penicillins (including ampicillin and synthetic penicillins) and cephalosporins are safe throughout pregnancy. Short-acting sulfonamides and nitrofurantoin may be used in the first two trimesters. The former can cause neonatal hyperbilirubinemia and the latter hemolytic anemia in newborn if used near term.

❏❏ **What is the incidence of bacteriuria in the elderly?**

Greater than 20% of women and >10% of men over 65 years have bacteriuria. The majority is asymptomatic.

❏❏ **What is the difference between bacterial persistence and unresolved bacteriuria?**

Unresolved bacteriuria implies that the urinary tract is not sterilized during therapy. Bacterial persistence means recurrence of infection with the same organism after initial clearance.

❏❏ **What is the significance of squamous cells in urine?**

Numerous squamous cells in the urine would indicate preputial, vaginal or urethral contamination.

❏❏ **Why is plasmid-mediated (R factor) resistance important?**

It is more common than selection of resistant clones. The resistance is transferable and produces multiple resistant strains making therapy difficult.

❏❏ **What problems do diabetics encounter with regard to urinary infections?**

Diabetic women appear to be more prone to UTIS. Diabetics often have glomerulopathy, with difficulty concentrating antimicrobials. They are also more prone to complications like papillary necrosis and emphysematous pyelonephritis.

❏❏ **What is the classic presentation of septic syndrome?**

Fever and chills followed by hypotension. But this occurs only in 30% of cases.

❏❏ **What is the earliest metabolic abnormality in septic syndrome?**

Metabolic alkalosis - as a consequence of hyperventilation. This occurs even before chills or fever.

❏❏ **What are the x-ray findings of malacoplakia?**

On IVU, enlarged kidneys with multiple filling defects (best appreciated on U/S or CT). On CT foci are less dense than parenchyma. Unifocal lesions are indistinguishable from other inflammatory lesions and neoplasia.

❏❏ **What is the added advantage in using low-dose TMP-SMX prophylaxis in renal transplant patients?**

In the immuno-suppressed patient, TMP-SMX not only prevents UTIS, but also provides protection against Pneumocystis carinii pneumonia, listeriosis and nocardiosis.

❏❏ **How do you treat candiduria in the renal transplant patient?**

As untreated candiduria can lead to formation of obstructing candidal fungal balls, they should be treated promptly with fluconazole or with low-dose amphotericin plus Rucytosine if it fails.

❏❏ **T/F: Steroids increase risk of UTI.**

True. The incidence of UTI increases about threefold in patients on steroid therapy.

❏❏ **Why are fluoroquinolones contraindicated in children and pregnant women?**

They have a potential to damage developing cartilage.

❏❏ **Why are trimethoprim and fluoroquinolones particularly suited for UTI prophylaxis?**

Both drugs are actively secreted in the vagina and bowel, thereby inhibiting growth of uropathogens at these sites.

❑❑ **What is the most reliable form of urine collection?**

Suprapubic aspiration is least prone to contamination.

❑❑ **What is the most common cause of recurrent UTI in women?**

Reinfection (new infection from bacteria outside the urinary tract) is the most common cause.

❑❑ **What is the basis for leucocyte esterase test?**

Leucocyte esterase is produced by neutrophils and catalyses the hydrolysis of an indoxyl carbonic acid ester to indoxyl. The latter oxidizes a diazonium salt on the dipstick to produce a color change.

❑❑ **How sensitive and specific is the nitrite dipstick test for bacteruria?**

Specificity is over 90% but sensitivity varies from 35-85%. The test is less reliable in detecting bacterial concentration $<10^5$. The most common cause of a false positive test is contamination.

❑❑ **Why is nitrofurantoin not suitable for treatment of pyelonephritis?**

Nitrofurantoin is rapidly excreted in the urine but does not achieve therapeutic levels in most body tissues including the kidney.

❑❑ **What constitutes significant bacteriuria in a catheterized patient?**

A count of $>10^2$ cfu/ml implies significant bacteriuria since these counts usually persist or increase in a catheterized patient within 48 hours.

❑❑ **What measures are useful in reducing catheter-associated UTIS?**

Use of closed-catheter drainage reduces catheter-associated UTIs from 90% at 4 days to 30-40%. Periodic instillation of a chemical e.g. hydrogen peroxide into the collecting bag may delay onset of infection.

❑❑ **How is Fournier's gangrene treated?**

Prompt treatment is critical, as the mortality is 20% or more. Intravenous hydration and antibiotics with adequate surgical debridement are mainstays of treatment. Hyperbaric oxygen has been useful in some cases. Orchiectomy is almost never needed.

❑❑ **Which antibiotics provide the best penetration into the prostate?**

Trimethoprim, Trimethoprim/sulfamethoxazole, fluoroquinolones all penetrate well into the prostate.

CYSTITIS, INTERSTITIAL, HEMORRHAGIC, RADIATION AND VIRAL

Eric S. Rovner, M.D. and Ricardo F. Sánchez-Ortiz, M.D.

❏❏ **How common is interstitial cystitis in the United States?**

Prevalence: 36.6 per 100,000 patients. Incidence: 2.6 per 100,000 women per year.

❏❏ **Are there racial/ethnic differences in the prevalence of interstitial cystitis (I.C.)?**

Yes. 94% of patients are Caucasian. There appears to be a slightly higher incidence in Jewish women.

❏❏ **What is the natural history of I.C.?**

Median presentation is at age 40. Spontaneous remission occurs in up to 50% of patients at a mean of 8 months following diagnosis. Patients may have complete and spontaneous relief from the symptoms, have a waxing and waning course, may be completely asymptomatic with intermittent "flares", or have a chronically progressive course of increasing symptoms over several years.

❏❏ **What is the exact etiology of I.C.?**

Unknown. The most common hypotheses include:

1. A pathogenic role of mast cells in the detrusor and/or mucosal layers of the bladder as a primary or secondary process.
2. A deficiency in the glycosaminoglycan layer (GAG) on the luminal surface of the bladder resulting in increased permeability of the surface layer and thus exposure of the underlying submucosal tissues to toxic substances in the urine.
3. An infectious process with a poorly characterized agent such as a slowly reproducing virus or extremely fastidious bacterium which cannot be cultured through conventional means.
4. The production of a "toxic" substance in the urine.
5. A neurogenic hypersensitivity or neurogenically mediated inflammation locally within the bladder or at the level of the spinal cord.
6. A manifestation of pelvic floor muscle dysfunction or dysfunctional voiding,
7. An autoimmune disorder.

❏❏ **What percentage of patients with I.C. are female?**

90%.

❏❏ **What other diseases have been associated with I.C.?**

Allergies (41%), irritable bowel (30%), inflammatory bowel disease (7%), Sjögren's syndrome, vulvar vestibulitis syndrome, systemic lupus erythematosus, fibromyalgia, and hypersensitive skin disorders.

❏❏ **What are the characteristic voiding symptoms of patients with I.C.?**

Irritative voiding symptoms including urinary urgency, urinary frequency (> 8/day by NIDDK criteria) with nocturia, and pain with negative urine cultures. Obstructive symptoms including a sensation of incomplete bladder emptying and double voiding may be present. Absence of nocturnal symptoms suggests an alternative diagnosis.

□□ What percentage of patients with I.C. experience dyspareunia?

50 to 75%.

□□ Do any of the following conditions exclude a diagnosis of I.C.: a) endometriosis, b) pyuria, c) hematuria, d) bladder instability on urodynamics, or e) ureteral calculus?

No. All of these conditions may co-exist in patients with I.C. Each of these may be related to a cause of lower urinary tract symptoms and should be properly investigated and treated prior to making a diagnosis of I.C.

□□ What urodynamic findings are common in I.C.?

There are no urodynamic patterns that are pathognomonic for I.C. On filling cystometry, most patients have detrussor hypersensitivity with a low volume at first sensation to void and a decreased capacity. Filling, even at 1 cc per second may be limited by an intense urge to void or pain. Bladder compliance, flow, and post-void residual are normal.

□□ What percentage of I.C. patients demonstrate detrusor instability on urodynamic testing? What is the significance of this finding?

Involuntary bladder contractions may be found in 14% of I.C. patients. This is not different from the general population. Other than excluding the patient from clinical trials adhering to the NIDDK criteria, there is no other significance.

□□ What are the common findings at cystoscopy in patients with I.C.?

Prior to hydrodistention – normal appearing bladder and urethral lumen, and rarely a Hunner's ulcer (found in <10% of patients).

Following hydrodistention under anesthesia – glomerulations (petechial hemorrhages), submucosal hemorrhages, mucosal cracking, and bloody effluent upon drainage (terminal pinking).

□□ What are the findings during cystoscopy in a patient with "classic" I.C. as compared to the non-ulcerative form of the disease?

Classic IC (10% of I.C. patients) - reduced capacity under anesthesia (<400 cc during hydrodistention), the presence of ulcers or scars.

Non-ulcerative disease (90% patients) - capacity >400 cc, no ulcers, scars, or mucosal cracking.

□□ What is the diagnostic utility of a bladder biopsy in I.C.?

Although a higher proportion of I.C. patients will have detrusor mastocytosis as compared to normal controls, there are no histologic findings on bladder biopsy which are pathognomonic of I.C. In general, bladder biopsy is performed on patients being investigated for I.C. in order to eliminate carcinoma in-situ or occult malignancy as a cause for their lower urinary tract symptoms.

□□ What is the significance of the NIDDK criteria for a diagnosis of I.C.?

These criteria were developed at an NIH sponsored consensus conference to ensure a relatively homogenous and uniform population of patients for accrual and inclusion into I.C. research studies. Fulfillment of these criteria is not necessary for the diagnosis of I.C. in clinical practice.

□□ What is the potassium chloride test?

This is an uncommonly performed in-office test used by some physicians in patients suspected of having a diagnosis of I.C. Following intravesical instillation of 45 ml KCl (400 meq/L) 70% of patients with a diagnosis of I.C. will experience pain, versus only 4% of normals. This is felt to be due to a defect in the GAG layer of the bladder in patients with I.C.

❏❏ What is the role of hydrodistention in patients with I.C.?

Hydrodistention can be both diagnostic and therapeutic in patients being evaluated for I.C. Following hydrodistention it is generally felt that many patients with I.C. will manifest glomerulations, submucosal hemorrhages, mucosal cracking and blood tinged effluent upon drainage ("terminal pinking"). Furthermore, a significant number of patients have relief of their symptoms following hydrodistention.

❏❏ Apart from I.C., which conditions may manifest glomerulations following hydrodistention?

Neoplasia, infectious cystitis, radiation cystitis, chemical cystitis, and a defunctionalized bladder (patients on dialysis or after urinary diversion).

❏❏ Name at least five oral agents which have been utilized clinically in the treatment of I.C.?

Tricyclic antidepressants, sodium pentosanpolyphosphate (Elmiron®), hydroxyzine (anti-histamines), L-arginine, nalmephene, anticholinergic agents (oxybutinin, hyoscyamine, etc.), corticosteroids, antispasmodics, immunosuppressives, anti-inflammatories, calcium channel blockers.

❏❏ What is the theoretical mechanism of action of amitriptyline in the treatment of I.C.?

The tricyclic antidepressants such as amitriptyline have a number of pharmacological properties which may be of some theoretical benefit in patients with I.C. including: anticholinergic effects, beta-adrenergic effects (smooth muscle relaxation), strong H_1-antihistaminic activity, and central nervous system sedative effects.

❏❏ How is bladder hydrodistention performed?

The bladder is filled to capacity at 80 cm H_2O under anesthesia for 8 minutes. The maximum pressure can be regulated by simply raising the height of the filling solution to 80 cm above the patinet's symphysis pubis.

❏❏ How effective is bladder hydrodistention in the management of I.C.?

Symptomatic improvement can be expected in up to 30-60% of patients.

❏❏ What is the mechanism by which hydrodistention relieves the symptoms of I.C.?

Unknown. Hypotheses include neuropraxis by mechanical trauma or epithelial damage from mechanical trauma.

❏❏ What is dimethylsulfoxide (DMSO) and how is it utilized to treat I.C.?

DMSO is a product derived from the wood pulp industry. It has a number of pharmacological properties which may have some theoretical benefit in patients with I.C. including anti-inflammatory, analgesic, muscle relaxant properties and mast-cell histamine release.   It is used as an intravesical lavage instilled on a weekly basis. It is sometimes administered in combination with steroids, alkalinizing agents and heparin.

❏❏ How effective is intravesical dimethylsulfoxide (DMSO) in I.C.?

Induces remission in up to 34% to 60% of patients. Progressive resistance may be seen after repeated treatments.

❏❏ What percentage of patients develop radiation cystitis after external beam therapy?

The incidence of early radiation cystitis is approximately 20% and it usually occurs 3 to 6 weeks following therapy. Late radiation induced hemorrhagic cystitis will occur in 3 to 12% of patients undergoing full course pelvic radiation.

❐❐ **What is the risk of transitional cell carcinoma of the bladder after pelvic radiation?**

Pelvic radiation has been associated with a two to fourfold increased risk of transitional cell carcinoma of the bladder over the general population. When diagnosed, the tumors tend to be high grade and locally invasive.

❐❐ **What are the approximate maximum radiation doses tolerated by the bladder?**

65 Gy to 70 Gy. Above 80 Gy, mucosal and/or full-thickness changes occur.

❐❐ **Which histopathologic changes lead to hematuria after pelvic radiation?**

Progressive endarteritis obliterans resulting in mucosal ischemia, telangiectasias, submucosal hemorrhage, and ulceration. Chronically, interstitial fibrosis ensues.

❐❐ **How effective is hyperbaric oxygen therapy for control of radiation cystitis?**

Resolution of hematuria has been reported in >90% of patients. Hyperbaric oxygen therapy promotes neovascularization and generalized vasoconstriction which can abate the bleeding process.

❐❐ **How many hyperbaric treatments are usually necessary for control of symptoms related to radiation cystitis?**

30 treatments at 2 atm for 2 hours per treatment.

❐❐ **What percentage of patients receiving cyclophosphamide will develop hemorrhagic cystitis in the absence of prophylactic measures?**

Up to 40% of patients undergoing "low dose" single agent or multi-agent chemotherapy protocols with cyclophosphamide will develop hemorrhagic cystitis. The risk increases in patients receiving high doses of cyclophosphamide in preparation for bone marrow transplantation.

❐❐ **When is the usual onset of hemorrhagic cystitis in patients treated with cyclophosphamide?**

Hematuria often develops acutely during therapy or shortly after a cycle has been completed.

❐❐ **Which metabolite of cyclophosphamide is thought to be responsible for hemorrhagic cystitis?**

Cyclophosphamide is metabolized to acrolein in the liver. Acroline is considered to be toxic to the urothelium.

❐❐ **Which agent(s) reduce the development of cyclophosphamide-induced hemorrhagic cystitis?**

Mesna - specifically binds acrolein. 20 mg/kg i.m. administered at 0, 4, 8, and 12 hours after cyclophosphamide dosing.

N-acetylcysteine (Mucomist) – oral, parenteral, or intravesical. Systemically, reduces the antineoplastic effects of cyclophosphamide.

❐❐ **What is the risk of bladder cancer after cyclophosphamide therapy?**

Studies suggest there is a nine-fold increased risk of bladder cancer in patients undergoing cyclophosphamide chemotherapy. The latency period can be 6-12 years. Published reports indicate a significant percentage of bladder tumors in these patients are muscle-invasive at the time of diagnosis.

❐❐ **What other drugs or derivatives are associated with hemorrhagic cystitis?**

Penicillins, danazol, busulfan, aniline dyes, toluidine, and ether have all been associated with hemorrhagic cystitis.

❑❑ **What is the mechanism of action of epsilon aminocaproic acid (EACA, AMICAR) in treating hemorrhagic cystitis?**

Epsilon aminocaproic acid acts by blocking plasminogen activation and fibrinolysis. Thus clot formation is promoted over bleeding surfaces. Amicar is contraindicated in patients with small vessel disease or patients at risk for thromboemolic events.

❑❑ **What is Alum and what is its mechanism of action in treating hemorrhagic cystitis ? How is it administered?**

Potassium or ammonium aluminum sulfate (Alum) forms a salt-protein precipitate over the bleeding surface of the bladder. It is administered as a 1% intravesical lavage at 5 ml/minute. Monitoring of serum aluminum levels is recommended in patients undergoing prolonged therapy with Alum.

❑❑ **What are the drawbacks of intravesical formalin for intractable hemorrhagic cystitis?**

Intravesical administration is quite painful requiring regional or general anesthesia. Reflux of formalin into the upper urinary tract may result in ureteral fibrosis, obstruction, and papillary necrosis.

❑❑ **What study should be performed prior to the initiation of intravesical formalin for hemorrhagic cystitis?**

A gravity cystogram with drainage views must be performed to exclude vesicoureteral reflux. If reflux is present an alternative therapeutic option should be entertained or ureteral balloon occlusion catheters must be used during installation to prevent reflux.

❑❑ **What is the mechanism of action of DDAVP (desmopressin) for intractable hemorrhagic cystitis?**

Increases factor VIII and von Willebrand factor levels.

❑❑ **Which parasites have been associated with hemorrhagic cystitis?**

Echinococcus, schistosomiasis.

❑❑ **Which viruses have been associated with hemorrhagic cystitis?**

Adenovirus types 11, 21, 35; papovarirus; influenza A; cytomegalovirus in immunodeficient states.

❑❑ **A 68-year-old female is referred with *de novo* urinary retention. Physical examination reveals a vesicular eruption over the mons pubis and right buttocks. What is your diagnosis?**

Herpes zoster may result in detrussor areflexia secondary to sacral root involvement. Characteristically, it involves a vesicular rash along sacral dermatomes. Intravesical vesicles may be seen. The condition often resolves spontaneously over 1 to 2 months.

❑❑ **What is eosinophilic cystitis and how does it present?**

Eosinophilic infiltrate of bladder lamina propria and detrusor. Non-specific presentation: urgency, frequency, hematuria. A history of allergies and peripheral eosinophilia may be present. Occasionally, a mass may be palpable, mimicking sarcoma in children.

❑❑ **What are the endoscopic findings in eosinophilic cystitis?**

Yellow raised plaques, necrotic ulcerated lesions, edema, erythema.

❑❑ **Which radiologic findings are associated with eosinophilic cystitis?**

Vesicoureteral reflux is seen in one-third of patients. Bladder wall thickening is a common finding on bladder sonography.

❑❑ How is eosinophilic cystitis treated?

Treatment is generally non-specific with steroids and antihistamines. The condition often has a self-limiting course.

❑❑ How do patients with malacoplakia present?

Chronic urinary tract infections. 40% have associated systemic diseases such as immunodeficiency, malignancies, or autoimmune disease.

❑❑ What are the characteristic pathologic findings of genitourinary malacoplakia?

Microscopically, infiltrates of bacteria-laden histiocytes (Michaelis-Gutmann bodies), lymphocytes, and plasma cells can be identified. Grossly, the lesions consist of raised yellow-brown plaques with hyperemic borders.

❑❑ What systemic diseases are associated with malacoplakia?

Immunodeficiency states (especially organ transplantation patients on immunosuppressants), carcinoma, and autoimmune diseases.

❑❑ What is the role of bethanechol in the management of genitourinary malacoplakia and what is the proposed mechanism by which it exerts it effect?

Along with antibiotics that have an intracellualr mechanism of action such as trimethoprim-sulfamethoxazole and the fluoroquinolones, bethanechol is the most commonly utilized agent for malacoplakia. Michealis-Gutmann bodies in malacoplakia are felt to represent incompletely digested bacterial material within the lysosomes of the histiocytes. Bethanechol increases the intracellular levels of cGMP promoting microtubule formation, which assists in lysosomal phagocytosis and digestion.

❑❑ Is there a gender difference in the incidence of emphysematous cystitis?

Yes, Two-thirds of patients are female.

❑❑ Which factors predispose patients to developing emphysematous cystitis?

Diabetes mellitus (50%), neurogenic bladder, chronic cystitis, bladder outlet obstruction, immunodeficiencies.

❑❑ What are the most common pathogens in emphysematous cystitis?

In decreasing frequency, E. coli, Enterobacter, Klebsiella, Clostridia and Candida.

PROSTATITIS

Durwood E. Neal, Jr., M.D.

❑❑ **The most common organism in acute bacterial prostatitis is:**

As in other types of urinary tract infections, E.coli is the most common.

❑❑ **T/F: Secretory activity of the prostate epithelium is increased in bacterial prostatitis.**

False. The secretory activity of the prostate gland, as in all other cellular / glandular functions is diminished in the setting of a bacterial infection.

❑❑ **What is Category IV prostatitis characterized by?**

The definition of Category IV prostatitis is based on the presence of inflammation by histology.

❑❑ **Differentiation between Category IIIa and IIIb prostatitis is by:**

The distinction between Category IIIA and IIIB is the presence of inflammation in the EPS or VB3 in IIIA.

❑❑ **What happens to proteins synthesis and citrate levels in the prostate in the face of acute bacterial prostatitis?**

Acute inflammation reduces the prostate gland's ability to synthesize proteins and acquire citrate. Therefore, both protein production and citrate levels will fall in the setting of acute inflammation.

❑❑ **What happens to serum PSA levels in the setting of acute bacterial prostatitis?**

Serum PSA is elevated in prostatitis, probably due to the enhanced release of PSA from the epithelial cells. There is no evidence of increased production of the protein in the setting of inflammation.

❑❑ **What happens to calcium and zinc levels in the prostate in the setting of acute bacterial prostatitis?**

Divalent cations are sequestered in the prostate gland by an active transport mechanism. These processes are reduced in the setting of acute infection.

❑❑ **What happens to the pH of the prostatic secretions in the setting of acute bacterial prosatitis?**

The prostatic secretions become more basic in the setting of acute infection.

❑❑ **What happens to prostatic PSA in the setting of acute bacterial prostatitis?**

There is no overall change in prostatic PSA with acute infection.

❑❑ **What happens to prostatic blood flow in the setting of acute bacterial prostatitis?**

Prostatic blood flow increases, up to a point, in acute infection as it does in any other organ. There is probably a redistribution of blood flow to the periphery due to edema in the more central portion of the gland.

❑❑ **Prostatic inflammation may result in infertility by which of the following mechanisms:**

Ductal obstruction, caused by a combination of the edema and scarring, reduces fertility in patients with prostatitis. Hypogonadism and anejaculation do not occur. Blood flow is actually increased and elevated PSA levels have not apparent effect on fertility.

❏❏ **T/F: The etiology of Category IIIb prostatitis may not involve the prostate.**

True. It is thought that Category IIIb prostatitis may be secondary to pelvic floor spasm or myalgia.

❏❏ **Which of the following are not considered part of the prostatitis symptom complex?**

Flank pain is not described by the majority of patients with prostatitis, unless there is concomitant upper urinary tract infection.

❏❏ **Are any of the following FDA approved for the treatment of Category III prostatitis: ciprofloxacin, terazocin, sulfamethoxazole-trimethoprim, oxybutinin?**

Currently, there are no medications that are FDA approved for Category III prostatitis. However, all listed have shown efficacy in the treatment of this disease process.

❏❏ **What is the most common form of prostatitis?**

The time incidence of prostatitis has been difficult to document due to under reporting, however, the most common variety is category IIIa, as most patients have inflammatory cells as well as sterile cultures.

❏❏ **Which of the following have been reported to be efficacious in non-bacterial prostatitis: terazosin, finasteride, pentosan polysulfonate, hydroxazine.**

All of these pharmacotherapeutics have been reported to be efficacious in prostatitis.

❏❏ **T/F: Receptors for uropathogenic bacteria include: P, Type I, and Dr.**

True. Uropathogenic bacteria have receptors (P, Type I, Dr, and others) that facilitate binding of bacteria to the urothelial cell surface.

❏❏ **T/F: P-fimbriated E. coli may be the most common organism in prostatitis.**

True. P-fimbriated E.coli are the most common organisms that are found in the setting of many acute UTI's, including prostatitis. Type I fimbriae are more commonly associated with simple cystitis.

❏❏ **T/F: Antibiotics for chronic prostatitis: should have high lipid solubility, be bacteriocidal, be given for 4 weeks or more, include the 5-fluoroquinolone group.**

True. For an antibiotic to be efficacious in acute prostatitis, there needs to be a mechanism for concentration in the prostate, one of which is lipid solubility. Since organisms tend to be sequestered there, bacteriostatic antibiotics, theoretically, should be less efficacious. The quinolones have the necessary properties.

❏❏ **Therapy for chronic prostatitis has included the following except: transurethral microwave thermotherapy, frequent prostate massage, allopurinol, cyclophosphamide, pelvic biofeedback.**

Cyclophosphamide, an antimetabolite has not been shown to be efficacious in chronic prostatitis. The literature suggests that the other listed treatments may benefit some patients.

❏❏ **Reported efficacious therapy for chronic bacterial prostatitis has included all of the following except: alpha interferon, radical TURP, 3-months of antibiotic therapy, a combination of antibiotics and alpha-blockade, intraprostatic injection of antibiotics.**

Alpha interferon, an immunomodulator, has not been tried in acute bacterial prostatitis. All the others have been reported to be efficacious.

❑❑ **T/F: Theories as to the etiology of non-bacterial prostatitis include all the following except: Autoimmunity, prostatic intraepithelial neoplasia (PIN), interstitial cystitis, chronic bacterial infection and fastidious microorganisms.**

False. There is no reported symptom complex for PIN. All the others have been implicated as etiologic in patients with Category III prostatitis.

❑❑ **T/F: The diagnosis of chronic bacterial prostatitis: requires a positive VB1 and bacteria in the VB3, is eliminated by a positive VB2, is established by leukocytes in the EPS.**

False. The hallmark of the diagnosis of Category II prostatitis is bacteria in the prostatic secretions and the post-prostatic massage urine. VB1 may be positive but not necessarily and VB2 is often positive for bacteria, although to a lesser extent than EPS or VB3.

❑❑ **What can one attribute the PSA elevation in prostatitis to?**

Prostatic epithelial cells release PSA after the stress of an inflammation. It is the same isoform as in prostate cancer and does not affect the ability to diagnose prostate cancer. It occurs prior to treatment, and is diminished with antibiotics.

❑❑ **T/F: Mechanisms of infertility in patients with prostatitis include: antisperm antibodies, asthenospermia, sperm agglutination, reduced semen volume.**

True. Antisperm antibodies cause asthenospermia as well as agglutination. Bacteria and leukocytes have the same effect on sperm. The reduced semen volume is a result of swelling (secondary to edema) in the prostate, and reduced passage of prostatic fluid through the attenuated ducts.

❑❑ **The antibiotic for prostatitis that has the most deleterious effect on fertility is:**

Doxycycline. Doxycycline both reduces sperm production and also reduces semen quality by toxic metabolites of the tetracycline component. The fluoroquinolones have only a mild negative effect on fertility, the most significant being ofloxacin. The macrolides have little effect on fertility.

❑❑ **Prostatic inflammation is found most commonly in which part of the prostate?**

In both human and non-human primates, the peripheral zone is most commonly involved with the inflammatory process. This is probably due to the straight orientation of the ducts themselves, as opposed to the ducts of the central zone.

❑❑ **T/F: Organisms typically found in Category II prostatitis include: diptheroids, E. cloi, Proteus sp. and Pseudomonas aeruginosa.**

False. Diphtheroids are not considered to be pathogenic in prostatitis, although they are frequently isolated in the urine (VB1 or VB3). The others are frequently isolated in bacterial (Category I or II) prostatitis.

❑❑ **Prostatic abscess risk factors include all the following: urethral stricture, steroid use, alcoholism, and AIDS.**

True. Each condition has been associated with prostatic abscess formation. Additional factors include obstructive uropathy and immunosuppression independently.

❑❑ **Prostatic sequestration with certain fungi causes reinfection by all the following except: poor penetration of some antifungals into the prostate, glycocalyx formation, ductal obstruction, poor prostate blood flow.**

True. All of these factors may contribute to the scenario wherein there is a recrudescence of infection after a presumptively adequate course of therapy with antifungals. The organism is often found in the prostate as a relatively protected site.

❑❑ **T / F: Saw palmetto extract has anti-inflammatory, antibacterial, and dimished blood flow activity on the prostate.**

False. Among all of the actions purported to be associated with saw palmetto, none of these have been reported. It may have estrogenic or antiandrogenic actions, as well as growth factor inhibitory properties.

☐☐ **T/F: The expressed prostatic secretions in category II prostatitis: have > five WBCs per high power field, have reduced zinc levels, have at least one log more organisms than the VB2.**

True. All of these points define Category II prostatitis.

☐☐ **T/F: Coliforms are found in prostatitis because of lymphatic spread from the colon.**

False. This is a common misconception regarding prostatitis. This disease entity is an ascending infection by the urethra.

☐☐ **Prostatic inflammatory conditions predispose to prostate cancer.**

False. There is no correlation of prostate cancer with prostatic inflammation. Some authors suggest a negative association.

☐☐ **T/F: Hematospermia usually indicates the presence of a bacterial infection and is a common side-effect of finasteride and / or alpha blocker use.**

False. Hematospermia is most commonly a benign, self-limited condition. Bacterial infection is uncommonly associated with it. Neither alpha-blockade nor five-alpha reductase inhibitors cause this condition. Cystoscopy is indicated only if there is concomitant hematuria.

☐☐ **What is the appropriate treatment for category I prostatitis?**

Alpha-blockade may be necessary to treat the urinary retention that results from auto prostatitis. One should avoid prostatic massage and urethral catheters. Most authors suggest that some evaluation of the upper urinary tracts is indicated in a male with a UTI. The VB, should be positive for bacteria.

☐☐ **T/F: Category IIIb prostatitis may be caused by: disordered voiding, pelvic floor myalgia, radiation therapy, obstructed ejaculatory ducts and afferent nerve dysfunction.**

False. Radiation therapy to the pelvis may cause symptoms suggestive of Category III b prostatitis, but the definition of this disease is precluded by radiation therapy.

☐☐ **T/F: Interstitial cystitis and chronic prostatitis have many common features.**

True. There are a number of correlation's of I.C. with prostatitis. The symptom complex is similar (pain, disordered voiding), the theoretical etiologies are similar, and the medications are frequently the same.

☐☐ **T/F: Prostatitis may be sexually transmitted.**

True. Surprisingly, this disease entity is quite common and described as severe by its sufferers. Dietary changes have been shown to mitigate symptoms on occasions. Some types of prostatitis may be associated with gonorrhea, Chlamydia, Chycoplasma, and Ureaplasma

GENITOURINARY TUBERCULOSIS

Peter Langenstroer, M.D.

☐☐ **What is tuberculosis?**

Tuberculosis is a bacterial infection caused by Mycobacterium tuberculosis. It spreads from person to person by a pulmonary route followed by hematogenous seeding to the genitourinary tract.

☐☐ **When was the first case of tuberculosis described?**

Tuberculosis is a disease that has been prevalent for many centuries. Dating back to 7000BC, human skeletal remains have revealed pathologic findings consistent with TB infections.

☐☐ **What are other historical names used for tuberculosis?**

Scrofula, consumption, phthisis, Kings-Evil.

☐☐ **What is the incidence of TB worldwide?**

The worldwide incidence of TB is 10 million cases per year with 3 million deaths per year.

☐☐ **What is the estimated number of people a TB infected person could subsequently infect?**

Thirty.

☐☐ **What are the two main mechanisms for eradication of TB?**

Case identification and treatment, and bacille Calmette-Guerin vaccination.

☐☐ **What are the problems associated with BCG vaccination?**

The duration of response is only 15 years. It has little effect on the incidence of infection and is ineffective in patients with prior TB infection. BCG also carries many potential side effects.

☐☐ **What are the unique microbiological characteristics of *Mycobacterium tuberculosis*?**

M. tuberculosis is an aerobic non-motile bacteria with a high propensity to develop drug resistance. Its doubling time is slow at 24 -hours. It can survive following phagocytosis in the lysosome of the macrophage.

☐☐ **Describe the inflammatory response associated with GU TB.**

The response is mainly via the cellular mediated immunity. Lymphocytes and Langhans' giant cells make up the typical histological findings of the TB granuloma.

☐☐ **Do non-tuberculosis mycobacteria cause pathogenic changes in the GU tract?**

This is very rare. Only a handful of cases have been reported. The mycobacterium involved include *M.kansasii, M. avium-intracellulare, M. xenopi* and *M. fortuitum.*

☐☐ **What test can be used to differentiate *M. tuberculosis* from non-tuberculosis mycobacteria?**

p-nitro-a-acetylamino-B hydroxypropriophenole, the NAP test.

❏❏ What populations are at highest risk for developing TB?

People living in underdeveloped countries, alcoholics, HIV patients, IV drug abusers, the homeless, and the elderly.

❏❏ What is the most common age group to develop GU TB?

GU TB is most commonly seen in the 20 – 40 year old age group with a 2:1 male to female predominance.

❏❏ What is the classic triad of TB infection?

Fatigue, weight loss, anorexia.

❏❏ What percent of extra-pulmonary TB is related to the GU tract?

Worldwide, 14% of all cases of extra-pulmonary TB are related to the GU tract.

❏❏ How is TB spread to the GU tract?

GU TB is the result of metastatic spread of the mycobacterium via the blood stream. It usually results from a primary pulmonary focus.

❏❏ What is the mechanism that leads to TB of the lower urinary tract?

Urinary excretion of the mycobacterium from the kidney causes seeding and infection of the lower urinary tract.

❏❏ What are some of the clinical findings associated with GU TB?

Sterile pyuria is the hallmark of GU TB. Other less specific signs are, painless urinary frequency, nocturia, hematuria, hematospermia, suprapubic pain and flank pain.

❏❏ How should one culture the urine of a patient suspected of having GU TB?

Five consecutive early morning urine specimens should be obtained and cultured on two separate media. Lowenstein –Jensen medium will isolate *mycobacterium tuberculosis,* BCG, and non-tuberculosis mycobacterium.

❏❏ A 41-year-old woman native of India is referred to her urologist with irritative voiding and sterile pyuria. What is the differential diagnosis?

Carcinoma in situ, genitourinary TB, interstitial cystitis.

❏❏ What genitourinary organs are spared from TB infections?

None, all organs of the genitourinary tract are targets for TB infections. However, TB of the penis, prostate and urethra are rare.

❏❏ What medications are currently used to treat GU TB?

Rifampin, Isoniazid, Pyrazinamide, Streptomycin and Ethambutol.

❏❏ Describe the usual medical treatment regimen for uncomplicated GU TB.

Pyrazinamide, 25 mg/kg/day, Isoniazid, 300 mg/day, and Rifampin, 450 mg/day for two months. Then, Isoniazid, 600 mg, and Rifampin, 900 mg, 3 times per week for two months. An alternative regimen would be to add Streptomycin, 1 gm/day to the first two months.

❏❏ **A 45-year-old woman has just completed her course of medical therapy for renal TB. She is asymptomatic and feels well. How should she be followed?**

She should be seen at 3, 6 and 12 - months following completed treatment. At each visit she should have 3 consecutive morning urine specimens sent for TB cultures. Radiographic examination of her upper urinary tract would also be indicated. She should also return if symptoms recur.

❏❏ **What is a nonspecific test that can be used to monitor the effectiveness of treatment for TB?**

Erythrocyte sedimentation rate (ESR), if elevated prior to therapy can be used to monitor the effectiveness of a specific treatment.

❏❏ **Of the five most commonly used anti-tuberculosis medications, (Rifampin, Isoniazid, Pyrazinamide, Ethambutol, and Streptomycin), which drugs are bactericidal?**

Rifampin, Isoniazid, Pyrazinamide, and Streptomycin.

❏❏ **Following institution of Isoniazid, Rifampin and Pyrazinamide for GU TB, the patient notices the development of a puritic macular rash. This is followed by generalized myalgias and conjunctivitis. Which drug is most commonly associated with this hypersensitivity reaction?**

Rifampin and Streptomycin are most commonly associated with hypersensitivity reactions.

❏❏ **Which anti-TB drugs are to be avoided in the presence of renal failure?**

Ethambutol and Streptomycin are primarily renally excreted and should be avoided in this situation.

❏❏ **A 62-year-old man receiving Isoniazid, Rifampin, Pyrazinamide and Ethambutol for GU TB has developed visual changes since the initiation of medical therapy. What is the most likely cause of his new symptoms?**

Ethambutol can lead to optic neuritis. It is recommended that all patients receiving the drug undergo monthly visual examinations.

❏❏ **Three weeks following initiation of medical treatment for GU TB, the patient is noted to have a rise in the liver enzyme panel. Jaundice is not present. How should this be managed?**

Most patients will have a transient elevation in the liver enzyme panel for the few weeks of therapy. If jaundice develops, the medications should be withdrawn until the jaundice resolves. Medical therapy can then be reinstituted.

❏❏ **Which of the anti-tuberculosis drugs is ototoxic?**

Streptomycin.

❏❏ **A 34-year-old woman on oral contraceptive medications becomes pregnant following the initiation of an anti-tuberculosis regimen. What is the likely cause for the failure of her contraceptive?**

Rifampin can affect the metabolism of estrogen in oral contraceptive preparations. This can lead to an increased failure rate of these contraceptives. Women of childbearing age should use an alternative means of contraception while taking anti-tuberculosis drugs.

❏❏ **A 40-year-old man with the new diagnosis of GU TB has severe cystitis secondary to bladder involvement. Anticholinergic medications did not improve his symptoms. What can be added to the usual drug regimen in order to improve his symptoms?**

Prednisone can reduce the symptoms of acute TB cystitis. It may also be of benefit if a distal ureteral stricture is present. Rifampin will significantly decrease the bioavailability of prednisone.

❏❏ **A 32-year-old man is being evaluated for left flank pain and sterile pyuria. What is the appropriate work up?**

This individual should have a repeat urine analysis, urine cytology, urine culture for TB, intravenous pyelogram and cystoscopy.

❏❏ **On plain film of the abdomen the patient is noted to have a large left upper pole calcification. The intravenous pyelogram (IVP) reveals he has minimal function of this kidney and blunting of his calices. His urine cultures reveal TB. What would be the indications for nephrectomy in this individual?**

A non-functioning kidney, associated renal cell carcinoma, uncontrolled hypertension, persistent severe flank pain, and patient noncompliance with the appropriate medical treatments are all indications for nephrectomy in the described setting.

❏❏ **When is the appropriate time to perform the nephrectomy?**

Four to six weeks after the initiation of medical therapy.

❏❏ **A 27-year-old woman with hypertension is found to have an atrophic right kidney from chronic renal TB. What is the likelihood she will have an improvement in her hypertension with a nephrectomy?**

Approximately 65% of patients with significant unilateral renal involvement will have improvement in their hypertension.

❏❏ **What are the common IVP (intravenous pyelogram) findings of renal TB?**

Calcification, parenchymal loss, distorted calices, calyceal loss, poorly or nonfunctioning kidneys.

❏❏ **A 21-year-old man with renal TB has a small renal calcification resulting from the infectious process. He has been adequately treated for his TB. How should his stone be managed?**

Calcification is associated with the normal tissue response from the destructive process and subsequent mineralization of the fibrous scar tissue. Small calculi can be observed. Larger calculi should be excised in a parenchyma sparing fashion.

❏❏ **What are the common radiographic findings of TB in the ureter?**

Ureteral strictures, beading of the ureter, hydroureterosis from distal stenosis, ureterovesical obstruction, and vesicoureteral reflux.

❏❏ **What is the most common area of the ureter to be affected by TB?**

The ureterovesical junction.

❏❏ **How does TB lead to vesicoureteral reflux?**

Scarring in the bladder at the level of the ureteral orifice can cause contraction of the surrounding tissue leading to a contracted rigid golf hole type ureteral orifice. This same process can also lead to stenosis of the ureteral orifice.

❏❏ **A 50-year-old man was diagnosed with a distal ureteral stricture secondary to GU TB. He is placed on the standard medical regimen for GU TB. After three weeks of medical therapy he has no improvement in his ureteral obstruction. What is the next appropriate step in management?**

The addition of prednisone to his regimen would be indicated and should improve his ureteral stenosis.

❏❏ **Following three more weeks of medical management his obstruction persists. What are the remaining options for the treatment of his distal ureteral stricture?**

Balloon dilation, psoas hitch re-implantation, Boari flap re-implantation, and transureteroureterostomy.

□□ Describe the usual features of TB cystitis.

The bladder lesions arise at the ureteral orifices. The lesions are velvety, red, inflamed and edematous with granulations as a later finding. More advanced disease can affect the entire bladder.

□□ When is a bladder biopsy indicated in GU TB?

Never. If the urine cultures are negative, the bladder biopsies will also be negative. If there is concern for an urothelial malignancy, then a bladder biopsy is indicated.

□□ A 55-year-old man was treated for severe GU cystitis with Isoniazid, Rifampin, Pyrazinemide and prednisone for six months. Following treatment, he remains disease free. However, he has severe persistent urgency, frequency and nocturia. His bladder capacity is 120 cc. What would be the next appropriate therapy?

Augmentation cystoplasty

□□ A 20-year-old man presents with a superficial ulcer of his glans penis. Biopsy of the lesion rules out a malignancy but reveals TB. How could he have contracted this disease?

Hematogenous spread from a primary pulmonary source, or direct inoculation from the female genital tract.

□□ How does TB orchitis develop?

TB orchitis is almost always a direct extension of TB of the epididymis. TB is spread to the epididymis is via the blood stream.

□□ A 22-year-old HIV positive man presents with scrotal swelling and a tender right testicle and epididymis. Upon palpation he has beading of his associated vas deferens. He has a poorly defined fullness to globus major of the epididymis that is directly associated the testis. What would be the next step in the management of this patient?

A scrotal ultrasound should be obtained to further delineate the fullness.

□□ The ultrasound reveals a solid mass involving the testis and epididymis and a small associated loculated hydrocele. What is the next step in the management?

The patient should have tumor markers drawn and undergo a radical orchiectomy. This lesion may represent a testicular malignancy.

UROLITHIASIS DIAGNOSIS AND MANAGEMENT

Manoj Monga, M.D.

❏❏ **How common is nephrolithiasis?**

The prevalence of stone disease is approximately 3%.

❏❏ **How many Americans experience a bout or renal colic due to nephrolithiasis annually?**

720,000.

❏❏ **Is nephrolithiasis more common in men or women?**

The male:female ratio is 3:1.

❏❏ **What type of calculus is more common in women then men?**

Struvite stones are twice as likely to occur in women than in men due to the higher incidence of urinary tract infections in the female population.

❏❏ **What is the most common age at presentation with nephrolithiasis?**

A peak incidence for nephrolithiasis occurs from 20-40 years old.

❏❏ **What is the risk for stone recurrence after an initial symptomatic episode of urolithiasis?**

The stone recurrence rate is 50% within five years from the first stone episode.

❏❏ **In what percentage of patients can a metabolic abnormality predisposing to urolithiasis be identified?**

A probable metabolic etiology of nephrolithiasis can be found in 97% of patients who are properly evaluated.

❏❏ **What is the most important mediator of intestinal absorption of calcium?**

The most important mediator of calcium absorption is calcitriol (1,25-dihydroxyvitamin D_3), which increases calcium transport across the intestinal lumen. The conversion of precursors to calcitriol is initiated by hypophosphatemia and parathyroid hormone (PTH).

❏❏ **What additional effects does PTH have on calcium homeostasis?**

PTH is a polypeptide that stimulates the osteoclasts to resorb bone, releasing calcium and phosphate into the bloodstream. PTH also acts upon the kidney to resorb calcium.

❏❏ **How much dietary calcium is absorbed on a daily basis?**

Approximately 33% of the total dietary calcium (600-1200mg or 15 mg/kg) is absorbed and 100-200mg is secreted into the intestinal tract, for a net absorption of about 100-300mg. Calcium ions that are complexed in the GI tract to phosphate, oxalate, citrate, and sulfate are not absorbed.

❏❏ **Citrate is an important inhibitor of stone formation. What drink is highest in citrate content?**

Grapefruit juice (14,500 mg/L of citrate).

❏❏ How does citrate supplementation affect citrate levels in the urine?

Citrate absorbed from the intestine is converted to bicarbonate in the liver. This increased alkali load stimulates renal excretion of citrate and higher urinary citrate levels.

❏❏ What type of crystal is depicted in this urine sample?

Figure A.

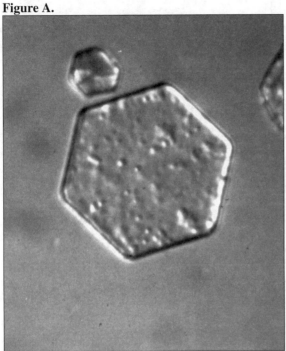

Cystine: hexagonal shape.

Figure B.

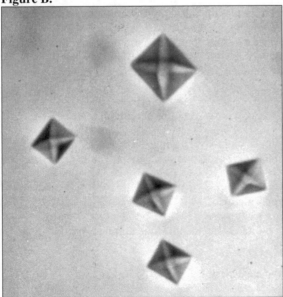

Calcium oxalate: star-box shape.

Figure C.

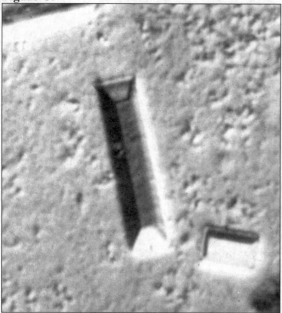

Calcium Phosphate: coffin-shape

❏❏ **How is Hypercalciuria defined?**

Hypercalciuria is defined as the excretion of greater than 200 mg / 24-hours in a patient taking a diet containing 400mg calcium and 100mEq sodium for a week. Approximately 50% of patients with calcium oxalate stones have hypercalciuria with normal serum calcium

❏❏ **What are the three types of hypercalciuria?**

1. Absorptive hypercalciuria due to increased intestinal absorption of calcium.
2. Renal hypercalciuria due to an abnormality in renal absorption of calcium.
3. Resorptive hypercalciuria due to augmented bone demineralization.

❏❏ **Is an elevated serum calcium an effective screening test for absorptive hypercalciuria?**

No. The increased absorption of calcium secondarily increases the filtered calcium presented to the kidney, thereby suppressing parathyroid function, and subsequently decreasing renal resorption of calcium. The hypercalciuria offsets the increased intestinal absorption, thereby keeping serum calcium in the normal range.

❏❏ **Is an elevated serum calcium an effective screening test for renal hypercalciuria?**

No. Renal leak of calcium results in a lowering of serum calcium levels, which stimulate PTH and 1,25-dihydroxy vitamin D_3. This results in an increase in intestinal absorption of calcium, which normalizes the serum calcium levels.

❏❏ **What is the medication of choice for renal hypercalciuria?**

Thiazide diuretics correct the renal leak of calcium by indirectly augmenting calcium reabsorption in the distal and proximal tubules.

❏❏ **Is an elevated PTH diagnostic of resorptive hypercalciuria?**

No. PTH is secondarily increased in renal hypercalciuria. An oral calcium load will suppress the hypersecretion of PTH in renal hypercalciuria. This can help differentiate this entity from primary hyperparathyroidism.

❏❏ **How does sodium cellulose phosphate work and what are the potential side effects?**

Sodium cellulose phosphate is a non-absorbable ion exchange resin that binds calcium and inhibits calcium absorption. Side effects include hypomagnesemia via binding of intestinal magnesium. Patients also get secondary hyperoxaluria since more divalent cations are bound in the gut and subsequently more oxalate is available for absorption. Lastly, there can be a negative calcium balance with consequent stimulation of PTH. Supplementation of magnesium and limitation of dietary oxalate are important adjuncts with the use of this agent.

❏❏ **How do orthophosphates work and what are their side effects?**

Orthophosphates exert their hypocalciuric effect by inhibiting $1,25\text{-}OH_2\text{-}D_3$ synthesis. Side effects include secondary PTH stimulation and soft tissue calcification. Orthophosphates are indicated in vitamin-D dependant absorptive hypercalciuria.

❏❏ **What is the drug of choice for absorptive hypercalciuria Type 1 in patients at risk for osteoporosis?**

Thiazides act by causing diuresis and increasing renal absorption of calcium. The main side effects include hypokalemia and hypocitraturia. These can be overcome by the addition of potassium citrate supplements.

❏❏ **Why is it important to limit sodium intake when taking thiazides for stone disease?**

Thiazides inhibit sodium reabsorption in the distal convoluted tubule, causing contraction of the extracellular volume. This leads to increased sodium and calcium reabsorption in the proximal convoluted tubule. Excess sodium intake would inhibit the ability of thiazides to contract the extracellular volume.

❏❏ **Is the hypocalciuric response to thiazides routinely permanent?**

No. If the response to thiazides is lost, a 6-month "drug holiday" during which time sodium cellulose phosphate therapy is utilized will often reinstate responsiveness to thiazides.

❏❏ **When are thiazides contraindicated with hypercalciuria?**

Thiazides should never be used in patients with hyperparathyroidism.

❏❏ **What is the most common cause of hypercalcemia in the outpatient setting?**

Hyperparathyroidism. It should be suspected in patients with high or high-normal serum calcium and urinary lithiasis.

❏❏ **How does one diagnose hyperparathyroidism?**

Assays that measure the carboxy-terminal portion of PTH are approximately 90% sensitive in detecting elevations in blood levels of PTH. PTH also causes an increase in cAMP, which can be measured in the urine.

❏❏ **What are alternative treatments for primary hyperparathyroidism if the patient cannot undergo parathyroidectomy?**

Orthophosphates or thiazides and potassium citrate can be used if surgery is contraindicated. Estrogen supplements can be tried in postmenopausal women.

❏❏ **What is the most common cause of hypercalcemia in the inpatient setting?**

Malignancy. Less than 1% of patients with urinary lithiasis have a malignancy. The most common tumors in descending order of occurrence are lung, breast, renal cell, head and neck, and hematologic.

❏❏ **Why does malignancy cause hypercalcemia?**

The mechanism for most hypercalcemia related malignancy is osteoclastic bone resorption stimulated by cytokines and other substances released by the tumor, such as PTH-related polypeptide, prostaglandins, tumor necrosis factors, and transforming growth factors.

❏❏ What are other causes of hypercalcemia?

Hyperthyroidism, glucocorticoid excess, pheochromocytoma, prolonged immobilization, familial hypocalciuric hypercalcemia, thiazides, lithium, milk-alkali syndrome, vitamin A toxicity, and granulomatous diseases such as sarcoidosis, histoplasmosis, tuberculosis, leprosy, silicosis, and coccidiomycosis. Sarcoid granulomas may produce calcitriol.

❏❏ How is hypercalcemia treated?

Hypercalcemia is treated by addressing the underlying cause, systemic hydration, bisphosphonates, calcitonin, and mithramycin.

❏❏ What calculi are radiolucent?

Uric acid, sodium urate, ammonium urate, xanthine, silica and 2,8-dihydroxyadenine calculi.

❏❏ How does hyperuricosuria lead to stone formation?

Stones secondary to hyperuricosuria are a result of the precipitation of sodium-urate crystals in the urine. These crystals can initiate both urate or calcium oxalate stones and also remove certain inhibitors of stone formation from the urine.

❏❏ Why are humans and dalmations the only mammals prone to uric acid urolithiasis?

Humans and dalmations lack uricase, a hepatic enzyme that converts uric acid to soluble allantom.

❏❏ What causes hyperuricosuria?

Hypersecretion of urate can be due to increased dietary purines, gout, or states of overproduction of purines such as malignancy, myeloproliferative diseases, and glycogen storage diseases. Urate stones may also be found in states of chronic diarrhea such as Crohn's disease, ulcerative colitis, or jejuno-ileal bypass, which produce a state of acidosis via bicarbonate loss and dehydration.

❏❏ What is another effect of systemic acidosis that promotes stone formation?

Systemic acidosis is the most important etiological factor for the development of hypocitraturia.

❏❏ What foods are high in purine content?

Beef, poultry, peanuts and fish.

❏❏ Does most of urinary oxalate come from dietary sources?

No. About half of the enteric oxalate is degraded by two luminal bacterium, Oxalobacter formigens and Pseudomonas oxaliticus. Most (80%) of the urinary oxalate comes from hepatic conversion.

❏❏ In what conditions does dietary oxalate contribute significantly to urinary oxalate?

Secondary hyperoxaluria (Enteric hyperoxaluria) occurs in patients with short bowel syndrome, inflammatory bowel disease, jejuno-ileal bypass or intestinal malabsorption. Intestinal fat malabsorption characteristic of ileal disease results in saponification of calcium and magnesium. This decreases the amount of calcium available to complex with oxalate in the intestinal lumen, raising the free oxalate pool available for intestinal absorption.

❏❏ What other conditions can lead to enteric hyperoxaluria?

Pyridoxine deficiency, excess ascorbic acid ingestion, ethylene glycol ingestion and methoxyflurane anesthesia.

❏❏ What is primary hyperoxaluria?

Primary hyperoxaluria is an extremely rare autosomal recessive disorder resulting in increased hepatic production of oxalate.

❏❏ What are some medical therapies for hyperoxaluria?

High doses of calcium .25-1.00 g/day are recommended. The calcium will complex the free oxalate in the intestinal tract thus preventing oxalate absorption. Large doses of pyridoxine 200-400mg/day are beneficial in primary hyperoxaluria. Side effects of pyridoxine include hypomagnesuria. Cholestyramine helps in enteric hyperoxaluria by binding free intestinal oxalate.

❏❏ What other stone disease is characterized by autosomal recessive inheritance?

Cystinuria is a rare autosomal recessive disorder characterized by a urinary excretion of >250mg / day of cystine. The urinary sediment contains flat hexagonal crystals, which increase in solubility as the urine pH rises (especially pH>7.5).

❏❏ What other dicarboxylic amino acids are affected by the inheritance of the above renal tubular absorption abnormality?

Ornithine, lysine and arginine. COLA is a useful mnemonic. These amino acids are more soluble than cystine, so they do not form calculi.

❏❏ What gene is responsible for cystinuria?

The dibasic amino acid transporter gene SLC3A1.

❏❏ What is a characteristic radiographic appearance of cystine stones?

Ground-glass. Less opaque than calcium stones.

❏❏ What is the first line of medical therapy for cystine stones?

Aggressive hydration (aiming for 3-4 liters of urine per day) and alkalinization to a pH of 7-7.5.

❏❏ What is a potential side effect of alkalinization beyond a pH of 7.5?

Calcium phosphate crystallization.

❏❏ What are advantages of potassium citrate over sodium bicarbonate as an alkalinizing agent?

Limits sodium intake, of special importance in patients with congestive heart failure. Does not promote calcium oxalate crystallization to the same degree.

❏❏ What other medications may be used to treat cystine stones?

Drugs that contain a disulfide structure can reduce cystine to form soluble cysteine. These include D-penicillamine, alpha-mercaptopropionylglycine and captopril. Penicillamine has been associated with frequent side effects including nephrotic syndrome, exfoliative dermatitis and pancytopenia. Alpha mercaptopropionylglycine has a more favorable safety profile, making it the drug of choice. Tiopronin can be used in patients who manifest adverse effects to above mentioned drugs. Dietary restriction of methionine should be instituted.

❏❏ What vitamin should be supplemented if D-penicillamine is utilized?

Pyridoxine (Vitamin B6). Deficiency of Vitamin B6 leads to gastrointestinal upset, glossitis, dermatitis and seizures.

❏❏ **What is the chemical composition of struvite stones (infection stones)?**

Struvite or infection stones consist of magnesium, ammonium and phosphate and carbonate-apatite.

❏❏ **What types of bacteria are associated with struvite stones?**

Urinary tract infection caused by urease producing organisms leads to the formation of struvite stones. The most common culprits include Proteus, Pseudomonas, Klebsiella and Staphylococcus saprophyticus. Escherichia coli does not produce urease.

❏❏ **Why is urease important?**

Urease splits urea in the urine to ammonia (contributes to ammonium in struvite stones) and bicarbonate. Bicarbonate creates an alkaline urine, promoting the crystallization of struvite stones. Struvite does not precipitate unless the pH is >7.

❏❏ **What is a staghorn calculus?**

Staghorn calculus describes the appearance of a calculus that has formed on a matrix cast of the pyelocalyceal system of the kidney. It is most commonly a struvite calculus, however cystine and uric acid calculi may form staghorn configurations.

❏❏ **What is the goal of medical therapy for struvite stones?**

Antibiotics to maintain a sterile urine. Amoxicillin suppression after clearance of the offending organism is useful.

❏❏ **What adjunctive medical therapies are useful for struvite stones?**

Urease inhibitors such as acetohydroxamic acid are useful. Acetohydroxamic acid reduces the urinary saturation of struvite and retards calculus formation. The recommended dosage is 250-mg three times per day. Deep venous thrombosis is a rare but serious complication associated with this medication. Limiting side effects include gastrointestinal upset, headaches, anxiety and hallucination.

❏❏ **Which type of Renal Tubular Acidosis is associated with nephrolithiasis?**

Renal tubular acidosis describes several conditions (types 1, 2, and 4) where defects in renal / urinary acidification lead to metabolic acidosis. Only Type 1 (distal) RTA is characterized by nephrolithiasis, hypokalemia, hyperchloremia, and non-anion gap metabolic acidosis. About 70% of adults with distal RTA (type 1) have renal calculi.

❏❏ **What is the metabolic defect in RTA type 1?**

Defective excretion of hydrogen ions by the distal tubule results in a high urinary pH. The urine remains relatively alkaline (pH>6.0) despite systemic acidosis due to the inability of the distal tubule to maintain a proton gradient. Systemic acidosis results in hypercalciuria due to decreased renal reabsorption, increased bone resorption and hypocitraturia.

❏❏ **When do you suspect RTA type 1?**

Clinical suspicion raised by hypocitraturia, hypokalemia, systemic acidosis (serum bicarbonate <23 mEq/L), nephrocalcinosis on radiographs or renal ultrasound, recurrent calcium phosphate stones (>30% of stone) and urine pH>6.

❏❏ **How do you diagnose RTA type 1?**

Ammonium chloride load test. Diagnostic if urine pH>5.5 after taking 100 mg NH_4Cl/kg body weight the day prior.

❏❏ **What medications may promote stone formation, and should be elicited in the history-taking?**

Indinavir, triamterene, carbonic anhydrase inhibitors (acetazolamide), vitamin C, vitamin D, calcium, antacids, calcium supplements, uricosuric agents, chemotherapeutics, theophylline, furosemide.

❑❑ When is allopurinol used and how does it work?

Allopurinol (300 mg/day) is used for hyperuricosuric calcium oxalate nephrolithiasis and uric acid nephrolithiasis. It decreases urate synthesis by inhibiting xanthine oxidase and lowers urinary urate. Allopurinol should be given with moderate sodium restriction.

❑❑ What type of stone may form as a result of allopurinol therapy?

Xanthine.

❑❑ What medications are associated with the formation of ammonium urate calculi?

Laxatives, acetazolamide, allopurinol, triamterene, sulfonamides.

❑❑ How is a urine pH helpful in guessing the stone composition?

Low pH (<5.5) suggests the presence of uric acid or cystine calculi while an alkaline pH (>7.5) suggests the presence of struvite or calcium phosphate calculi. .

❑❑ What is the sodium nitroprusside test?

Examination of a spot urine sample for cystine can be performed by the nitroprusside test. The cyanide-nitroprusside colorimeter test gives a magenta ring at urinary cystine levels of greater than 75mg/L.

❑❑ What is the therapy for gouty diathesis?

The mainstay of treatment is to alkalinize the urinary pH to approximately 6.5. Potassium citrate has been demonstrated to provide adequate alkalinization. Potassium citrate 30-60-mg / day given in two divided doses. Sodium bicarbonate is a less expensive option, however it should be used with caution in patients with congestive heart failure. Elevation of the urinary pH above 7 should be avoided to prevent precipitation of calcium phosphate. Allopurinol is also recommended irrespective of the presence or absence of hyperuricemia.

❑❑ What is an intravenous alternative for alkalinization?

Sodium lactate (1/6 M). Infuse 500 ml every 8 hours. Sodium lactate is completely converted to bicarbonate within 1-2 hours.

❑❑ What diseases are calcium phosphate stones associated with?

Primary hyperparathyroidism, renal tubular acidosis, sodium alkali therapy.

❑❑ What dietary restrictions would you recommend for enteric hyperoxaluria?

Leafy green vegetables, rhubarb, spinach, cocoa, okra, potatoes, peanuts, turnips, chocolate, pecan, carrots, berries, tea, powdered coffee, broccoli.

❑❑ What tests should be obtained prior to percutaneous chemolysis of calculi?

Stone composition should be known. Urinary tract infection should be excluded by urine culture. Urinary extravasation should be excluded by antegrade contrast study.

❑❑ What is the solution of choice for chemolysis of uric acid calculi?

Sodium bicarbonate (50 mEq in 1L of 0.45% NaCl, pH 8).

❑❑ What is the solution of choice for chemolysis of cystine calculi?

Acetylcysteine (0.3M) in Tromethamine E (Tham E, pH 10).

☐☐ **What are the main ingredients in Suby G's solution and hemiacidrin solution, utilized for struvite calculi dissolution?**

Citric acid and magnesium citrate. Both these solutions maintain a pH of 4.

☐☐ **What was a potentially lethal complication of irrigation with hemiacidrin?**

Hypermagnesemia. Magnesium is added to the solution to decrease uroepithelial irritability. With high intrapelvic pressures (>25 cm H20), hypermagnesemia can occur, leading to respiratory depression.

☐☐ **What laboratory studies should be monitored during hemiacidrin irrigation?**

Daily magnesium levels, creatinine and phosphorus levels. Urine culture every 3 days.

☐☐ **What is a finding on physical examination suggestive of a high magnesium level?**

Depressed deep tendon reflexes.

☐☐ **How would hypermagnesemia be treated?**

Intravenous calcium, furosemide and saline.

☐☐ **What are some changes during pregnancy that could alter stone formation?**

Placental production of $1,25\text{-}(OH)_2$ vitamin D can stimulate hypercalciuria. This may be off-set by increased renal excretion of citrate and nephrocalcin.

GENITOURINARY TRAUMA

James M. Cummings, M.D., F.A.C.S.

❏❏ **What are the indications for imaging of the kidneys following blunt trauma?**

Gross hematuria or microhematuria combined with shock defined as systolic BP< 90 at any time following the injury are an absolute indication for GU tract imaging.

❏❏ **Staging of renal trauma is best accomplished with what radiographic test?**

CT scanning of the kidneys provides detailed images of the kidneys that allow for delineation of most renal injuries and their severity.

❏❏ **A small cortical laceration in the kidney with a small perirenal hematoma would be classified as what grade injury?**

Grade II

❏❏ **What are the absolute indications for renal exploration following blunt trauma?**

An expanding or pulsatile retroperitoneal hematoma must be explored. Initial control of the involved renal pedicle prior to opening of the hematoma must be achieved by means of a retroperitoneal incision medial to the inferior mesenteric vein and anterior to the aorta. The dissection is carried cephalad until the involved renal pedicle is encountered. Vascular control is achieved and the hematoma can now be entered.

❏❏ **An attempt to repair a main renal artery injury should be pursued under what circumstances?**

In a hemodynamically stable patient who has no other associated major organ system injuries, an ischemia time less than 8-10 hours, and / or bilateral renal injuries or injury to a solitary kidney one should entertain repair of the main renal artery.

❏❏ **The treatment of choice for renal arteriovenous fistulas is?**

Angiographic arterial embolization.

❏❏ **A 1-cm segment of left ureter is damaged during an elective left colectomy. The injury is recognized intraoperatively. The best choice for management at that time is?**

Debridement of any devitalized tissue, mobilization of the 2 ends of the ureter and a spatulated ureteroureterostomy over a stent. The area must be adequately drained post operatively.

❏❏ **Following a ureteral reimplant with a psoas hitch, a patient complains of anterior thigh numbness. What is the most likely etiology for this complaint?**

The genitofemoral nerve lies on the anterior aspect of the ileopsoas muscle. Injury to this never can occur during suturing of the bladder to the tendon of the psoas minor muscle.

❏❏ **Options for closing a large gap between the proximal end of a damaged ureter and the bladder when a psoas hitch will not reach include?**

Initially, the bladder should be mobilized on the contralateral side to the injury. This often involves division of vascular structures (superior vesical artery, obliterated umbilical artery etc…). A Boari bladder flap can gain considerable length and / or one may have to do a caudal nephropexy which can gain additional length to allow for closure of the defect. When these maneuvers are unsuccessful a transureteroureterostomy can be performed in the patient with unprepared bowel, otherwise an ileal interposition graft may need to be employed.

❑❑ **The arterial vascular supply of the ureter comes most commonly from what sources?**

Upper ureter – renal artery
Middle ureter – iliac artery
Lower ureter – superior vesical artery

❑❑ **A retrograde pyelogram done at the end of a difficult ureteroscopic stone extraction shows moderate extravasation at the previous location of the stone. Visual inspection reveals a perforation of the ureter, and a wire placed initially is still in place in the renal pelvis. Appropriate management at this time is?**

Placement of a ureteral stent along with a Foley catheter to maximally drain the system and allow for healing of the ureter. A follow up retrograde pyelogram should be performed at approximately 6-weeks postoperatively to assess healing of the involved area.

❑❑ **A woman presents with continuous urinary leakage 2-weeks following an abdominal hysterectomy. On physical examination, urine is identified in the vaginal vault. A cystogram is normal. What test should be done next?**

An IVP should be performed to rule out ureterovaginal fistula.

❑❑ **In an adult suspected of having bladder trauma, what volume of contrast should be instilled into the bladder?**

The bladder should be filled under gravity with up to 400 cc of contrast, or until a bladder contraction occurs. Following adequate AP filling views, oblique views need to be obtained as well as drainage views of the anatomic pelvis.

❑❑ **A pitfall of CT cystography in the evaluation of bladder injury is?**

If done with IV contrast only, the bladder may not be adequately distended to reveal the injury and thus give a false-negative result.

❑❑ **Extraperitoneal bladder ruptures may be managed non-operatively under what circumstances?**

If adequate bladder drainage via a large Foley catheter or suprapubic catheter can be achieved, there is no perforating bony fragment in the bladder wall and the injury does not involve the bladder neck, non-operative management can be successful. Close clinical follow up is mandatory in this situation.

❑❑ **Intraperitoneal bladder ruptures should be managed in what manner?**

Intraperitoneal bladder ruptures should be managed with surgical exploration, a multilayered closure, adequate bladder drainage and possible drainage of the space of Retzius.

❑❑ **In the United States, the most common event leading to vesicovaginal fistula is?**

Iatrogenic injury during gynecologic surgery (particularly hysterectomy) is the most common etiology of ureteral injury. Fistulas from childbirth are more common in underdeveloped countries.

❑❑ **Vesicovaginal fistulas following hysterectomy are a result of what etiologic event?**

An unrecognized bladder injury during hysterectomy with subsequent urinary extravasation into the surgical field and drainage via the vaginal cuff suture line leads to formation of the fistula.

❑❑ **What is the best time to repair a vesicovaginal fistula following an uncomplicated hysterectomy?**

Timing of the repair depends largely on the time interval to the diagnosis of the injury as well as the clinical condition of the patient. Although 3-6 months has been recommended in the past, early intervention can be successful if there is minimal inflammation in the tissues and there are no other complicating factors.

❑❑ **Tissues commonly used for interposition grafts in surgical repair of vesicovaginal fistulas include?**

Labial fat pad (Martius graft), gracilis muscle, peritoneum and omentum.

❑❑ **When used for interposition for vesicovaginal fistula repair, the omentum is mobilized on which vessel?**

The omentum is mobilized off the greater curvature of the stomach and the right gastroepiploic arterial supply is preserved. This is usually the dominant vessel supplying the omentum and mobilization in this manner often allows the omentum to reach the deep pelvis.

❑❑ **Physical findings of posterior urethral injury include?**

Blood at the meatus, a distended bladder, and a high-riding prostate gland on rectal exam are all consistent with a posterior urethral injury.

❑❑ **How does one diagnose a posterior urethral injury?**

Retrograde urethrography with the patient in a semioblique position is an effective method of diagnosing this injury. Extravasation of contrast is diagnostic. Attempted catheterization is controversial and can covert a partial urethral disruption into a complete disruption.

❑❑ **A 32-year-old male victim of a motor vehicle accident suffers a pelvic fracture. Retrograde urethrography shows extravasation at the level of the membranous urethra. He is otherwise stable and no other immediate management is planned by the trauma team or orthopedics. The best urological management at this point is?**

Management of a posterior urethral injury is controversial. In an otherwise stable patient, options include immediate realignment and delayed repair. Primary realignment may be possible in patients with limited pelvic bleeding. In this scenario every attempt is made to avoid the pelvic hematoma and a urethral Foley catheter is placed as well as a suprapubic catheter. In delayed repair a suprapubic catheter is placed and plans are made for a possible urethroplasty after convalescence from the injures.

❑❑ **Steps to gain length for an end-to-end bulboprostatic urethral anastomosis for repair of a stricture from membranous urethral injury include?**

Mobilization of the urethra up to the penoscrotal junction
Division of the intercavernosal septum
Inferior pubectomy
Routing of the urethra over one of the cavernosal crura

❑❑ **The best candidates for penile revascularization for traumatic impotence have what characteristics?**

1. Demonstration of a focal arterial obstruction without diffuse atherosclerosis
2. Young patients and otherwise healthy
3. Patient has strong sexual desire and highly motivated

❑❑ **A man presents with priapism. He gives a history of falling on a ladder and straddling one of the rungs 2 months ago. What are the likely characteristics of the blood aspirated from the penis?**

Blood gas determinations will show high oxygen levels since the likely etiology is arteriovenous fistula from the straddle injury.

❑❑ **The next step in treating the above patient with traumatic priapism is?**

Arteriography with selective embolization of the fistula.

❑❑ **A 24-year-old male suffers a gunshot wound to the penis. On examination there is an entrance wound in the lateral mid-shaft with an exit wound at the ventral penoscrotal angle. The next step should be?**

Performance of a urethrogram to check for urethral injury is mandatory prior to planned surgical intervention.

❑❑ **A urethrogram in a male with a gunshot wound to the penis demonstrates stretching and elongation of the urethra in the penile urethra but no extravasation. The best management for this injury is?**

The best management for this patient is careful placement of a small urethral catheter, and leave it indwelling for 10-14 days followed by a voiding cystourethrogram.

❑❑ **A urethrogram in a male with a gunshot to the penis shows extravasation in the mid-penile urethra. There is minimal swelling on physical examination. The patient is stable without other significant injuries. Management of the injury should consist of?**

Exploration, debridement and if the defect is small, primary repair.

❑❑ **In penile amputation injuries, how should the amputated portion of the penis be preserved for transport?**

Wrapped in saline soaked gauze, placed within a plastic bag which is then immersed in a cooler with ice slush surrounding the bag.

❑❑ **Penile reimplantation is performed with what anastomoses?**

The corpora cavernosa are anastomosed, as is the urethra. Attempts are made to microscopically anastomose the dorsal neurovascular structures. Finally, the skin edges are sutured together.

❑❑ **The clinical signs reported by the patient with penile fracture are?**

A "cracking" sound followed by pain, detumescence and swelling.

❑❑ **The diagnostic test recommended for patients presenting with penile fracture is?**

Urethrography. Approximately 10% of these patients will have an associated urethral injury.

❑❑ **The best management of penile fractures is?**

Surgical exploration, identification of the tunical injury and closure of the defect.

❑❑ **A male presents with the skin of the penis dark from ischemia from a constricting ring left on at the base of the penis for 24 hours. Management should be?**

Excision of ischemic penile skin as first step. Following resolution of the inflammatory process, split thickness, unmeshed skin grafts can be applied to cover the penis.

❑❑ **Testis ruptures from blunt trauma should be managed by?**

Exploration, debridement of nonviable tissue, reconstruction of the tunical defect.

❑❑ **Major scrotal skin loss can be managed by?**

Meshed split thickness skin grafts covering the testes and sutured to the remaining skin at the groin and perineum.

ADRENAL PHYSIOLOGY

Michael S. Cookson, M.D. and David J. Grossklaus, M.D.

❑❑ **Embryologically, does the adrenal arise from a single structure?**

No, the adrenal cortex and medulla are derived from embryologically distinct structures. The cortex develops from embryonic mesoderm and the medulla from embryonic neurectoderm The hormonal secretions of each have different actions. Regulation of cortical and medullary secretions are independent of each other. Despite their anatomic proximity there is virtually no functional relationship between the adrenal cortex and medulla.

❑❑ **What are the three zones of the adrenal cortex?**

Zona glomerulosa lies immediately beneath the capsule of the gland, the zona fasciculata is the middle zone and is the largest portion of the cortex, the zona reticularis is the innermost zone.

❑❑ **Is there a functional significance between the anatomic zonations of the adrenal gland?**

Yes, each anatomic zone is also a functional zone with aldosterone being produced exclusively in the zona glomerulosa, cortisol is produced in the two inner zones, zona fasciculata and the zona reticularis, adrenal androgens are produced in the inner cortical zone, the zona reticularis.

❑❑ **What are the building blocks of adrenal hormones?**

Adrenal cells are capable of synthesizing cholesterol *de novo*, but most of the adrenal cholesterol used for steroidogenesis is derived from circulating lipoproteins and in particular from low-density lipoproteins (LDL).

❑❑ **Adrenal androgen production is limited by what factors?**

Many steroid compounds can be synthesized by the adrenal cortex, however, the enzymes required for the production of testosterone and estrogen are found in low concentration in the cortical cells. Consequently, androgens are normally produced in only very small quantities.

❑❑ **What is the first step in the production of adrenal steroid hormones?**

The first step is the production of pregnenolone from cholesterol via two hydroxylations followed by cleavage of the cholesterol side chain. Pregnenolone has no known biologic activity but it is an intermediate in the production of all the biologically active steroid hormones.

❑❑ **What is the most important mineralocorticoid produced by the adrenal cortex?**

Aldosterone, although produced in small quantities is the most physiologically important mineralocorticoid. Other mineralocorticoids such as 11-deoxycorticosterone (DOC) have both glucocorticoid and mineralocorticoid properties but are secreted in such small quantities that they are physiologically unimportant.

❑❑ **Does the androgen precursor dehydroepiandrosterone (DHEA) have any androgenic activity in males?**

Only minimal; DHEA is secreted in large quantities by the adrenal cortex in males. DHEA has much less activity than testosterone, and in males the overall effect of DHEA as an androgen is negligible. In females both DHEA and androstenedione may be converted to testosterone at extra-adrenal sites, thus it has more androgenic activity in females.

❒❒ How are adrenal hormones stored?

Adrenal hormones are steroid hormones and as all biologic steroid hormones adrenal hormones are not stored but are secreted immediately upon synthesis. The rate of steroid hormone secretion can be controlled by regulation of synthesis.

❒❒ Are active forms of adrenal hormones free or bound in serum?

Only the free hormone is biologically active, however, all steroid hormones are largely protein bound when they circulate in plasma. Because of the limited solubility of steroid hormones in water, protein binding acts to increase the amount of hormone that can circulate in the blood. Since the protein bound fraction of hormone is relatively resistant to metabolism, protein binding also increases the plasma half-life of steroid hormones.

❒❒ What is the weight of a normal adult adrenal gland?

5 grams.

❒❒ What percentage of the adrenal gland is made up of the adrenal cortex?

The cortex constitutes 90% of the gland.

❒❒ What are the main physiologic functions of aldosterone?

To regulate sodium resorption in the kidney, gut, salivary gland and sweat glands.

❒❒ What is the site of action of aldosterone within the kidney?

The principle site of aldosterone action is the distal tubule of the nephron.

❒❒ What are the three endocrine glands required for regulation of cortisol synthesis and release?

The hypothalamus, pituitary and adrenal glands.

❒❒ Where is corticotropin releasing hormone (CRH) produced and what is its function?

CRH is synthesized in the hypothalamus and is carried to the anterior pituitary via the portal blood. CRH stimulates ACTH release.

❒❒ What are secondary stimulants of ACTH?

Vasopressin, oxytocin, epinephrine, angiotensin II, vasointeractive peptide, gastrin releasing peptide, atrionaturetic factor, and gamma-aminobutyric acid are all secondary stimulants.

❒❒ What complex is ACTH derived from?

ACTH is a 39 amino acid polypeptide produced from the protein proopiomelanocortin (POMC). Other POMC derivatives include; beta-lipotropin, alpha-melanocyte stimulating hormone, beta-melanocyte stimulating hormone, beta-endorphin, methionine, and enkephalin.

❒❒ Is ACTH produced constantly throughout the day?

No, ACTH secretion is characterized by an intermittent diurnal rhythm leading to parallel changes with cortisol and ACTH.

❒❒ What is the relationship between ACTH and circulating cortisol?

ACTH and circulating cortisol are reciprocally related.

❒❒ Is adrenal hormone production in the zona reticularis and fasiculata regulated by ACTH?

Yes, there is some influence of ACTH on the zona reticularis and fasiculata. After administration of ACTH both precursors, DHEA and DHEAS rise, thus leading to androgen production.

❑❑ What is the most significant regulator of aldosterone secretion?

Angiotensin II is the primary physiologic control of aldosterone secretion. Angiotensin II directly stimulates production of aldosterone by the zona glomerulosa. A second less important stimulus is an elevated serum potassium level. Hypokalemia blunts the adrenal gland's ability to synthesize aldosterone thus causing a decrease in production and secretion.

❑❑ What is the basis of aldosterone production and its role in the renin, angiotensin, aldosterone system (RAAS)?

In response to multiple stimuli, but primarily hypovolemia and decreased renal perfusion, renin is released from the juxtaglomerular apparatus (JGA) of the afferent arteriole. Renin cleaves angiotensin I (AI) from angiotensinogen. Angiotensin converting enzyme converts AI, to angiotensin II (AII) primarily in the pulmonary vasculature. Secretion of aldosterone results from direct stimulation of the adrenal gland by AII. The actions of aldosterone include: a) increased renal conservation of sodium, b) increased glomerular filtration fraction by increasing efferent arteriole tone, c) increased peripheral vasomotor tone, d) increased thirst. The overall effect is an increase in plasma volume and renal perfusion.

❑❑ What effects do glucocorticoids have on cellular metabolism?

Glucocorticoids are essential for life and affect a wide spectrum of cellular metabolism including increased glycogen synthesis, increased gluconeogenesis, impaired peripheral glucose utilization, muscle wasting, myopathy, osteopenia, and decreased immune mediated inflammation and hormonal interaction.

❑❑ What is the primary laboratory test to identify Cushing's syndrome if it is clinically suspected?

A 24-hour urine to measure cortisol and creatinine. The 24-hour urine collection commences following the first morning void, and continues throughout a 24-hour period until completion of the next morning void. The urine should remain refrigerated in an opaque container until transported to the lab.

❑❑ Urinary free cortisol can be used as a screening test for what adrenal disorder?

Cushing's Syndrome. Although 3.3% of individuals without Cushing's syndrome will have elevated values this test is 95% specific for Cushing's syndrome.

❑❑ What tests are used to distinguish adrenal tumors in women with hirsutism?

Serum testosterone and DHEA.

❑❑ What is the half-life of plasma aldosterone?

20-30 minutes.

❑❑ What are the major catecholeamines secreted by the adrenal medulla?

Epinephrine, Norepinephrine, Dopamine.

❑❑ Why is epinephrine secretion localized to the adrenal medulla?

The enzyme phenylethanolamine-N-methyltransferase (PNMT), is located exclusively in the adrenal medulla, catalyzes the methylation of norepinephrine to epinephrine. This can be clinically significant in patients with extraadrenal pheochromocytoma, in which case only norepinephrine is produced due to the absence of PNMT at the extraadrenal site.

❑❑ Are glucocorticoid and epinephrine production related?

Yes, high levels of glucocorticoids are necessary to maintain levels of PNMT and thus epinephrine production. This may explain the proximity of the adrenal medulla to the venous drainage system within the adrenal gland.

❏❏ **What are the substrates of Epinephrine and Norepinephrine?**

Dietary tyrosine and phenylalanine.

❏❏ **What is the major regulation of catecholamine biosynthesis?**

Activation of tyrosine hydroxylase activity, which combines phenylalanine and tyrosine to form dopa as a precursor to Norepinephrine. Tyrosine hydroxylase activity may be regulated by the adrenal cortex.

❏❏ **How are catecholamines stored?**

They are stored in separate vesicles within nerve terminals.

❏❏ **What causes preganglionic sympathetic nerves to release catecholamines?**

Stress, pain, cold, heat, asphyxia, hypotension, hypoglycemia, and sodium depletion all cause catecholamine release.

❏❏ **What is the serum half-life of catecholamines?**

Less than 20 seconds.

❏❏ **How are catecholamines degraded?**

They are degraded by the action of catechol-O-methyltransferase (COMT) and monoamine oxidase (MAO), following re-uptake by nerve terminals.

❏❏ **How are catecholamine breakdown products measured?**

The primary metabolite of catecholamine breakdown is urinary vanillylmandelic acid (VMA) with metanephrine and nor-metanephrine being secondary breakdown products. These are best measured by means of a 24-hour urine collection.

❏❏ **What is Cushing's syndrome?**

A symptom complex caused by excess glucocorticoid production.

❏❏ **What is Cushing's disease?**

Pituitary hypersecretion of ACTH, usually secondary to a pituitary adenoma, which results in increased production and secretion of glucocorticoids.

❏❏ **What percentage of patients with Cushing's syndrome actually have Cushing's disease?**

75-85% of Cushing's syndrome is due to Cushing's disease. Other causes of Cushing's syndrome include adrenal adenomas, adrenal carcinomas and ectopic secretion of either CRH or ACTH.

❏❏ **What is the most common cause of ectopic or exogenous glucocorticoid excess causing Cushing's syndrome?**

Exogenous steroid administration.

❏❏ **With respect to the normal diurnal variation with circulating cortisol levels, is the level higher in the morning or evening?**

Healthy subjects have a peak of cortisol levels in the morning with a fall throughout the day and into the evening. Patient's with Cushing's syndrome lose the diurnal variation of circulating cortisol.

❏❏ **What is Nelson's syndrome?**

Ten to 20% of individuals undergoing bilateral adrenalectomy for severe Cushing's syndrome will suffer from growth of a pituitary adenoma (usually a chromophobe adenoma). Growth of the space occupying lesion is attributed to the lack of hypothalamic/pituitary feedback and high levels of ACTH. With the development of treatments for Cushing's disease other than bilateral adrenalectomy, Nelson's syndrome is rarely encountered today.

❏❏ **What are the treatments of Cushing's disease?**

Treatments for Cushing's disease include: transphenoidal hypophysial microsurgery to remove the pituitary adenoma. This treatment is effective in 85-95% of patients. Other treatments include pituitary external beam radiation and heavy particle proton beam therapy.

❏❏ **If Cushing's syndrome is diagnosed during pregnancy, is immediate treatment warranted or should it wait until the post-partum period?**

Both maternal and fetal morbitiy have been reduced with treatment of Cushing's syndrome during pregnancy, either by surgical removal of an adrenal adenoma during the second trimester or by transphenoidal adenomectomy or with medications such as metyrapone.

❏❏ **What is Addison's disease?**

Addison's disease is an inadequate production of corticosteroids by the adrenal cortex caused by a defect within the adrenal cortex rendering them unable to synthesize normal amounts of steroid hormones.

❏❏ **What is the most common cause of adrenal insufficiency?**

The most common cause of Addison's disease is withdrawal of exogenous steroid therapy. Additional causes include: adrenal tuberculosis or lymphocytic adenitis with adrenal fibrosis, malignant infiltration of the adrenal, sarcoidosis, histoplasmosis, blastomycosis, and coccidioidomycosis. Additionally, Addison's disease may occur with administration of aminoglutethimide, ketoconazole, mitotane or suramin.

❏❏ **What is the classic triad of Addison's disease?**

Hyponatremia, hyperkalemia, and azotemia are the classic triad, however, the entire triad is present in only 50-60% of cases. Other disorders associated with Addison's disease may include hypercalcemia, hyperthyroidism, hypothyroidism and diabetes.

❏❏ **What symptoms are associated with Addison's disease?**

Symptoms associated with Addison's disease are weakness, prostration, dehydration and coma.

❏❏ **How does one diagnose Addison's disease?**

The clinical test for Addison's disease is failure to increase plasma or urinary corticosteroid levels in response to an ACTH infusion. The simple screening test is a cosyntropin stimulation test.

❏❏ **What can cause acute adrenal insufficiency?**

Acute adrenal insufficiency can be caused by withdrawal of exogenous steroids, sepsis, bilateral adrenal hemorrhage, surgical bilateral adrenalectomy, or surgical removal of a functional adenoma in a patient with an atrophic contralateral adrenal.

❏❏ **What is the treatment of acute adrenal insufficiency?**

The treatment is administration of glucocorticoids along with replacement of saline.

❏❏ **What is the treatment of chronic Addison's disease?**

Maintenance with chronic glucocorticoids and mineralocorticoids.

❏❏ **What is Conn's syndrome?**

Conn's syndrome is primary hyperaldosteronism.

❏❏ **What are the clinical features of Conn's syndrome?**

The clinical features of Conn's syndrome include hypertension, hypokalemia, hypernatremia, alkalosis and periodic paralysis.

❏❏ **What is the phenomenon of renal escape?**

In primary aldosteronism after a gain of 1.5Kg of extracellular fluid there is a decrease in absorption of sodium at the proximal tubules. Escape is associated with an increase in renal artery pressure and an increase in atrial naturetic factor (ANF). Renal escape limits the clinical hypertensive response in patients with primary hyperaldosteronism.

❏❏ **What is the most common cause of primary hyperaldosteronism?**

The most common cause is an aldosterone producing adenoma of the adrenal gland.

❏❏ **What is the most common cause of secondary hyperaldosteronism?**

The most common cause is renal arterial disease or renal parenchymal disease. This disease is a disorder with over secretion of aldosterone secondary to excess production of angiotensin II and the renin, aldosterone, angiotensin system (RAAS).

❏❏ **In treatment of an aldosterone producing adrenal adenoma, adrenalectomy should be preceded by what preoperative measure?**

Adequate clinical treatment of hypertension and correction of hyperkalemia or other metabolic abnormalities.

❏❏ **What is the treatment of primary aldosteronism caused by bilateral hyperplasia?**

The treatment is medication with the drug spironolactone, which is a competitive antagonist of the aldosterone receptor.

ADRENAL TUMORS

Christopher P. Evans, M.D.

❑❑ **What are the 2 general questions one needs to answer when working up an adrenal mass?**

Whether it is functional or nonfunctional and whether it is malignant or benign.

❑❑ **What is the differential diagnosis of a benign, incidental adrenal mass?**

The more common adrenal lesions are adrenal adenomas, myelolipomas and adrenal cysts. Less commonly one encounters ectopic tissue, pheochromocytoma, hyperplasia, aldosteronomas and adrenal hemorrhage. Adrenal hemorrhage can occur following difficult childbirth and more often affects the right side. This phenomenon has been attributed to an increase in intraabdominal pressure that is transmitted through the short right adrenal vein and into the parenchyma resulting in hemorrhage.

❑❑ **What is the differential diagnosis of a malignant adrenal mass?**

Adrenocortical carcinoma, pheochromocytoma, neuroblastoma, and metastatic disease.

❑❑ **What is the most direct and reliable index of glucocorticoid function?**

The 24-hour excretion of cortisol in the urine. Patients with Cushing's syndrome often lose the diurnal variation or show higher basal levels than healthy subjects.

❑❑ **In the dexamethazone suppression test, what serum and urine endpoints should change?**

There should be a fall in 17-hydroxycorticosteroid, urinary free cortisol, or plasma cortisol.

❑❑ **How does one determine if a patient has ACTH-dependent or independent hypercortisolism?**

The simultaneous measurement of both plasma ACTH (corticotropin) and cortisol by 2-site immunoradiometric assay.

❑❑ **When using the metyrapone-stimulation test to differentiate between pituitary Cushings and ectopic ACTH secretion, what result does one look for?**

Metyrapone blocks the conversion of 11-desoxycortisol to cortisol. As plasma cortisol concentrations fall, the pituitary gland secretes more ACTH, thus increasing urinary 17-hydroxy corticosteroid levels. Patients with Cushing's disease have a normal or supranormal increase in 17-hydroxy corticosteroid urinary excretion. Patients with ectopic ACTH-secreting tumors will have little or no increase in urinary 17-hydroxy corticosteriod levels since ectopic ACTH production will not be influenced by plasma cortisol feedback on the pituitary gland.

❑❑ **What is the radiographic appearance of a solitary adrenal adenoma?**

Adrenal adenomas are usually larger than 2 cm, associated with atrophy of the opposite gland, and are of low density due to the high lipid concentration.

❑❑ **Why is the size cut-off for an adrenal carcinoma reported to be both 5 and 6cm?**

Studies have shown that tumors <6 cm in size pathologically are unlikely to be adrenal carcinomas. However, CT scanning underestimates the size of the adrenal glands, so a 5cm cut-off is used radiographically as the equivalent of the 6cm pathologic size.

❏❏ **Name 3 agents used to reduce the secretion of functional steroids in patients with Cushing's syndrome.**

Aminoglutethimide blocks the conversion of cholesterol to pregnenolone. Patients given aminoglutethimide must be observed for adrenocortical insufficiency, since aldosterone production is also impaired. Metyrapone blocks the conversion of 11-desoxycortisol to cortisone. Ketoconazole blocks cytochrome P-450 mediated side-chain cleavage and hydroxylation at both the early and late steps in steroid biosynthesis.

❏❏ **What is Nelson's syndrome and when has it been seen in the treatment of Cushing's disease?**

Historically, patients with Cushing's disease often were treated with bilateral adrenalectomy. 10-20% of these patients subsequently developed pituitary tumors, usually chromophobe adenomas, secondary to the lack of hypothalamic/pituitary feedback and high ACTH production. This could occur years after bilateral adrenalectomy and can be treated by prophylactic pituitary radiation.

❏❏ **What is the currently accepted treatment of choice for Cushing's disease and what are the cure rates?**

Presently, transphenoidal hypophysial microsurgery for the removal of pituitary adenomas results in cure rates of approximately 90%.

❏❏ **How do functional adrenal carcinomas present?**

Functional adrenal lesions typically present as Cushing's syndrome, virilization in females with either increased DHEA-17 ketosteroid or increased testosterone, feminizing syndrome in the male, hyperaldosteronism, or a combination of the above.

❏❏ **What can one do to further work up an incidentally discovered nonfunctional adrenal mass, measuring between 3 cm and 6 cm in size?**

One can perform a fine-needle aspirate of the mass under ultrasound or CT guidance. Studies have supported a 96% incidence of obtaining significant cytologic material and an 86% incidence of accurately differentiating benign from malignant disease processes. Additionally, one can perform an MRI and a high signal-intensity ratio on T2 images suggestive of a malignant lesion.

❏❏ **What primary cancers metastasize to the adrenal gland?**

The most common metastatic lesions to the adrenal gland include melanoma and carcinoma of the breast and lung. Additionally, carcinomas of the kidney, contralateral adrenal gland, bladder, colon, esophagus, gall bladder, liver, pancreas, prostate, stomach, and uterus can metastasize the adrenal gland.

❏❏ **Virilization in the absence of elevated urinary 17-ketosteroids in a female patient should raise the suspicion of what other lesion?**

In addition to adrenocortical tumors that secrete testosterone, one should also consider testosterone-secreting ovarian tumors.

❏❏ **A male patient with a functional adrenocortical tumor presents with gynecomastia, testicular atrophy, and impotence. What is the presumed diagnosis?**

This patient likely has an estrogen-secreting adrenocortical tumor that secretes androstenedione, which is converted peripherally to estrogens. Eighty percent of these lesions are malignant, with the 3-year survival being <20%.

❏❏ **Can primary hyperaldosteronism be due to adrenal carcinoma?**

Yes. While primary hyperaldosteronism is usually due to small, benign, solitary adenomas, in Conn's syndrome or bilateral adrenal hyperplasia it also can be caused by adrenocortical carcinoma.

❏❏ **How does the presentation of adrenocortical carcinoma in children differ from that in adults?**

The majority of these tumors are hormonally active, usually presenting with Cushing's syndrome, virilization in the female, and isosexual precocious puberty in males.

□□ **What syndromes can be associated with adrenocortical carcinoma in children?**

Beckwith-Wiedemann syndrome (exomphalos, macroglossia, gigantism and neonatal hypoglycemia), isolated hemihypertrophy, and Li-Fraumeni syndrome.

□□ **What is the 5-year survival of adrenocortical carcinoma?**

Approximately 45%, with the most common metastatic sites being lung, liver, and lymph nodes.

□□ **What is the standard management of adrenocortical carcinoma?**

Surgical removal of the primary tumor, with an attempt to remove the entire lesion with contiguous organs (spleen, kidney) *enbloc* if necessary, and a regional lymphadenectomy.

□□ **What drugs are available for the medical management of advanced adrenocortical carcinoma?**

Mitotane, a DDT-derivative, has been shown to induce a tumor response in 35% of patients. Ketoconazol has an adrenolytic effect. However, these compounds, in addition to metyrapone, have not been shown to improve long-term survival.

□□ **Do calcifications in adrenal cysts suggest that these are actually malignant?**

No. Fifteen percent of adrenal cysts contain calcifications and this does not imply malignancy.

□□ **What findings constitute the diagnosis of primary hyperaldosteronism?**

Hypokalemia with metabolic alkalosis, suppressed peripheral renin activity, elevated urinary and plasma aldosterone levels in hypertensive patients.

□□ **What is the most sensitive diagnostic test for hyperaldosteronism?**

Urinary excretion tests are more sensitive than serum studies. A 24-hour urine for aldosterone and sodium under conditions of prolonged sodium loading (> 10 gm / day diet for 5-7 days) with urinary aldosterone > 14 micrograms and urinary sodium > 250 mEq confirms the diagnosis.

□□ **What plasma aldosterone to renin ratio is suggestive for primary aldosteronism?**

A plasma aldosterone to renin ratio >50 (aldosterone ng/dl to PRA ng/ml/hr) is more common in primary aldosteronism than either essential hypertension or renal vascular disease.

□□ **What is the best test to lateralize functional aldosterone-producing adenomas?**

Adrenal vein sampling of aldosterone is very sensitive lateralizing these lesions.

□□ **What is the management of a solitary unilateral adrenal mass identified on CT scan with biochemical criteria consistent with primary aldosteronism?**

After confirming functional status of the lesion surgical extirpation would be appropriate. Adrenal vein sampling is not essential to lateralize the tumor, but can be helpful.

□□ **In patients with primary aldosteronism secondary to bilateral adrenal hyperplasia, what is the medical management of choice and how does it work?**

Medical therapy consisting of Spironolactone (aldactone), which is a competitive antagonist of the aldosterone receptor is sufficient for many patients.

□□ **Is the pattern of hypertension with pheochromocytomas sustained or paroxysmal?**

Sustained hypertension is found in 37% of patients with pheochromocytomas, and is a more common finding in children and patients with multiple endocrine adenoma Type-2 (MEA-2). Paroxysmal hypertension affects approximately 47% of patients, females > males. A third pattern, sustained hypertension with superimposed paroxysms, is found in 50-65% of patients.

❏❏ Is it possible to have a pheochromocytoma in a normotensive patient?

Yes. Approximately 10% of pheochromocytomas are found in normotensive patients. It is important not to eliminate pheochromocytomas from your differential diagnosis in a normotensive patient with an adrenal mass.

❏❏ Pheochromocytomas may be part of what familial syndrome?

Pheochromocytomas occur in MEA-2, which is a triad including pheochromocytoma, medullary carcinoma of the thyroid, and parathyroid adenomas. In addition, pheochromocytomas are part of the MEA-3 which includes medullary carcinoma of the thyroid, mucosal neuromas, thickened corneal nerves, alimentary tract ganglioneuromatosis, and frequently a Marfanoid habitus. Pheochromocytomas may also be a component of MEA-2a or von Hippel Lindau disease. Finally, pheochromocytomas may be associated with neuroectodermal dysplasias, including Von Recklinghausen's disease (neurofibromatosis), tuberous sclerosis, and Sturge-Weber syndrome.

❏❏ How do the manifestations of pheochromocytoma in children vary from those in adults?

Children manifest a higher incidence of familial pheochromocytomas (10%) and bilaterality (25%). Additionally, there is a 15% -30% incidence of multiple pheochromocytomas in children and a 15% -30% incidence of extra-adrenal location as well.

❏❏ What laboratory tests confirm the diagnosis of pheochromocytoma?

Elevated levels of catecholemines in the blood or urine occurs in 95-100% patients with pheochromocytomas. Specifically, plasma norepinephrine, epinephrine, and dopamine levels and urinary catecholemines should be used as an initial test.

❏❏ What is the utility of CT scanning for detecting pheochromocytomas?

CT scanning detects >90% of pheochromocytomas of adrenal origin, and approximately 75% of extra-adrenal pheochromocytomas. Computed tomography alone cannot differentiate between pheochromocytomas and other adrenal lesions nor can one delineate malignant potential based upon the CT scanning alone.

❏❏ What is the characteristic appearance of pheochromocytoma on MRI scanning?

They appear as a characteristically bright image on T2-weighted studies. MRI is considered the best scanning procedure for patients with biochemical findings suggestive of pheochromocytoma.

❏❏ What is an MIBG scan and how is it useful?

The metaiodobenzylguanidine (MIBG) scan images adrenal medullary tissue and is particularly useful for identifying pheochromocytomas of extra-adrenal origin or multiple pheochromocytomas. The MIBG scan has an overall sensitivity and specificity of 87%, and 99% respectively.

❏❏ What is the preoperative medical preparation for patients with pheochromocytomas?

All patients must be vigorously hydrated in preparation for surgery since elevated catecholamines levels lead to significant dehydration. Additionally, patients are started on an alpha-adrenergic blocker such as phenoxybenzamine, with an initial divided dose of 20-30 mg orally, increasing to 40-100 mg as needed. Secondly, beta-adrenergic blockers can be added to the alpha-blockers to protect against arrhythmias and permit reduction in the alpha blocker requirement. Beta-blockers are usually only added when cardiac arrhythmias are identified.

❏❏ **What problem can arise if beta-blockers are initiated prior to alpha-blockers?**

There can be a marked rise in the total peripheral vascular resistance secondary to unopposed alpha adrenergic activity which can lead to circulatory collapse.

❏❏ **What additional drug might be used in the preoperative preparation of patients with pheochromocytomas who have cardiomyopathies, multiple catecholemine-secreting paragangliomas, or resistance to alpha blockers?**

Alpha-methylparatyrosine (metyrosine) decreases the rate of catecholemine synthesis (the conversion of tyrosine to Dopa).

❏❏ **How should the surgeon and anesthesiologist be prepared for fluctuations in blood pressure at the onset of anesthetic induction in surgery?**

The patient must be volume-expanded with several liters of intravenous crystalloid prior to induction of anesthesia. In addition, alpha and beta-adrenergic blocking agents should be readily available for IV use. Phentolamine, a short-acting alpha-blocker (50 mg per 500 cc of ringers lactate), or sodium nitroprusside (50 mg per 250 cc of 5% dextrose in H_2O) should be on hand. Esmolol or propranolol should be available for persistent tachycardias or arrhythmias.

❏❏ **What are the indications, advantages, and disadvantages for using a modified posterior incision for adrenal tumors?**

A modified posterior lumbotomy may be utilized in patients with right-sided adrenal aldosterone-secreting tumors or benign adenomas <5 cm. The main advantage over a flank or transabdominal incision is the excellent exposure of the vena cava in the region of the short right adrenal vein. The disadvantages include a limited visual field and compression of the abdominal contents and thoracic cavity that may impair respirations in the jack-knife position. This approach is not recommended for pheochromocytomas or malignant adrenal tumors.

❏❏ **Following surgical exposure of a pheochromocytoma, what anatomic structure must be initially addressed?**

The adrenal vein should be divided initially to avoid systemic release of catecholemines during manipulation of the adrenal gland.

❏❏ **When is laparoscopic adrenalectomy indicated?**

Laparoscopic adrenalectomy is a well established technique that can be applied to small adrenal tumors and even pheochromocytomas. Large tumors, especially adrenal carcinomas, are not well suited to this technique.

RENAL PHYSIOLOGY

Marc Beaghler, M.D. and Gregory Stewart, M.D.

❑❑ **The juxtaglomerular apparatus is composed of three cell types, the macula densa cells, the granular cells and the extraglomerular mesangial cells. Which cell type contributes to control of renin secretion?**

Macula densa cells. While the granular cells contain secretory granules containing renin, the macula densa contributes to control of renin secretion as well as control of glomerular filtration rate.

❑❑ **What are the three layers of the filtration barrier in the renal corpuscle?**

Capillary endothelium, basement membrane, and single celled layer of podocytes lining Bowman's capsule in contact with the glomerulus.

❑❑ **Glomerular filtration rate is in part determined by glomerular-capillary hydraulic pressure. What three factors determine this pressure and what is their influence on GFR.**

Increasing renal arterial pressure tends to increase GFR, increasing afferent arteriole resistance tends to decrease GFR, and increasing efferent arteriole resistance tends to increase GFR. The latter is clinically significant with respect to ACE inhibiting drugs. ACE inhibitors cause vasodilation of both the afferent and efferent arterioles; however, efferent arteriolar dilation is proportionally more than afferent arteriolar dilation. This results in a drop in hydrostatic pressure at the glomerulus and reduces GFR.

❑❑ **T/F: With regard to tubular resorbtion, glucose will not begin to appear in the urine at plasma concentrations substantially below the transport maximum concentration.**

False. Glucose will first appear when it reaches its threshold concentration which is significantly below transport maximum concentration. This difference is known as splay and is due to enzymatic induction of the glucose transporter as well as variability among the different individual nephrons.

❑❑ **Inulin is freely filtered at the glomerulus and is neither secreted nor resorbed. Calculate the GFR based on a urine inulin concentration of 500 mg / L, urine volume of 0.1 liters over 1 hours and a plasma inulin concentration of 5 mg / L.**

Amount filtered / time = amount excreted / time.
Amount filtered / time = GFR x plasma concentration.
Amount excreted / time = urine concentration x urine rate.
GFR = urine concentration x urine rate/plasma concentration.
GFR in this case = (500mg/L x 0.1L/1hr) / 5mg/L = 10 L/hr

❑❑ **Para-aminohippurate is freely filtered at the glomerulus, and when the plasma concentration is low, the remainder is secreted and none is resorbed. Because of these properties PAH can be used to measure what renal parameters.**

PAH can be used to estimate effective renal plasma flow as well as effective renal blood flow.

❑❑ **Increased plasma flow past the macula densa primarily affects what area of the renal vasculature?**

Increased plasma flow past the macula densa results in afferent arteriole vasoconstriction thereby reducing blood flow to the kidney which helps preserve the filtration fraction.

❏❑ **Renal autoregulation fails to maintain constant blood flow below what pressure?**

70mm Hg

❏❑ **The majority of sodium, chloride and water is reabsorbed in which portion of the tubule?**

Proximal, including straight and convoluted portions, driven by active processes.

❏❑ **What is the mechanism of action of the osmotic diuretic mannitol in the proximal tubule?**

Mannitol is freely filtered but not reabsorbed thus inducing the diffusion of water, followed by sodium and chloride into the lumen.

❏❑ **Which cells of the collecting ducts are targets for vasopressin, and what is the mechanism of action of vasopressin?**

Vasopressin acts on receptors located in the basolateral membrane of the principal cells. This induces migration and insertion of water permeable protein channels to the luminal membrane. Vasopressin is synthesized in the hypothalamus and secreted from the posterior pituitary in response to small changes in tonicity as well as in response to hypovolemia.

❏❑ **Compare obligatory water loss with insensible water loss.**

Obligatory water loss is the minimal amount of water necessary to dissolve waste products eliminated in the urine. It is determined by the maximum concentrating capability of the kidney and represents the minimum amount of urine, which must be produced. Insensible loss is the water lost though evaporation from the skin and respiratory tract unrelated to renal losses.

❏❑ **The countercurrent multiplier system relies on active sodium transport in which portion of the loop of Henle?**

The ascending portion of the loop of Henle contains active sodium transporters and is impermeable to water.

❏❑ **With regard to calcium homeostasis, what effect does increased parathyroid hormone levels have on renal phosphate handling?**

Increased serum parathyroid hormone levels act to increase urinary phosphate excretion by reducing proximal tubule reabsorbtion of phosphate.

❏❑ **Given that tubular reabsorbtion of calcium is increased in primary hyperparathyroidism, what is the net effect on urinary calcium excretion?**

Urinary calcium excretion is increased due to the overwhelming effect of increased filtered calcium load.

❏❑ **Which step in the synthesis of 1,25 dihydroxyvitamin D3 is the major physiological control point?**

The second hydroxylation at the 1 position occurs in the kidney and is subject to control by parathyroid hormone levels. The first step in hydroxylation at the 25 position occurs in the liver and is not a physiological control point.

❏❑ **Hydrogen ion secretion is accomplished by which cell type in the collecting ducts?**

Intercalated cells secrete hydrogen ion and reabsorb potassium.

❏❑ **What effect does extracellular volume contraction have on metabolic alkalosis?**

Hydrogen ion secretion is increased via aldosterone and other unknown mechanisms, thereby maintaining the preexisting metabolic alkalosis.

❏❏ **High plasma aldosterone levels in combination with potassium depletion can lead to what acid-base disturbance?**

Metabolic alkalosis is generated by excessive secretion of hydrogen ion. This condition can occur with use of potassium wasting diuretics.

❏❏ **Define tubuloglomerular feedback.**

The negative feedback system in which glomerular capillary pressure varies inversely with fluid delivery to the distal nephron.

❏❏ **By what mechanism does atrial natriuretic peptide increase GFR without increasing renal blood flow?**

Simultaneous afferent arteriolar vasodilatation and efferent arteriolar vasoconstriction. ANP also suppresses renin secretion and blocks secretion of aldosterone.

❏❏ **T/F: Creatinine clearance is always less than GFR at all levels of renal function.**

False, creatinine clearance always overestimates GFR due to tubular secretion of creatinine.

❏❏ **What is the mechanism of action of aldosterone on principal cells in the collecting duct?**

Aldosterone stimulates sodium reabsorption by increasing sodium conductance.

❏❏ **What are the four major effects of angiotensin II?**

Arteriolar vasoconstriction, decreased renal blood flow with increased filtration fraction, sodium retention, and stimulation of aldosterone synthesis.

❏❏ **T/F: Short-term response to changes in serum potassium levels are handled primarily by the cortical collecting duct.**

False, short-term potassium fluctuations are corrected by redistribution between intracellular and extracellular fluid compartments and do not involve the kidney.

❏❏ **Name the four classes of diuretics which are potassium wasting.**

Loop diuretics, thiazide diuretics, carbonic anhydrase inhibitors and osmotic diuretics.

❏❏ **What effect does magnesium deficiency have on potassium homeostasis?**

Magnesium depletion promotes potassium wasting and must be corrected prior to potassium replacement.

❏❏ **What is the most common electrolyte disturbance seen in clinical practice?**

Hyponatremia.

❏❏ **Define pseudohyponatremia.**

A lower reported value of sodium concentration associated with dilutional effects of hyperlipidemia or hyperproteinemia.

❏❏ **Hyponatremia occurs primarily with what type of diuretic?**

Thiazides, which inhibit NaCl reabsorbtion in the distal tubule.

❏❏ **In the setting of hypokalemic, hyperchloremic metabolic acidosis, how might one use the urinary anion gap to distinguish between GI losses and renal tubular acidosis as the etiology of the acidosis?**

In the absence of disease, urinary anion gap is normally close to zero. During GI bicarbonate loss, the increased ammonium excretion produces a markedly negative urinary anion gap. With renal tubular acidosis the gap is close to zero.

❏❏ **What effect does proximal (Type II) renal tubular acidosis have on serum potassium levels?**

Hypokalemia is present due to high rates of potassium excretion secondary to hyperaldosteronism and increased delivery of bicarbonate to the collecting duct. Calcium excretion is also elevated.

❏❏ **Which of the renal tubular (type I/type II) acidoses is self-limited?**

Type II, proximal RTA is self-limited because of equilibration of acid production and excretion at a lower plasma bicarbonate level. In type I, distal RTA excretion of titratable acid is impaired due to impaired secretion of hydrogen ion in the collecting ducts. Acidosis is progressive in this case.

❏❏ **What acid-base disorder is seen with severely decreased GFR?**

At a GFR of 20-30 ml / min hyperchloremic metabolic acidosis develops; when GFR decreases to below 15-20 ml / min an anion gap acidosis results.

❏❏ **What is the mechanism of action of loop diuretics within the kidney?**

Loop diuretics inhibit the $Na^+/K^+/Cl^-$ transport system on the luminal membrane of the thick ascending portion of the loop of Henle. The result is a reduction in the reabsorption of Na^+ and Cl^- in this portion of the tubule.

❏❏ **With regard to calcium handling, how does a loop diuretic compare to a thiazide?**

Loop diuretics promote excretion of calcium and may be used to treat hypercalcemia. In contrast, thiazide diuretics actually decrease the excretion of calcium.

❏❏ **What is the mechanism of action of thiazide diuretics.**

Thiazide diuretics inhibit NaCl reabsorption from the luminal side of the early segments of the distal convoluted tubule resulting in a diuresis. The resulting "dehydration" causes a compensatory increase in proximal tubule absorption of calcium and NaCl.

RENOVASCULAR HYPERTENSION

Jay L. Bloch, M.D.

❏❏ **T/F: Gadolinium- DTPA enhanced magnetic resonance angiography will not detect accessory renal arteries any better than non-enhanced images.**

False. Contrast images allow better visualization of accessory renal arteries. Studies are highly accurate in detecting R.A.S. >50%, with a sensitivity of 93% and specificity of 98%. M.R.A. is particularly useful in patients with impaired renal function who are at increased risk for contrast induced nephropathy.

❏❏ **Given a group of hypertensive patients on at least 3 anti-hypertensive medications, with a diastolic BP ≥ 95 mm Hg – What is the prevalence of R.A.S.?**

25%. This maybe a simple, but useful set of criteria by which to select patients for diagnostic studies. Renovascular hypertension accounts for approximately 5% of all hypertensive patients, yet it is the most common cause of secondary hypertension. Not only can R.A.S. cause hypertension, but it may also lead to progressive renal failure. Modern, less invasive diagnostic techniques, combined with percutaneous transluminal angioplasty and renal stenting, has stimulated a renewed interest in this subject.

❏❏ **T/F: Ischemic nephropathy accounts for ≤ 5% of patients with ESRD on dialysis.**

False. 17% of patients are dialysis dependent because of ischemic nephropathy. Significant R.A.S. has been demonstrated in >50% of patients with a creatinine clearance <50 ml/min. Particularly at risk are patients with DM, hypertension, and generalized atherosclerosis. Median survival of patients on dialysis due to ischemic nephropathy is 27 months vs. 56 months for other etiologies.

❏❏ **T/F: Fibromuscular dysplasia progresses to occlusion in 15% of patients.**

False. Nonatheromatous causes of R.A.S. do not commonly progress to occlusion, conversely, 15% of atherosclerotic R.A.S. cases progress to occlusion. The time to occlusion is brief (13 months) in patients presenting with > 75% occlusion.

❏❏ **T/F: Atherosclerotic R.A.S. progresses from less than 60% to greater than 60% within 1 year in 30% of patients.**

True. The lumen narrows most rapidly from <60% to >60%, 44% of patients progress by 2 years and by 3 years 48% progress. The progression occurs bilaterally in 20-50% of these patients.

❏❏ **In patients undergoing cardiac catheterization, risk factors for R.A.S. include each of the following except which one: extent of CAD, female sex, smoking, hypertension?**

Hypertension. Both multivariate and univariate analysis of patients undergoing cardiac catheterization failed to identify hypertension as a risk factor for significant R.A.S. Other risk factors that were identified include increasing age, CHF, PVD, Creatinine > 1.06 mg/dl.

❏❏ **T/F: Renal angiography is the gold standard for screening for R.A.S.**

False. Although angiography remains the gold standard for identifying R.A.S., risks include nephrotoxicity and possible complications of arterial puncture (hematoma, cholesterol embolization). Digital subtraction angiography may preclude the need for arterial puncture, but in so doing, requires a larger dose of contrast. CO_2 angiography obviates the need for iodinated contrast, but is not readily available and is more operator dependent. Lastly, conventional angiography may miss stenoses en face, requiring oblique imaging to project stenoses (as opposed to CT or MRI imaging)

❏❏ **T/F: A decrease in renal length of >1 cm is seen in most patients with R.A.S. > 60%.**

False. Renal dimensional changes of this magnitude are seen in only 26% of such patients. More important is doppler interrogation of the extrarenal and intrarenal (segmental, interlobar) arteries. Extrarenal doppler parameters include peak systolic velocity >200 cm/s, renal aortic ratio > 3.3 – 3.5, end diastolic velocity >150 cm/s. Intrarenal doppler parameters include resistive index < 0.45 – 0.59, difference of resistive index with contralateral kidney > 0.05 – 0.08, pulsatility index < 0.93 (difference of PI with contralateral kidney > 0.14), acceleration time > 60 – 120 ms and acceleration > 7.4 m/s^2.

❏❏ **Doppler renal sonography is highly accurate in screening for R.A.S.**

True. Five independent studies evaluating a total of 597 patients demonstrated a sensitivity of 89 – 93% and a specificity of 92-98%. Positive predictive value of 88-98% and negative predictive values of 92-98% were reported. The lumbar approach to evaluating the intraparenchymal arteries is unaffected by the number of accessory arteries, bowel gas, or obesity. DRS is operator dependent and may not yield accurate results regarding multiple renal arteries or branch occlusions. A galactose microbubble based agent may enhance the doppler signal but is generally not necessary.

❏❏ **T/F: Spiral CT angiography no longer requires contrast since predictions regarding R.A.S. can be made by evaluating renal arterial calcifications.**

False. 17% of patients with no calcification, 30% of patients with <3 mm calcification, and 44% of patients with >3 mm calcification had ≥75% R.A.S. However, the data does not preclude the use of contrast for accurate diagnostic information. Contrast enhanced CT studies may visualize vessels as small as 1 mm.

❏❏ **T/F: Captopril challenge tests and renal vein sampling are poor screening tools for ischemic nephropathy.**

True. These tests are most useful in differentiating renovascular hypertension from other etiologies. Ischemic nephropathy is often secondary to artherosclerotic R.A.S. The tests are less sensitive in the situation of bilateral disease and renal compromise.

❏❏ **T/F: Revascularization is considered primary treatment for R.A.S. (vs. medical therapy).**

True. Angiotensin converting enzyme (ACE) inhibitors have been shown to protect nonstenotic kidneys from nephrosclerosis due to hyperfiltration. Although angiotensin II may have a role in the progression of glomenular sclerosis and atherosclerosis, the effect on efferent arterioles and subsequent diminution of GFR may have a deleterious effect on renal function.

❏❏ **T/F: Surgical revascularization for ischemic nephropathy virtually always results in substantial improvement in serum creatinine.**

False. 55% of patients improved (ie. 20% decrease in serum creatinine), 32% of patients revascularized remained stable, 14% of patients worsened, and 6% died peri-operatively (accumulated data from 8 studies involving 352 patients from 1983-1992).

❏❏ **List 3 pre-operative criteria indicative of renal improvement following revascularization for total occlusion of the renal artery.**

Any of the following – collateral vessels with nephrogram on angiography, swift pre-op deterioration of GFR, patent vessels distal to proximal occlusion (back bleeding during revascularization surgery), viable nephrons on biopsy, renal length >9 cm, lateralization of renin secretion, and differential urinary concentration on split function tests. The criteria need to be used together as a guide as individual parameters lack predictive value.

❏❏ **Percutaneous transluminal angioplasty (P.T.A.) has failed to replace surgical revascularization for atherosclerotic lesions.**

True. Although P.T.A. has been as successful for nonostial lesions as surgery, 80-85% of atherosclerotic R.A.S. is an extension of aortic atherosclerosis involving the ostia. Dilation of ostial lesions is often unsuccessful.

❑❑ **Overall, 10% of renovascular operations for hypertension and renal insufficiency fail.**

True. Post-operative management following revascularization should include routine evaluation of blood pressure, serum creatinine, and periodic non-invasive radiologic assessment of renal blood flow (eg. doppler renal sonogram, nuclear renography, M.R.A.). Approximately 10% of patients following revascularization will demonstrate recurrent hypertension or a diminution of renal function. This may be due to re-stenosis of the operated vessel, stenosis of the contralateral renal artery, or progressive nephrosclerosis.

❑❑ **T/F: Splenorenal bypass is an ideal operation following a failed left aortorenal bypass.**

True. The success of the operation depends on the celiac trunk, which is visualized on the lateral aortic film of conventional angiogram, or by less invasive means. The splenic artery is divided proximally to avoid distal splenic atherosclerosis, and anastamosed end to end to the left renal artery. The spleen will remain viable as collateral blood flow is derived from the gastroepiploic and short gastric vessels.

❑❑ **T/F: Hepatorenal bypass is an ideal operation following a failed right aortorenal bypass.**

True. Patency of the celiac axis needs to be ascertained pre-operatively. A saphenous vein graft is interpositioned between the common hepatic artery (where it divides into the main hepatic artery and gastroduodenal artery, thus forming a trifurcation) and the renal artery. The proximal anastamosis is performed end to side and the hepatic artery is not divided because of ischemic risk to the gallbladder (ischemic risk to the liver is minimal due to portal venous circulation). An end to end anastamosis is performed to the kidney to reduce turbulent flow.

❑❑ **Iliorenal bypass or supraceliac aortorenal bypass are the operations of choice following a failed aortorenal bypass.**

False. If the celiac axis is involved by advanced disease or is inaccessible due to prior surgery, the operations above are indicated. Iliorenal bypass is limited by possible progressive disease involving the iliac vessel, and requires a long graft (saphenous vein or synthetic) directed cephalad. Supraceliac aortorenal bypass often requires a thoracic as well as an abdominal incision, and is much more difficult to tunnel to the right renal artery.

❑❑ **T/F: Renovascular surgery patients are commonly hypertensive post-operatively.**

True. Post-operatively these patients are hypertensive due to hypervolemia, hypothermic vasoconstriction, or pain, despite a patent arterial anastamosis. Management is with nitroprosside infusion to maintain the diastolic BP at approximately 90 mmHg to insure adequate renal perfusion (avoiding graft thrombosis) yet, not so high to prevent anastamotic hemorrhage.

❑❑ **T/F: Risk of hemorrhage following re-operation for renovascular disease is no different than that following the primary operation.**

False. Due to dense retroperitoneal fibrosis from the primary operation, hemorrhage is more likely to occur as embedded lumbar vessels are more difficult to secure and the anastamosis itself is more arduous. Other likely sources of hemorrhage include the ipsilateral adenal and an untied branch of a saphenous vein graft. Extra-aortic techniques during secondary operations avoid the potential complication of aortic hemorrhage requiring aortic clamping.

❑❑ **Renal artery thrombosis post-operatively following renovascular surgery occurs because of (list 2 reasons) _____ and _____.**

Hypotension, hypovolemia, arteriolar nephrosclerosis, or a hypercoagulable state may result in thrombosis. Kidneys with severe nephrosclerosis are best managed by nephrectomy. Technical problems are the most likely cause of post-operative thrombosis (mishandling, kinking, distortion, or angulation of the bypass graft, or atheromatous emboli).

❏❏ **T /F: Secondary revascularization results in cure or improvement in BP in 97% of patients.**

True. The operative mortality in one series was 1.4% with the incidence of nephrectomy being approximately 40% at re-operation. Nephrectomy will control BP as well as revascularization, and is indicated for the nonsalvageable kidney producing renin.

❏❏ **T/F: Renal arterial bypass grafting (RABG) is more likely to normalize serum creatinine in patients with renovascular hypertension vs. percutaneous transluminal renal angioplasty (PTRA) or percutaneous transluminal stent placement (PTSP).**

False. Actually all three failed to substantially alter creatinine in a study involving 130 patients. In comparing these modalities the results are as follows:

	PTRA	PTSP	RABG
Technical Success	91%	98%	92%
Complications	13%	16%	38%
Decrease in mean arterial BP at 12-months following procedure	21 mmHg	20 mmHg	20 mmHg
Initial treatment costs	$1,400	$2,600	$15,000

❏❏ **T/F: Results of percutaneous transluminal stent placement (PTSP) are dismal when utilized for atherosclerotic lesions within 5 mm of the renal artery ostium.**

False. Although serum creatinine did not improve significantly, the findings of this study of 108 patients are as follows:

Methods: 125 stents deployed (82 ostial stenoses, 43 ostial adjacent stenoses ie. <5 mm from renal ostium)

Results:	cured or improved	no change	worse
Renovascular hypertension	68%	27%	5%

Patency Rate:	primary	secondary @ 36 months
	74%	85%

Complications:	Contrast induced renal insufficiency	1
	Preinephric hematoma	1
	Death secondary to myocardial infarction	2
	Death secondary to progressive renal failure	2

❏❏ **T/F: Percutaneous transluminal stent placement is highly successful in preventing congestive heart failure and pulmonary edema in patients with bilateral renal artery stenosis or stenosis in a solitary functioning kidney.**

True. In this study 23 of 56 patients (41%) had a history of the above referenced co-morbidity prior to PTSP of one or both arteries. Following the procedure, 77% of these patients remained free of congestive heart failure and pulmonary edema (mean follow up 18.4 months). In contradistinction, only 4 of 34 subjects (12%) with unilateral stenosis and a normal contralateral kidney had a history of congestive heart failure or pulmonary edema, and only 1 of 3 (33%) subjects were free of CHF and pulmonary edema following PTSP.

❏❏ **Percutaneous transluminal renal angioplasty (PTRA) for ostial atherosclerotic renal artery stenosis yields results similar to percutaneous transluminal stent placement (PTSP).**

False.

	PTRA	PTSP
Primary success rate (<50% residual stenosis)	57%	88%
Secondary patency rate at 6 months	29%	75%
Re-stenosis following initial success	48%	14%

Secondary stent placement following early or late failure of PTRA resulted in success rates similar to patients undergoing primary PTSP. Despite the potential cost savings in stents using PTRA, the need for reintervention is greater. Therefore, PTSP is currently a better approach for ostial atherosclertotic stenosis.

RENAL TRANSPLANTATION

Nic Muruve MD, F.R.C.S.C.

❑❑ 36-year-old female under went a cadaveric renal transplant 2-days ago. Her donor was a 57-year-old male hypertensive who died of a stroke. Cold ischemia time was 26 hours. Her most recent creatinine is 7.8 mg/dl. Her current immunosuppressive agents include anti-thymocyte globulin (ATG) at 10 mg/kg, Mycophenolate mofetil 1 g bid, and Prednisone 50 mg bid. Her urine output has been ranging from 5-10cc an hour. A renal scan was obtained. Figure 1 demonstrates the transplant kidney 30 minutes after injection of isotope. The diagnosis is?

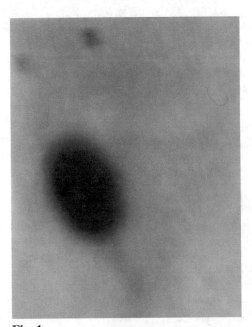

Fig. 1

The above history is suggestive of delayed graft function or acute tubular necrosis (ATN). Factors that contribute to ATN post-operatively include cadaveric donors, donor age, prolonged cold ischemia, unwitnessed cardiac arrest, pressor agents in the management of the donor, and poor perfusion of the kidney (low blood pressure). The renal scan demonstrates uptake of isotope but no excretion. This may also be seen in acute rejection and cyclosporine toxicity, however rejection 2 days post operatively is rare as immunosuppression is often maximized early on.

❑❑ 18-year-old female with a history of reflux nephropathy and neurogenic bladder receives a living related kidney transplant from her mother. Her creatinine has come down from a pre operative value of 10.8 mg/dl to 4.7 mg/dl on post-operative day number 2. She develops some mild lower abdominal pain over the incision and a temperature of 38.1° C. Cyclosporine level is normal. A renal scan is obtained. Figure 2a shows the transplant kidney 4 minutes after injection of isotope, and figure 2b is the same study 24 minutes after injection. The diagnosis is?

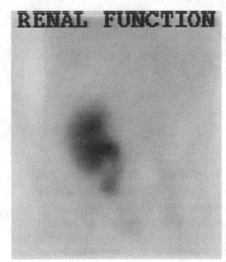

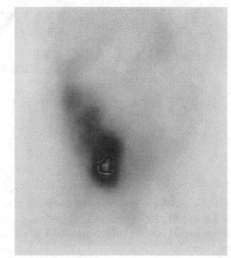

Fig. 2a   **Fig. 2b**

The scan demonstrates extravasation of isotope beyond the ureter and likely into the para-colic gutter supporting a diagnosis of a urine leak. If present, urine leaks are usually identified early in the post-operative course and often within the first week since surgery. Early clinical findings include wound leakage, pain, fever, and deterioration of renal function. The most common causes for leakage include ureteral damage during retrieval, ischemic ureter, surgical technique, and urinary retention. This patient was voiding with a large residual urine volume after surgery and likely disrupted her anastamosis. Treatment, in this case, consists of surgical repair of the leak with intermittent catheterization to prevent future recurrence.

❑❑ **A 40-year-old diabetic male received a cadaveric renal transplant 6-weeks ago. He presents in clinic with a swollen right leg and a rise in his creatinine from 1.5 mg/dl to 2.2 mg/dl. Cyclosporine level is 186 ng/ml. A renal ultrasound and CT scan were obtained (fig.3a, 3b). Diagnosis?**

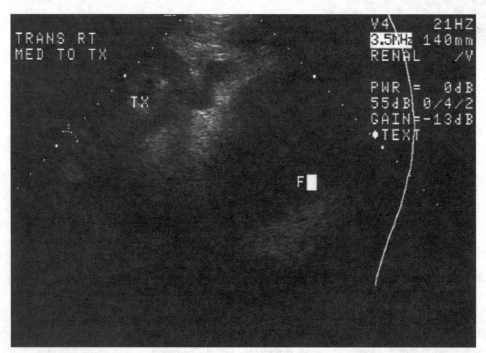

Fig. 3a

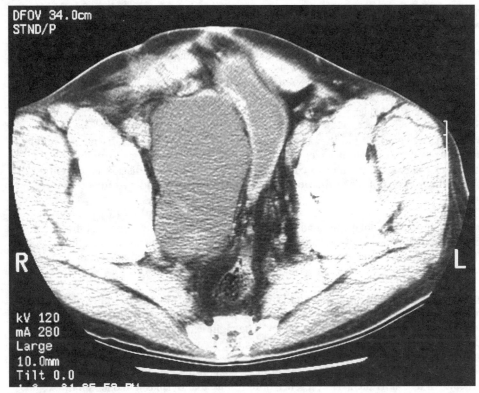

Fig. 3b

The ultrasound demonstrates a fluid collection with mild hydronephrosis of the transplanted ureter. CT scan confirms the fluid collection is separate from the bladder. Fluid aspiration for creatinine level will determine whether it is lymphatic or urine. Lymphoceles are more common 6-weeks out from surgery and in this case the fluid had a creatinine level of 2.6 mg/dl supporting a diagnosis of lymphocele. These occur from lymphatic leaks from the donor kidney or surrounding iliac lymphatics of the recipient. Treatment is marsupialization into the peritoneal cavity either laparoscopically or with an open procedure.

❑❑ **A patient received a renal transplant 10-days ago. The post-operative course was complicated by wound drainage and a urine leak was diagnosed. He is taken to the operating room to repair the leak and upon exposing the ureteral-vesical anastamosis site, the distal one third of the ureter is found to be ischemic. What is the best management option?**

Pyelovesicostomy offers the best option for a successful outcome. Ischemic necrosis of the ureter is due to damage to the arterial supply usually during the kidney harvest. The arterial supply to the ureter comes solely from the renal hilar vessels. Therefore, minimizing the amount of ureter used by trimming it back to the renal pelvis will improve the chance of obtaining viable tissue. Another option would include pyelo-ureterostomy to the patient's native ureter on that side. If his urine output is marginal in the native kidney, the proximal native ureter may be tied off and an end to end anastamosis over a stent can then be done from the donor renal pelvis to the native distal ureter.

❑❑ **An 18-year-old female with end stage renal disease secondary to vesicoureteral reflux presents for evaluation for a possible renal transplant. She makes about 1 liter of urine a day. A urinalysis demonstrates bacteriuria and 5-10 WBC's /hpf. She is asymptomatic. The next step in her evaluation would include:**

A urine culture to confirm an infection as well as a voiding cystourethrogram is needed to further evaluate the extent of her disease. High-grade reflux may act as a reservoir for persistent bacteria and infection in the post transplant period. These should be addressed prior to transplantation.

❑❑ **A 35-year-old male with a T6-7 cord injury from an MVA 19 years ago presents for renal transplant evaluation. He has developed end stage renal disease secondary to vesicoureteral reflux.**

He is on intermittent catheterization but despite q2h caths, he is still incontinent. His pre-transplant management would include:

A cystometrogram and a leak point pressure will confirm that he has a small volume, high pressure bladder. This needs to be corrected prior to transplantation or the renal allograft will fail similarly to his native kidneys. Anticholinergic therapy may help but he will likely require a bladder augmentation prior to transplantation. This is preferable over an ileal conduit as the risk for pyelonephritis is less and you preserve the use of the patient's bladder.

❏❏ **A 45-year-old farmer requires a kidney transplant. He has end stage renal disease secondary to diabetes. During your evaluation you discover that he was recently treated for a squamous cell carcinoma on the back of his neck, which was completely excised. No nodal disease is present on examination. Assuming the rest of his evaluation is normal, can he be considered for transplantation?**

Yes, nonmelanotic skin lesions are not a contraindication to transplantation. Recurrences of those tumors can be effectively followed clinically and treated as they arise. Prophylaxis with sunscreen after transplantation should also be recommended. Contraindications would include untreated malignancies or recent treatment (less than 2 years) of other non-skin (except melanoma) cancers.

❏❏ **A 48-year-old mother is willing to donate a kidney one of her kidneys to her daughter with end stage renal disease. During her evaluation, a renal angiogram of her kidney is obtained. She is found to have 2 left renal arteries and one right renal artery. The right renal artery is also found to have evidence of mild fibromuscular dysplasia. The best choice is:**

None, the mother is not a candidate for donation. The primary goal during the evaluation of a living donor is not to risk the health of that individual. The presence of fibromuscular dysplasia in one kidney excludes her rules as a donor since the potential exists for her to develop the same condition in the contralateral kidney. Angioplasty or vascular reconstruction can be considered but only after thorough discussion with all involved. Renal donation is not a good option in this case as it could jeopardize the donor's health in the future.

❏❏ **A patient with rising creatinine gets a transplant renal biopsy. The histology shows proliferative endarteritis, interstitial fibrosis, and tubular atrophy. This is consistent with:**

Chronic renal rejection is a slow inflammatory process resulting in renal damage. It is associated with gradual dysfunction and eventual graft loss, and does not respond to current anti-rejection therapies. The only treatment is re-transplantation.

❏❏ **T-cell activation is an important step in the initiation of a rejection response. In order for T-cells to proliferate what 2 events need to occur at the cellular level between the T-cells and antigen presenting cells?**

T-cell activation requires the interaction of the T-cell receptor and the antigen, MHC class II complex on the antigen presenting cell. This is termed signal 1. However, this alone will not cause T-cell expansion. Interaction between CD28 and B7-1, or –2 is necessary to start the inflammatory process. This is termed the second signal (signal 2, costimulation) and without it, it will cause anergy of the T-cells to the antigen.

❏❏ **A 23-year-old female undergoes cadaveric renal transplant. She receives anti-thymocyte globulin (ATG) at 10 mg/kg as induction, Azathioprine 1.5 mg/kg, and Prednisone. Post-operatively her urine output is adequate and creatinine is decreasing. A white count was obtained which was 4.2 thou/mm^3 and a platelet count was 78 thou/mm^3. The most likely cause is:**

ATG is known to cause thrombocytopenia. Management of this involves lowering the dose of ATG and at times even stopping the drug if the former doesn't work. Azathioprine is a purine analogue and antiproliferative agent. It is associated with bone marrow suppression and can affect all cell lines.

❏❏ **A 48-year-old male underwent cadaveric renal transplant 7-months ago. His immunosuppression consists of Prednisone, Mycophenolate mofetil, and Cyclosporine. His post-transplant course had been unremarkable until one week ago when he developed lethargy, lack of** energy, and a temperature of 38.1 degrees C. Lab tests revealed a WBC of 3.1 thou/mm^3, platelet count of 103 thou/mm^3 and a hemoglobin of 12.9 g/l. His evaluation should include:

Cytomegalovirus (CMV) is a common infection of transplant recipients. It can present clinically with lethargy, leukopenia, thrombocytopenia, hepatitis, gastrointestinal ulceration or inflammation, chorioretinitis, and pneumonia. The diagnosis can be confirmed by culture of the buffy coat, PCR analysis, or inferred by changes in CMV IgG or IgM titers. Treatment consists of decreasing immunosuppressive medications, antivirals (Ganciclovir), and gamma globulin.

❑❑ **A recipient of a renal transplant develops fever, rising creatinine and peripheral adenopathy. A transplant renal biopsy demonstrates a lymphocytic infiltrate and node biopsy reveals a B cell lymphoma. This condition is seen in patients with which risk factors?**

Post-transplant lymphoproliferative disorder (PTLD) is associated with primary Epstein-Barr virus (EBV) infection, excessive immunosuppression, and preceding symptomatic CMV infection. Level of EBV replication appears to have predictive value in assessing the risk of the disease.

❑❑ **A 75 kg patient is diagnosed with post-transplant lymphoproliferative disorder. He was transplanted 7 months prior to the diagnosis and his immunosuppression consists of Cyclosporine 250 mg bid, Azathioprine 125 mg qd and prednisone 10 mg qd. Management of this problem should include.**

Decrease or even withdrawal of immunosuppression is an important part of curing this condition. PTLD is often the result of excessive immunosuppression associated with a positive EBV serology. Other areas of possible treatment include anti-viral therapy, adoptive immunotherapy, chemotherapy and/or radiation.

❑❑ **A 28-year-old 65 kg female with a stable renal graft for 3 years wishes to get pregnant. Her creatinine is 1.9 mg/dl and her medications include Cyclosporine 125 mg bid, Azathioprine 75 mg qd and Prednisone 5 mg qd. Your advice to her on whether to proceed with pregnancy is?**

Successful pregnancies in renal transplant recipients have been extensively reported. The incidence of birth defects in neonates from mothers on immunosuppressive medication is no different than in the non-transplanted population. Patients on Cyclosporine may see higher rates of hypertension (20-60%) and preeclampsia (30%) and about 50% of babies are born prematurely or of low birth weight. There appears to be no increase risk of injuring the transplant kidney during vaginal delivery, however cesarean section rates remain high for fear of renal damage during delivery.

❑❑ **Organ preservation solutions are designed to mimic what fluid type?**

Prolonged preservation of organs became possible with the development of solutions that resembled intracellular fluid. This prevented cellular edema and the loss of intracellular potassium. Other items deemed necessary in preservation fluids include osmotic agents, such as mannitol, free radical scavengers (glutathione), adenosine (ATP precursor and vasodilator), membrane stabilizers (steroids) and pH buffers.

❑❑ **A 27-year-old male with end stage renal disease secondary to obstruction from posterior urethral valves presents for transplant evaluation. He had an ileal conduit placed at the age of 7 years, and he still drains urine through it. The rest of his evaluation is essentially negative. Part of his pre-transplant should include:**

People with prior urinary diversions should have their native bladders considered for transplant ureteral implantation. This evaluation should include urodynamic studies, (to assess for capacity, flow rate, filling pressure, compliance and continence) as well as a VCUG to assess the extent of residual valve tissue. Undiversion, if possible, offers a better option by decreasing the risk of infection and urologic complications. If the bladder is not usable, the existing diversion can be used.

❑❑ **A 47-year-old female is diagnosed with allograft failure and has been placed back on dialysis. She is still on Cyclosporine 125 mg bid, Azathioprine 75 mg qd and Prednisone 10 mg qd. Her nephrologist starts to decrease her immunosuppression by stopping her azathioprine and cyclosporine and tapering her prednisone over 2 weeks. After 10 days the patient presents with pain over her graft, fever and microhematuria. Management would include:**

This patient is experiencing an acute rejection of her kidney from too rapid a decrease in her immunosuppression. Azathioprine can be stopped immediately. Cyclosporine can be reduced by 50% and discontinued after 2 months. Prednisone should be tapered gradually over 2 to 3 months. This patient should be treated with a steroid bolus to reverse the rejection and then placed on a longer taper. If the symptoms cannot be reversed, then a transplant nephrectomy is indicated.

❑❑ **A 12-year-old girl underwent a cadaveric renal transplant. She received anti-thymocyte globulin induction therapy and then was started on steroids and Azathioprine. Her post-operative course was unremarkable and her creatinine decreased to 2.8 mg/dl on day 3 after surgery. She should now be started on:**

A calcineurin inhibitor should be added at this point. Her renal function is satisfactory and should tolerate it. The choice is between Cyclosporine and Tacrolimus. Although the experience with tacrolimus is limited in pediatric patients, it may be a better choice than Cyclosporine because of its side effect profile. Tacrolimus has no hypertrichosis and minimal gingival hyperplasia, and, because of this improved cosmetic side effect profile, may be a better choice in the adolescent age group.

❑❑ **A 6-year-old boy has end stage renal disease secondary to chronic obstruction from recurrent renal calculi. A metabolic work up for his stones reveals high serum and urinary oxalate levels consistent with type 1 hyperoxaluria. He has no evidence for urinary tract infection. Your recommendation regarding his candidacy for a renal transplant is:**

Type 1 hyperoxaluria has been considered as a contraindication to renal transplantation due to the deleterious effect of oxalate deposition in the graft. However, a combined kidney and liver transplant would provide the deficient enzyme and thus prevent further stone formation. Intensive hemodialysis to reduce plasma oxalate prior to surgery and post-operative diuresis will also decrease the risk of oxalate deposition in the new kidney.

❑❑ **A 34-year-old diabetic undergoes kidney-pancreas transplantation. Three months post-operatively he presents with frequency, urgency, dysuria, and hematuria. Urinalysis shows a pH of 5.5, mild proteinuria, numerous RBC's and WBC's. Urine culture is negative. The cause and management of this condition is:**

Urinary drainage of the exocrine function of the pancreas can lead to activation of the enzyme trypsinogen. This can be brought on by acid urine, volume depletion or bladder dysfunction and can result in a chemical cystitis, urethritis or balanitis. Treatment involves analgesics, hydration, alkalinization of urine, and Foley catheter drainage. Antibiotics are useful if concomitant infection is present. If symptoms are refractory to treatment, conversion to enteric drainage of the pancreas is indicated.

❑❑ **A 53-year-old diabetic female received a living related kidney from her brother. Her post-operative course is unremarkable and she is discharged on Prednisone, Azathioprine and Cyclosporine. Two weeks later, she sees her local doctor who notices some of her medications were not renewed after surgery. He places her back on Famotidine for her acid reflux, Allopurinol for her gout, and Trazadone for her "mood swings". Four weeks later she presents with lethargy, fever, and a white count of 1.3 thou/cu.mm. Management should include:**

This patient has leukopenia and likely developed an infection as a result. Once appropriate cultures are obtained and broad spectrum antibiotics started, her low count needs investigation. A likely cause was the addition of Allopurinol. This, in combination with Azathioprine, can cause significant marrow suppression. The Allopurinol should be stopped to see if it restores her white count. If Allopurinol is essential in her care, then it can be restarted with a decrease in the Azathioprine dose and careful monitoring of her cell counts.

❑❑ **A 27-year-old male with an ileal conduit and renal failure secondary to neurogenic bladder presents for transplant evaluation. He has had his conduit for 18 years, and his bladder is still in place. During his evaluation, you order a urodynamic assessment of his bladder and find his bladder volume to be 250 cc's, no hyperreflexia and a urine flow rate of 9 ml/min with a post-void residual of 175 ml. His best option for drainage is:**

Although he has a low flow rate and poor emptying of his bladder, he will likely do better with undiversion to his bladder. He will likely need to do intermittent catheterizations but this is associated with a lower infection rate than conduit drainage. He will need to have this reviewed with him prior to transplantation and if the patient is motivated, he can start to learn the procedure prior to his surgery. His low bladder volume may also improve with time once a normal urine flow returns to the bladder.

❑❑ **A 46-year-old 75 kg female receives a cadaveric renal transplant. She has end stage renal disease secondary to diabetes. Post operatively her urine output is > 100cc's an hour and her creatinine has dropped from a pre-op value of 7.6 mg/dl to 3.8 mg/dl over 2 days. Her medications at this point include Basilixumab 20 mg IV on day 1 post surgery, Cyclosporine 250 mg bid, Mycophenolate mofetil 1 g bid and Prednisone 50 mg bid on a taper. Her Cyclosporine level is 395 ng/ml. Her serum potassium is 6.5 meq/L. She receives Kayexalate, Sodium bicarbonate and insulin with IV dextrose but her potassium only drops to 6.2 meq/L. Another management option should include:**

Cyclosporine is known to produce hyperkalemia in the face of improving renal function. She did not respond to standard treatment in this case and her Cyclosporine level is high (normal 200-250). Reduction of her Cyclosporine dose may improve her potassium or at least make it more responsive to treatment. This should be combined with a decrease in her dietary potassium plus discontinuation of any potential potassium sparing diuretics.

❑❑ **A renal biopsy is obtained from a renal transplant patient with a rising creatinine. The histology is read out as interstitial lymphocytic invasion, mild tubulitis with normal glomeruli and vessels. The diagnosis is:**

This biopsy demonstrates mild acute rejection. The cellular infiltrate and tubular changes are characteristic for rejection. In more severe cases, lymphocytic infiltration of vessels and a larger interstitial inflammatory response is seen.

❑❑ **A 31-year-old renal transplant recipient develops a persistent cough and low-grade fever. She sees her local doctor who diagnoses mycoplasma pneumonia and starts her on Erythromycin 500 mg tid. Her renal function is normal (creatinine = 1.7 mg/dl) and she is on Cyclosporine, Mycophenolate mofetil and Prednisone. Five days later she presents with hypertension (BP 180/110), tremors, and an elevation of her creatinine to 2.3 mg/dl. The best method to resolve these abnormalities is:**

This patient is demonstrating signs of Cyclosporine toxicity. The best way to confirm this is to obtain a Cyclosporine level. The likely cause of this sudden elevation is the Erythromycin. Erythromycin will inhibit the elimination of Cyclosporine through the P450 enzyme system. The best course of action here is to lower her Cyclosporine dose and monitor her Cyclosporine levels. Once she stops the Erythromycin, she can return to her normal Cyclosporine dose.

❑❑ **A renal transplant recipient presents with new onset hypertension. He is one year out from his transplant and his medications include Tacrolimus, Mycophenolate mofetil, and Prednisone. His Tacrolimus level is normal; his most recent creatinine level is 1.8 mg/dl. On examination his blood pressure is 192/105, pulse 86. Abdominal exam reveals no masses, no tenderness, normal bowel sounds and a bruit over the right lower quadrant. Pulses are normal to palpation. Diagnostic options for the hypertension include:**

Transplant renal artery stenosis usually presents between 3 and 24 months after surgery. Hypertension is the usual mode of presentation but this can also be seen with graft dysfunction. This diagnosis is made more difficult in patients with existing hypertension and/or marginal renal function. Deterioration of renal function after being placed on angiotensin-converting enzyme inhibitors may suggest the diagnosis, but to confirm its presence, doppler ultrasound and/or angiography are required.

❑❑ **The same patient from the previous question undergoes angiography and confirms renal artery stenosis in the transplant kidney. Treatment options include:**

There are 3 options available for treatment. First is medical management. If he can be controlled with a reasonable level of medications and his creatinine remains stable, then no further treatment is required. The second option is angioplasty. This can often be done at the time of angiography but is associated with a recurrence rate as high as 16% and response rates are variable. In general lesions 1 cm away from the anastamosis respond better than lesions located at the site of anastamosis. The latter have a higher chance of rupture at the time of angioplasty. Finally surgical repair can be done but should be approached cautiously as the degree of fibrosis around the vessels and kidney make this a very difficult undertaking.

☐☐ **A patient undergoes cadaveric renal transplantation and is treated initially with anti-thymocyte globulin, Prednisone and Azathioprine. Once his renal function drops below 4.0 mg/dl he is started on Cyclosporine. One week after his transplant he experiences a rise in his creatinine and a diagnosis of acute rejection is made by biopsy. He responds to pulse steroids with normalization of his creatinine. Two weeks later he returns again with an elevation of his creatinine and an ultrasound demonstrates a large fluid collection in the pelvis with hydronephrosis. Treatment would include:**

Pelvic fluid collections in a transplant patient can be either lymphatic or urine. This can be confirmed by needle aspiration of the fluid and sending a sample for creatinine level. This patient was found to have a urine leak, as the creatinine level of the fluid was 64 mg/dl. Urine leaks can present late especially when associated with a history of rejection or other conditions that can affect its blood supply. Management this far out from transplantation is best carried out percutaneously as surgical treatment is more difficult. Percutaneous nephrostomy tube insertion and nephrostogram will confirm the site of leakage and also allow for antegrade stent placement. Percutaneous drain placement is also required and this will usually allow the leak to resolve. If it fails to repair itself, then surgical intervention is required.

☐☐ **A 39-year-old female with a living related renal transplant done 2 years previously presents with a rising creatinine. An ultrasound study demonstrated hydronephrosis of the transplant kidney and a 2 cm stone in the renal pelvis. No other abnormalities are detected. Treatment options include.**

Calculus disease in a transplant kidney can be treated in the same fashion as stones in non-transplant kidneys. Percutaneous nephrolithotomy is easily performed in transplant kidneys due to their superficial location and is probably the best option in this case. Other options include ESWL in the prone position, and ureteroscopy. Ureteroscopy is often the most difficult option due to the position of the transplant ureter. Flexible ureteroscopy is a better choice to gain endoscopic access to the ureter if needed.

☐☐ **A 52-year-old diabetic male undergoes cadaveric renal transplantation. Post-operatively he is placed on Prednisone, Tacrolimus, and Mycophenolate mofetil. During his hospital stay his blood glucose levels run high ranging 300-400 mg/dl. He is placed on an insulin pump but his glucose level remains difficult to control. Another option to be considered for the management of his hyperglycemia would be:**

Tacrolimus is known to cause insulin resistance in transplant patients. Lowering the dose of this drug or even stopping it in favor of Cyclosporine may make his glucose levels easier to control since there is a lower incidence of steroid induced diabetes with Cyclosporine.

☐☐ **A 51-year-old 80 kg male receives a cadaveric renal transplant. He is placed on Cyclosporine, Azathioprine and Prednisone. His post-operative course is unremarkable. Three months after his transplant his creatinine is noted to rise and a biopsy confirms acute rejection. His medications at this point include Prednisone 10 mg a day, Cyclosporine 225 mg bid, and Azathioprine 100 mg a day. His cyclosporine level was 235 ng/ml at the time of diagnosis. His rejection responds to 3 days of IV Solumedrol 500 mg. Appropriate management of his immunosuppression at this point should include:**

This patient developed a rejection episode on what appears to be adequate immunosuppression. A normal Cyclosporine level and appropriate doses for his weight confirm this. Now that his rejection is treated, he should not be placed on the same regimen that brought on the rejection. An appropriate alternative would be switching Cyclosporine to Tacrolimus and changing Azathioprine to Mycophenolate mofetil. This should decrease his risk of future rejections.

☐☐ **A kidney transplant recipient is diagnosed with acute rejection. He is initially treated with steroids but fails to respond. He then is started on OKT3 5 mg a day for treatment of steroid resistant rejection. On the first day of his treatment he develops fevers, hypotension and shortness of breath. The most likely cause for this is:**

OKT3 is a monoclonal antibody directed at the CD3 antigen on T cells. It depletes circulating T cells and modulates or removes the CD3 molecule from the cell surface making the cell nonfunctional. A side effect of OKT3 is cytokine release syndrome seen usually within the first 30 to 60 minutes of the first or second dose. It presents with fevers, chills, nausea, vomiting, diarrhea, weakness, myalgia, bronchial spasm or hypotension. It is believed to be mediated through cytokine release, mainly TNF and INF-γ. Premedication with anti-histamines, steroids and non-steroidal anti-inflammatory drugs will reduce the symptoms.

❒❒ **Daclizumab, a novel immunosuppressive agent, was recently approved for use in transplant recipients. Its mechanism of action is:**

Daclizumab is a humanized murine monoclonal antibody directed towards CD25, the IL-2 receptor. It competitively inhibits IL-2 from binding to its receptor on the T cell and has been shown to be a useful agent when used with other immunosuppressive drugs for induction therapy.

❒❒ **A renal transplant recipient elects to undergo surgical drainage for a recurrent pelvic lymphocele. During the procedure, while opening the lymphocele sac, the transplant ureter is accidentally cut. The best method of repair is:**

A new ureteroneocystostomy is the procedure of choice. If the ureter is not long enough then a psoas hitch or boari flap would be required. The blood supply of the transplant ureter comes entirely from the renal artery. Therefore only the proximal portion is viable. Attempts at uretero-ureterostomy will fail due to the now ischemic distal portion.

❒❒ **A patient is preparing to receive a cadaveric renal transplant from a 27 year old MVA donor that has recently become available. During the evaluation you get a phone call saying the crossmatch is positive. This means:**

A crossmatch is performed by mixing donor lymphocytes with recipient serum. A positive result means that the donor cells were lysed and thus indicates that the recipient serum had pre-formed anti-donor-HLA antibodies. Anti-HLA antibodies are developed through exposure to foreign HLA. This can occur through previous transplants, blood transfusions, and pregnancy. Transplantation in this setting will result in hyper-acute rejection and therefore the next available candidate should be evaluated.

❒❒ **A 47-year-old diabetic female has undergone 2 previous renal transplants. Both failed due to rejection, one after 2 years and the most recent one after 4 years. She wishes to be placed on the waiting list for a third kidney and during her evaluation her PRA (panel reactive antibody) is found to be 99%. This result means:**

A PRA is obtained by testing a recipient's serum against a panel of lymphocytes from different volunteers. Volunteers are selected based on their HLA type so that as many HLA antigens as possible are present in the panel. If someone has a PRA of 99% that means that they reacted (lysed the cells) with 99% of the panel and therefore has numerous anti-HLA antibodies and a high probability of a positive crossmatch to any future donor. This has prognostic significance in that the chance of finding a donor for her that will yield a negative crossmatch is around 1%.

❒❒ **An example of a xenograft would be:**

A xenograft is a tissue graft from one species to another. Examples would include pig to monkey, or baboon to human transplants. An allograft is the transplantation of tissues within the same species but to genetically non-identical individuals (e. g. standard renal transplant). An autograft would be a transplant of tissue from the same person or animal to a different site (e.g. skin graft, saphenous vein graft).

❒❒ **A father wants to donate his kidney to his dialysis dependant son. Both he and his son complete the evaluation and are found to be healthy for the proposed living related kidney transplant. As an aside, the father asks how many antigens match between him and his son. Your reply with:**

A parent to offspring transplant is a 3 antigen, or haplotype, match. The genes that encode the HLA proteins are located on the short arm of chromosome 6 and one allele comes from each parent. Each allele has a locus for a -DP, -DQ, -DR, -C, -B, and -A antigen. We routinely type for HLA-A, -B, and –DR antigens therefore the son in this example will match 3 antigens. Simply put, he will have 3 antigens from his father's allele and 3 from his mother. The only time you have more than three is if there is a coincidental match in antigens from the mother's allele in the son to the father's other non-inherited allele present in the renal tissue donated.

BENIGN RENAL CYSTIC DISEASE

John Chandler Williams, MD

❏❏ **Describe the radiographic characteristics of a simple cortical cyst.**

On intravenous pyelography, a simple cyst is a well circumscribed lucent mass, which may distort the contour of the kidney and may show a "beak sign" with normal parenchyma. Computed tomography demonstrates a mass with water density (-10 to +20 HU) with an imperceptible wall, sharp margins with the renal parenchyma and no enhancement after intravenous contrast administration. On T1 weighted MRI the mass is homogenous with low signal intensity (less than liver or renal cortex), and on T2 weighted images the lesion is homogenously hyperdense. There is no enhancement following intravenous administration of Gadolinium DTPA.

❏❏ **Describe the radiographic characteristics of a complicated cyst.**

A complicated cyst has an unusual contour, internal septations, calcifications or evidence of enhancement on a contrasted CT scan.

❏❏ **What are the Bosniak criteria for cyst classification?**

Delineates four categorizes of renal cysts. The categorizations have management implications associated with risk of malignancy.

❏❏ **What is Bosniak I?**

Bosniak I cysts are solitary, and fulfill the sonographic and CT criteria for simple cysts.
Sharp, thin, smooth walled, spherical or ovoid, water density lesions (-10 to +20 Hounsfield units) with no internal echoes and no enhancement after intravenous contrast administration on CT.

❏❏ **What is Bosniak II?**

Considered benign 90% of the time, these cysts can have thin central septations, thin peripheral calcifications, or they can be hyperdense non-enhancing lesions with Hounsfield units between 50 to 100.

❏❏ **What is Bosniak III?**

These are complicated cysts with extensive calcification, thickened walls, and irregular borders. There should be a high level of suspicion for malignancy in these lesions.

❏❏ **What is Bosniak IV?**

A complex cystic renal mass with thick septae and / or thick walls, thickened calcifications that can be central or peripheral, and / or an enhancing component on contrasted images. These lesions can be found in association with solid tumor.

❏❏ **What is the current classification of cysts based upon?**

Several classifications have been proposed based upon microscopic findings, clinical presentation or radiographic appearance. Most recent publications in the Urologic literature follow the 1987 the Committee on Classification, Nomenclature and Terminology suggestions of the American Academy of Pediatrics, Section on Urology. The primary distinctions are genetic and nongenetic.

❏❏ **What are the genetic renal cystic diseases?**

Autosomal dominant (adult) polycystic kidney disease.
Autosomal recessive (infantile) polycystic kidney disease.
Juvenile nephronophthisis-medullary cystic disease complex.
Juvenile nephronophthisis (autosomal recessive).
Medullary cystic disease (autosomal dominant).
Congenital nephrosis (familial nephrotic syndrome) autosomal recessive.
Familial hypoplastic glomerulocystic disease (autosomal dominant).
Rare multisystemic disorders (von Hippel-Lindau, Tuberous sclerosis, etc.).

⬜⬜ What are the nongenetic renal cystic diseases?

Multicystic dysplastic kidney.
Benign multilocular cyst.
Simple cysts.
Medullary sponge kidney.
Sporadic glomerulocystic kidney disease.
Acquired renal cystic disease.
Calyceal diverticulum.

⬜⬜ What is Autosomal Dominant Polycystic Disease (PKD)?

Also, known as adult polycystic kidney disease, this is an important cause of renal failure and accounts for almost 10% of all dialysis patients. The incidence is approximately 1 in 500 to 1 in 1000. While this condition typically presents in the 3rd to 5th decades of life, it has been identified in newborns. Large irregular cysts of varying sizes appear diffusely throughout the renal cortex and the medulla. Renal function is impaired and hyptenison and microscopic hematuria are common.

⬜⬜ What is Autosomal Recessive Polycystic Kidney disease (RPK)?

RPK is typically diagnosed during infancy and carries a 50% mortality rate in the first few hours to days of life. This disease has a spectrum of severity with the most severe form being diagnosed at birth and the less severe forms are diagnosed later in infancy / childhood. The affected newborn has massively enlarged kidneys that are hyperdense on sonography due to the presence of multiple subcapsular cysts. All patients have some degree of hepatic fibrosis with lesions in the periportal region of the liver. This pathologic entity can be readily diagnosed by the gross appearance of the kidneys.

⬜⬜ What is Juvenile Nephronophthisis?

Juvenile nephronophthisis and medullary cystic disease both cause polydipsia and polyuria in more than 80% of cases. The cysts are medullary in position. There is a severe renal tubular defect associated with the inability to conserve sodium. The polyuria is refractory to vasopressin and a large salt intake diet is required to maintain sodium balance. There is associated growth retardation in Juvenile nephronophthisis.

⬜⬜ Describe the renal cysts associated with tuberous sclerosis?

The renal cysts of tuberous sclerosis are unique in that they have a lining of hypertrophic, hyperplastic eosinophilic cells.

⬜⬜ Describe the renal cysts associated with von Hippel-Lindau Disease?

The cysts usually resemble simple benign cysts with flattened epithelium that some investigators consider precancerous.

⬜⬜ What is the sonogrphic appearance of RPK in the newborn?

Bilateral, symmetrically enlarged, homogenously hyperechoic kidneys, usually without evidence of large discrete cysts.

⬜⬜ In what polycystic kidney disease would you suspect liver pathology?

Both. Autosomal dominant polycystic kidney disease is associated with hepatic cysts that become evident in adulthood and increase in incidence with age. Autosomal recessive polycystic kidney disease is associated with congenital hepatic fibrosis in all affected individuals.

❑❑ **What is the essential histopathologic finding to diagnosis dysplasia?**

Primitive ducts.

❑❑ **In what renal cystic diseases is there a high incidence of renal cell carcinoma?**

The highest incidence, 35%, is in von Hippel-Lindau disease. Tuberous sclerosis has a 2 % incidence of associated renal malignancy. All others carry the same incidence of renal cell carcinoma as the general population.

❑❑ **How do patients with medullary sponge kidney present?**

Renal colic, gross hematuria and urinary tract infections.

❑❑ **Can UPJ obstruction be differentiated from multicystic Kidney disease based on sonographic findings?**

In Multicystic Kidney Disease, the cysts are arranged in a random fashion. In UPJ obstruction, the largest cyst like structure is medial or central representing the renal pelvis and communications can be demonstrated between the central "cyst" or renal pelvis and the "peripheral cysts" which are actually the calyces.

❑❑ **In unilateral multicystic kidney disease what is the contralateral urologic finding?**

Twenty to 40% of patients have contralateral vesicoureteral reflux. Three to 10% of patients have a contralateral UPJ obstruction.

❑❑ **What is acquired renal cystic disease (ARCD)?**

Acquired renal cystic disease is a feature of end-stage renal disease rather than a response to dialysis. The cysts are predominately in the cortex, generally less than 1.0 cm in diameter. And are associated with a six-fold increase risk of renal cell carcinoma.

❑❑ **What is the most common presentation of acquired renal cystic disease?**

Loin pain, hematuria or both.

❑❑ **What is the incidence of renal cell carcinoma in acquired renal cystic disease?**

Three to 6 times higher than the general population.

❑❑ **What is the incidence of Autosomal Recessive Polycystic Kidney Disease (RPK)?**

Incidence is 1 in 40,000 births.

❑❑ **What is the presentation of RPK?**

Large kidneys or flank mass. Oligohydramnios, oliguria, cysts of the renal tubules, congenital hepatic fibrosis of varying degrees.

❑❑ **What genetic abnormality is associated with autosomal dominant polycystic kidney disease (DPK)?**

95% Caused by a gene located on short arm of chromosome 16. 50% of the patient's offspring will be affected. 5% caused by a defect on chromosome 4

❑❑ **What is the usual presentation of DPK?**

DPK usually presents between the ages of 30 and 50; occurs uncommonly in newborns. The presentation is with hypertension, flank pain, hematuria and urinary tract infection.

❑❑ **What other systemic anomalies are associated with DPK?**

Aneurysm of the circle of Willis (10% to 40%). Cysts in the liver, spleen, pancreas and lung. Diverticula of the colon. Mitral valve prolapse.

❑❑ **What is the differential diagnosis for a neonate with bilateral renal enlargement and homogenous hyperechoic kidneys?**

Autosomal recessive polycystic kidney disease.
Autosomal dominant polycystic kidney disease.
Sporadic glomerulocystic kidney disease.
Contrast nephropathy.
Renal vein thrombosis.

❑❑ **What is the genetic defect in RPK?**

Chromosome 6.

❑❑ **What is the histology of RPK?**

Collecting duct ectasia; cysts derived principally from the collecting duct.

❑❑ **What is the histology of DPK?**

Micro- and macrocysts derived from the entire nephron.

❑❑ **What percentage of renal failure in children is due to juvenille nephronophthisis?**

10 to 20%.

❑❑ **What is the genetic defect of juvenille nephronophthisis?**

Chromosome 2

❑❑ **What is the inheritance pattern for juvenille nephronophthisis and for Medullary cystic disease?**

Juvenille nephronophthisis is autosomal recessive on chromosome 2. Medullary cystic disease is autosomal dominant with an unidentified chromosomal abnormality.

❑❑ **What are the mainfestations of von Hippel-lindau disease?**

VHL is an autosomal dominant condition manifested by cerebellar hemangioblastomas, retinal angiomas, cysts of the pancreas, kidney and epididymis. It is also associated with pheochromocytomas and renal cell carcinoma.

❑❑ **What are the manifestations of tuberous sclerosis?**

Tuberous sclerosis is part of a triad of epilepsy, mental retardation and adenoma sebaceum. The hallmark lesion is a superficial cortical hamartoma of the cerebrum. Although renal cysts have been associated with tuberous sclerosis, angiomyolipomas are more common than cysts.

❑❑ **What is Multicystic kidney?**

Multicystic kidney (multicystic dysplastic) is a severe form of dysplasia in which there is no functioning renal parenchyma. The kidney does not have a reniform shape and calyceal drainage is not present. A "bunch of grapes" has been used to describe the kidney grossly. Renal size is variable. Multicystic kidney is the most common type of renal cystic disease and one of the most common causes of an abdominal mass in infants.

❏❏ **What are the characteristics of medullary sponge kidney?**

Medullary sponge kidney is characterized by the dilatation of the distal portion of the colllecting ducts with many associated cysts and diverticulae. The dilated collecting tubules have a distinct appearance on pyelography and look as if they were brushed on with the "bristles of a paint brush". One third of patients have hypercalcemia.

RENAL TUMORS, ADULTS

Matthew T. Gettman, M.D. and Horst Zincke, M.D.

❏❏ **What is the most common benign solid renal tumor?**

Renal medullary fibroma. These tumors are seen in up to 35% of autopsies and frequently cause no symptoms. Symptomatic lesions occur more commonly in females and are best treated with partial nephrectomy. Most of these lesions are less than one centimeter in diameter and 50% of these tumors occur bilaterally.

❏❏ **Can information from a percutaneous needle biopsy of a renal mass be considered reliable?**

Analysis of biopsies on permanent section is significantly more reliable than frozen section analysis. With experienced pathologists and radiologists, the expected sensitivity and specificity of a percutaneous needle biopsy is 97% and 100%, respectively. Percutaneous biopsy is advocated only when clinical or radiologic evidence suggests a diagnosis other than renal cell carcinoma.

❏❏ **What is the incidence of renal cell carcinoma (RCC)?**

RCC accounts for 3% of adult malignancies. Approximately 30,000 new cases of RCC are anticipated each year with approximately 12,000 RCC related deaths. RCC accounts for up to 90% of all kidney tumors.

❏❏ **Synchronous metastasis occur in what percentage of RCC patients?**

Up to one-third of patients will have synchronous metastases. Metachronous metastases occur in 30-50% of patients at five-year follow up. The prognosis is much worse for patients with synchronous metastasis.

❏❏ **How frequently does RCC invade adjacent organs?**

RCC invades adjacent organs in about 10% of cases. Invasion of adjacent organs is associated with a very poor prognosis with reported 5-year survival rates of less than 5%. In many cases surgical intervention can require partial resection of contiguous structures including: colon, pancreas, liver, or spleen. Preoperative imaging overstates the possibility of direct liver invasion in many cases.

❏❏ **A patient undergoes partial nephrectomy for organ-confined RCC. What recurrence rate would be expected in the ipsilateral kidney? Contralateral kidney?**

Recurrence in the ipsilateral kidney would be 5-10% and 3-5% in the contralateral kidney.

❏❏ **What percentage of RCC occur bilaterally?**

1-2% of RCC patients have tumors present in both kidneys simultaneously. Metachronous appearance of RCC occurs in 3-5%. The 5-year survival for synchronous bilateral RCC is better than asynchronous bilateral RCC.

❏❏ **What is the incidence of the different histologic types of RCC?**

Clear cell (70%) followed by papillary (15%), granular (7%), chromophobe (5%), sarcomatoid (2%), collecting duct cancer (1%), and renal medullary carcinoma (<1%).

❏❏ **T/F: 50% of renal cell carcinomas are vimentin-positive on immunohistochemical analysis.**

True. In addition, high-grade tumors and sarcomatoid RCC are more commonly vimentin-positive. Almost all renal cell carcinomas stain positively for keratin 8 and 18 and the majority stain positively for epithelial membrane antigen.

❏❏ What cystic renal diseases are associated with an increased incidence of RCC?

Acquired renal cystic disease is associated with a 4 to 6 fold increased risk of RCC over the general population. von Hippel-Lindau disease has a known incidence of bilateral renal cysts in 76% of affected individuals with a 35% - 38% incidence of RCC in affected individuals. Tuberous sclerosis is associated with a 2% increased risk of RCC over the general population.

❏❏ Which types of RCC are more aggressive?

Sarcomatoid, renal medullary carcinoma, and collecting duct carcinoma are more aggressive subtypes. The behavior of granular and clear cell types are best predicted by stage and grade.

❏❏ Which type of RCC is associated with psammoma bodies?

Papillary type RCC, which is also associated with a 15% incidence of multifocality within the affected kidney.

❏❏ What is the predominant group of patients in whom the renal medullary type of RCC appears?

Renal medullary carcinomas occur almost exclusively in association with sickle cell trait or hemoglobin SC disease. These are very aggressive tumors and tend to occur in younger patients.

❏❏ What is the cell type of origin of many RCC?

Proximal convoluted tubule. However, while recent immunohistochemical findings have linked clear cell tumors with the proximal convoluted tubule (89%), granular cell tumors reacted in 88% with a distal convoluted tubule or collecting duct origin. Furthermore, the origin of the Bellini tumors is the collecting duct and renal medullary carcinomas are thought to arise from the calyceal epithelium.

❏❏ What are the risk factors for RCC?

Tobacco use, male gender, urban dwellers. The majority of RCC occur in the fifth to seventh decade of life, however a recent trend suggests a higher incidence in younger females and adolescents. RCC is more commonly seen in patients with von Hippel-Lindau disease, horseshoe kidneys, and acquired renal cystic disease.

❏❏ What is von Hippel-Lindau disease?

A rare, autosomal dominant, multiorgan syndrome associated with a 25-35% incidence of RCC, 75% incidence of renal, epididymal and pancreatic cysts, cerebellar hemangioblastomas, retinal angiomas, and pheochromocytoma. Typically, RCC in this instance tends to be multiple and bilateral (80%). Historically, one-third of patients dies from RCC.

❏❏ What is the most common cause of hereditary pheochromocytoma?

VHL syndrome.

❏❏ Can the size or appearance of renal lesions in VHL disease predict presence of RCC?

No. No correlation exists between the size of a lesion and the diagnosis of RCC. 25-35% of RCC in VHL occur in cystic lesions.

❏❏ A patient with VHL has diffuse, high-volume, bilateral renal lesions. What treatment is best?

The best treatment in this case would be bilateral nephrectomy with subsequent transplantation. Nephron-sparing surgery, while technically feasible in many cases, is best reserved for patients with cystic and low-volume non-diffuse solid lesions.

❐❐ **What type of RCC typically is observed in patients with hereditary forms of RCC?**

Patients with von Hippel-Lindau disease most commonly have low-grade, clear-cell RCC. Familial forms of RCC have also been associated with papillary RCC. In general hereditary forms of RCC do not show a male predominance and occur at much earlier ages.

❐❐ **What is the function of the VHL gene?**

Tumor suppressor gene.

❐❐ **Where are the most common chromosomal changes observed in RCC?**

Consistent chromosomal deletions and translocations have been localized to chromosome 3p: familial tumors, breakpoint at 3p13-14.2; sporadic tumors, breakpoint at 3p21-24; and VHL, breakpoint at 3p25-26. The high incidence of clear cell carcinoma in VHL has been linked to a balanced 3:8 translocation. In hereditary papillary RCC, linkage analysis has suggested a possible chromosome-1 translocation to the X chromosome t(X;1) (p11.2;q210). Papillary RCC can also exhibit trisomy of chromosome 17 and trisomy or tetrasomy of chromosome 7.

❐❐ **T/F: Renal cell carcinomas have a true histologic capsule.**

False

❐❐ **What accounts for the yellowish gross appearance of many clear cell renal cell carcinomas?**

The presence of cholesterol causes the gross yellow appearance of these tumors. The lipid substances tend to dissolve during histologic preparation creating the microscopic appearance of clear cells.

❐❐ **T/F: Nuclear grade is a predictor of survival that is independent of pathologic stage.**

True. Tumors with bizarre nuclei generally have a worse prognosis. The exception to this idea occurs when spindle cells are present. Spindle cells indicate a poor prognosis independent of nuclear grade. A general relationship exists between DNA ploidy and nuclear grade: aneuploid cells are more common in anaplastic tumors.

❐❐ **What is the typical clinical presentation for most RCC?**

Incidental in the modern era. Hematuria (gross or microscopic), mass, and flank pain are not uncommon. The classic triad of pain, hematuria, and flank mass occurs in only 10-15% of patients. Presenting symptoms can often be attributed to metastasis or paraneoplastic syndromes.

❐❐ **Differentiate between the Bosniak classification of renal cysts and their relationship to malignancy.**

Category I-   a simple cyst, with through transmission on ultrasound and a clearly defined wall. There are no internal septae, echoes or calcifications. This portends a remote chance for cancer.

Category II-   a septated, non-enhancing cyst that can have thin peripheral calcifications, and minimally thickened wall. This lesion carries roughly a 15% chance of malignancy.

Category III-   a complex cyst, with a thickened wall, a hyperdense cyst that shows no enhancement with contrast administration, can have thick calcifications, or thickened septae that carries roughly a 50% cancer

Category IV-   an enhancing thick walled cyst, with irregular borders, thick calcifications that may be central, and carries roughly a 95% chance of malignancy.

❐❐ **What is the likelihood of missing a small RCC (< 3 cm diameter) on intravenous urography?**

Thirty percent. Smaller RCC have previously been referred to as Bell's adenomas; this description is outdated. Any lesion 1.5 cm or larger and registering more than 25 Hounsfield units on CT should be treated as a carcinoma. Lesions smaller than 1.5 cm in unsuitable candidates may be observed with serial imaging studies as long as the interval growth is slow.

☐☐ **What are the indications for partial nephrectomy?**

Solitary kidney, bilateral renal masses, renal insufficiency or anticipated renal insufficiency secondary to a comorbid disease process are imperative indications. An elective indication for partial nephrectomy is a small tumor (≤ 4.0 cm) in the presence of a normal contralateral kidney.

☐☐ **Intraoperatively, what maneuver is imperative prior to proceeding with partial nephrectomy?**

Complete exposure of the kidney to exclude multifocality. Intraoperative ultrasound is a valuable adjunct in this regard.

☐☐ **How commonly are paraneoplastic syndromes associated with RCC?**

Paraneoplastic syndromes are seen concurrently with or develop in 30% of patients with RCC.

☐☐ **Describe Stauffer syndrome.**

Reversible hepatic dysfunction in the absence of metastatic disease. Patients have abnormal liver function tests, fever, and hepatic necrosis which typically resolves after nephrectomy. Persistence or recurrence of disease is a poor prognostic sign.

☐☐ **What other disease is associated with Stauffer syndrome.**

Xanthogranulomatous pyelonephritis.

☐☐ **What type of RCC is frequently observed in patients with Stauffer syndrome?**

Clear cell type.

☐☐ **What is the etiology of hypercalcemia in patients with RCC?**

Osteolytic bone metastasis or paraneoplastic syndrome frequently cause hypercalcemia. Stromal cells of RCC are thought to produce a parathyroid hormone-like peptide responsible for the paraneoplastic syndrome.

☐☐ **What is the incidence of venous involvement by tumor thrombus in RCC?**

Renal vein only, up to 25%; inferior vena cava, 5-10%; atrial, 1%.

☐☐ **What clinical findings are suggestive of an increased risk for venous involvement by RCC?**

The presence of a varicocele, leg edema, deep vein thrombosis, recurrent pulmonary emboli, and caput medusae are reported manifestations but are found infrequently. A high index of suspicion for patients with larger centrally located tumors is an important finding.

☐☐ **What is the blood supply of the vena cava tumor associated with RCC?**

When vascularized, parasatised vessels from the renal artery typically feed the tumor thrombus.

☐☐ **What is the differential diagnosis of vena cava tumor thrombus?**

Wilms' tumor, transitional cell carcinoma, sarcoma, lymphomas, primitive neuroectodermal tumors, adrenal cortical carcinoma, testis tumors, and pheochromocytoma.

☐☐ **Where are the most common sites of metastasis from RCC?**

The most common sites are the lung, bone, lymph nodes, liver, adrenal glands, brain, heart, spleen, and skin. Liver metastasis are associated with an ominous prognosis, however, solitary liver metastasis occur infrequently. Adrenal metastasis occur in 1-10% of patients. Adrenal metastases are more common with large upper pole tumors in patients with other sites of metastatic disease.

❑❑ **Describe general five-year survival for RCC with tumor confined to the kidney, with perinephric fat involvement, with vena cava thrombus, with node-positive disease, or metastasis.**

The 5-year survival for organ-confined RCC is 85-90%, 70-75% for perinephric fat involvement, 40-60% for vena cava thrombus, 10-20% with node involvement, and 0-5% for metastatic disease.

❑❑ **What is the role of nephrectomy for patients with metastatic RCC?**

Nephrectomy is completed for palliation, prior to enrollment in experimental protocols, or in conjunction with resection of select solitary metastasis. For example, nephrectomy in conjunction with resection of a solitary pulmonary metastasis has yielded 5-year survival rates of 30-35%.

❑❑ **List the various forms of contemporary immunotherapy for metastatic RCC.**

Active specific immunotherapy - stimulation of T-cell by immunization of patient with inactivated autologous tumor cells, limited proven benefit.

Adoptive immunotherapy - typically involves either in vitro or in vivo interleukin stimulation (usually IL-2) of peripheral lymphocytes (lymphocyte-activated killer cells or LAK cells), reported response rates up to 20%.

Cytokines - typically alpha interferon therapy with direct or indirect cytotoxic effects on the tumor, response rates of 5-25%.

❑❑ **What are the typical characteristics of RCC in children?**

RCC accounts for only 3-5% of renal tumors in children. The tumors typically present around 9-years of age more commonly with an abdominal mass. No sex predilection exists. Survival for RCC in children is worse than Wilms' tumor survival.

❑❑ **What is the most common renal sarcoma in adults?**

Leiomyosarcoma accounts for 60% of renal sarcomas and is best treated with surgical removal. Other less common tumors include osteogenic sarcoma, liposarcoma, carcinosarcoma, fibrosarcoma, rhabdomyosarcoma of adults, and malignant fibrous histiocytoma.

❑❑ **T/F: Malignant fibrous histiocytoma is the most common soft tissue sarcoma of late adult life.**

True.

❑❑ **What renal tumors contain fat?**

Angiomyolipomas are the most common. Less common tumors that contain fat include lipomas, liposarcoma, some Wilms' tumors, an occasional oncocytoma, and very rarely renal cell carcinoma.

❑❑ **A 35-year old female with Klippel-Trenaunay syndrome has intermittent gross hematuria with bloody efflux from the right ureteral orifice. What benign renal tumor is most likely?**

Hemangioma. These present with intermittent gross hematuria 95% of the time. No gender or side predilection. 12% are multifocal and a few bilateral. Sometimes the lesions are seen in the renal pelvis. Most tumors have a 1-2 cm diameter. Treatment with embolization, laser ablation, or partial nephrectomy can be effective but is dependent on location and size.

❑❑ **Can multifocal renal hemangiomas be associated with syndromes exhibiting other vascular lesions.**

Yes. Renal hemangiomas can present in patients with Klippel-Trenaunay and Sturge-Weber syndromes.

❑❑ **What age group is most commonly associated with the presence of a lymphangioma?**

Young adults and children. Most occur in a peripelvic location. A rare presentation is a honeycombed or multicytic appearance.

❏❏ **Do mesoblastic nephromas only occur in early infancy?**

No. Reported cases have occurred in adults 18 to 50 years. While the infantile variety is monophasic, mesenchymal and epithelial components are seen in the adult type. These tumors are distinguished from sarcomatoid RCC by lack of malignant morphologic features.

❏❏ **What is the characteristic substance secreted by juxtaglomerular cell tumors?**

Renin. These are extremely rare, profusely vascular benign tumors that not uncommonly are difficult to locate because of the small size. They occur in young adults and adolescents. Patients typically present with sever hypertension. A partial nephrectomy should be considered if the diagnosis is made preoperatively.

❏❏ **T/F: Patients with juxtaglomerular cell tumors typically have hyperkalemia.**

False. The hyperreninemia causes a secondary hyperaldosteronism followed by hypokalemia.

❏❏ **At autopsy, what percentage of leukemia cases will have renal involvement?**

Up to 50%. Usually malignancies of the lymphoid type appear in the kidney as part of the systemic disease process. Non-Hodgkin's lymphoma is more common than Hodgkin's disease. Multiple, bilateral renal masses are common. The treatment is systemic for the most part. Lymphoid malignancies are the most common secondary tumors of the kidney.

❏❏ **A 60-year old man with plasmacytoma has an incidental diagnosis of a right renal mass. What is the best treatment?**

Surgical exploration and if feasible partial nephrectomy. While extramedullary plasmacytomas have been reported in the kidney, renal cell carcinoma is the more likely diagnosis.

❏❏ **Besides lymphoid malignancies, where are the sites of primary tumors that metastasize to the kidney.**

Virtually any solid neoplasm can metastasize to the kidney. Lung cancer (squamous cell) frequently metastasizes to the kidney as well as breast cancer and uterine cancer. Up to 20% of patients with lung cancer have occult renal metastases. Malignant melanoma is also frequently noted in the kidneys at autopsy.

❏❏ **What syndrome is associated with angiomyolipomas?**

Tuberous sclerosis. This is an autosomal-dominant inherited disease associated typically with multiple and bilateral AML, mental retardation, and adenoma sebaceum. AML in these patients develop frequently in late childhood. Although AML occur in 80% of patients with tuberous sclerosis, less than 40% of patients with AML have features of tuberous sclerosis.

❏❏ **What is another name for angiomyolipoma (AML)?**

Renal hamartoma. These tumors contain fat, smooth muscle, and blood vessels. The incidence is 0.3-2%. Isolated AML are commonly seen in middle-aged women. The majority of AML appear as single asymptomatic lesions and are not associated with tuberous sclerosis.

❏❏ **Does AML occur in other locations besides the kidney?**

Angiomyolipoma (harmartoma) have been reported to occur in the bone, heart, lung, brain, and eye.

❏❏ **What is the name of the pulmonary condition that can be seen concurrently with AML?**

Pulmonary lymphangiomyomatosis.

❑❑ **Are any other renal tumors associated with tuberous sclerosis?**

Renal cell carcinoma has been observed concurrently with angiomyolipoma in patients with tuberous sclerosis.

❑❑ **What percentage of renal cancers result in spontaneous perinephric hemorrhage?**

Up to 60% of cases of spontaneous perinephric hemorrhage are caused by renal cancers.

❑❑ **How do patients with AML typically present?**

Tumor size correlates well with symptoms. Most small lesions are asymptomatic. Lesions larger than 4 cm are at increased risk for hematuria, spontaneous rupture, retroperitoneal bleeding, pain, and possibly fever. At least 10% of patients with AML develop acute hemorrhage requiring intervention.

❑❑ **What hormone receptor is associated with AML?**

Some angiomyolipomas have progesterone receptors present in the tumor smooth muscle cells.

❑❑ **What chromosomal abnormalities are associated with angiomyolipomas?**

Loss of heterozygosity at chromosome 16p13 has been observed in 50% of AML occurring in association with tuberous sclerosis and 10% of sporadic AML. Changes in chromosome 9q have also been linked to tuberous sclerosis.

❑❑ **What are the treatment options for AML?**

Observation, angioinfarction, and partial nephrectomy. Asymptomatic patients with small tumors are often followed with serial imaging unless renal function decreases or tumor diameter increases. It has been suggested that asymptomatic tumors larger than 4 cm be treated. All symptomatic tumors should be treated.

❑❑ **What features are rarely seen with oncocytoma?**

Hemorrhage, cystic degeneration, and necrosis.

❑❑ **What is the characteristic organelle seen in oncocytomas on electron microscopy?**

Mitochondria. The abundant mitochondria are responsible for the eosinophilic cytoplasm seen in the polygonal, uniform cells of oncocytomas. Mitotic figures are rare.

❑❑ **What is the incidence of multifocal or bilateral oncocytomas?**

Oncocytomas are multifocal in 3-5% of cases. Bilateral oncocytomas can occur in approximately 3-5% of cases.

❑❑ **Do oncocoytomas ever occur concurrently with renal cell carcinoma?**

Yes. 10% of oncocytomas occur concurrently with a renal cell carcinoma in either the ipsilateral or contralateral kidney.

❑❑ **What chromosomal changes are associated with oncocytoma?**

Oncocytomas are characterized by loss of the Y chromosome and translocations involving the long arm of chromosome 1.

❑❑ **What are the classic radiographic signs associated with the appearance of oncocytomas?**

Oncocytomas can have a "spoke wheel" appearance on angiography created by the vessels, whereas on CT the presence of a stellate scar has been reported. Both of these findings lack adequate sensitivity to preclude exploration. Oncocytomas are also sharply demarcated, with no calcification, and isodense with a homogeneous pattern of enhancement.

❏❏ **T/F: Oncocytomas occur exclusively in the kidney.**

False. Oncocytomas have also been reported in the parathyroid and thyroid glands, salivary glands and the adrenal glands.

❏❏ **How common are renal oncocytomas?**

They account for 10% of all renal tumors. They are more common in men with a peak incidence in the sixth to eighth decade. Paraneoplastic syndromes and spontaneous rupture are uncommon. The radiographic differentiation from RCC is difficult.

❏❏ **What is cell type of origin for oncocytomas?**

Proximal convoluted tubule.

❏❏ **T/F: Wilms' tumor in adults typically is associated with a better prognosis than presence of Wilms' tumor in children.**

False. The prognosis is generally not as good as children stage for stage and adults typically present with more advanced stage.

❏❏ **What is the most common malignant tumor observed in a horseshoe kidney?**

RCC followed by Wilms' tumor. The incidence of Wilm's tumor in horseshoe kidneys, however, is much higher than normal kidneys.

❏❏ **What are classic features for cystic nephroma?**

An uncommon multicystic tumor that is solitary, unilateral, and multilobular. Predilection for middle-aged women, frequently in the upper pole.

RENAL TUMORS, CHILDREN

Matthew T. Gettman, M.D. and Stephen A. Kramer, M.D.

❑❑ **What is the North American incidence of Wilms' tumor in children less than 15 years old?**

The estimated incidence approaches 7 per 1,000,000. Wilms' tumor is the most common malignant renal tumor of childhood.

❑❑ **What percentage of Urologic cancer in patients under 15 years of age does Wilms' tumor represent?**

80%.

❑❑ **What percentage of solid tumors in children does Wilms' tumor represent?**

8%.

❑❑ **Where are Wilms' tumors thought to originate?**

Although controversial these tumors are thought to originate as a failure of differentiation of the nephrogenic blastema.

❑❑ **How often are congenital anomalies associated with Wilms' tumor?**

15% of cases. Congenital anomalies are much more common in patients with bilateral or simultaneous multifocal tumors.

❑❑ **What is the relationship of aniridia to Wilms' tumor?**

Aniridia is noted in 1.1% of cases with a frequency of 1 in 70 Wilms' tumors.

❑❑ **What genitourinary abnormalities are associated with Wilms' tumor?**

Renal hypoplasia, ectopia, duplications, hypospadius, crytporchidism, and cysts have been reported in 4% of cases.

❑❑ **How frequently does hemihypertrophy occur with Wilms' tumor?**

3% of cases. Hemihypertrophy can be complete, partial, unilateral, or crossed. It is more common in females than males.

❑❑ **What skin lesions are associated with Wilms' tumor?**

Hemangiomas, cafe au lait spots, neurofibromas, and nevi are seen in 3% of cases.

❑❑   **What is Beckwith-Wiedemann syndrome?**

A rare, congenital syndrome associated with exomphalos, splenomegaly, hepatomegaly, macroglossia, hyperinsulinemic hypoglycemia, and gigantism. Hemihypertrophy can also be present. Most cases are sporadic; 15% have autosomal dominant inheritance.

❑❑ **What is the incidence of Wilms' tumor in patients with Beckwith-Weidemann syndrome?**

10%.

◻◻ **What other syndromes are associated with increased incidence of Wilms' tumor?**

Microcephaly, retardation, spina bifida, intersex, trisomy 13 and 18, pseudohermaphroditism and nephrotic syndrome.

◻◻ **Has a familial basis for Wilms' tumor been described?**

Yes, approximately 1% of patients have a positive family history for Wilms' tumor. This is thought to be inherited in an autosomal dominant manner.

◻◻ **What chromosomal abnormalities have been associated with Wilms' tumor?**

Deletions in chromosome 11p13 are most commonly reported. The gene at this locus has been cloned and designated the WT1 tumor suppressor gene. A second Wilms' tumor locus, WT2, has been also identified on chromosome 11p15.5. 20% of Wilms' tumor patients have loss of heterozygosity on chromosome 16q and 11% of Wilms' tumor patients have loss of heterozygosity on chromosome1p.

◻◻ **What is WAGR syndrome?**

The WAGR syndrome is seen in children with Wilms' tumor, aniridia, genitourinary malformation, and mental retardation. Most children with WAGR syndrome have a chromosomal deletion on chromosome 11p13.

◻◻ **What is Denys-Drash syndrome?**

A syndrome of ambiguous genitalia, renal mesangial sclerosis, renal failure, and Wilms tumor. Associated with mutations of WT1, the Wilms' tumor suppressor gene on chromosome 11p13

◻◻ **What is the incidence of bilateral Wilms' tumors?**

Bilateral disease occurs in 5% of patients (4% synchronous, 1% metachronous).

◻◻ **Do sporadic, heritable, and bilateral cases of Wilms' tumor have varying mean ages of presentation?**

Yes. Bilateral and heritable cases of Wilms' tumors present with a mean age of 2.5 years, whereas sporadic cases have a mean age of presentation at 3.5 years.

◻◻ **How common is Wilms' tumor in neonates?**

Wilms' tumor is very uncommon in the newborn. The more likely solid renal tumor in this age group is congenital mesoblastic nephroma.

◻◻ **T/F: Wilms' tumor occurs most commonly after the age of 6 years.**

False. 50% of patients are 1-3 years old, 75% are 1-5 years old, and 98% are 1-10 years old at diagnosis. The peak incidence occurs between 1 and 3 years.

◻◻ **What is the prognostic significance of Wilms' tumors occurring in older children?**

Patients presenting at an older age typically have a more advanced tumor that is less responsive to treatment.

◻◻ **What are the common presenting symptoms for patients with Wilms' tumors?**

Abdominal mass is most common (90%) followed by hypertension (0-60%), pain (20-30%), nausea and vomiting (15%), fever (10-20%), and gross hematuria (5-10%).

◻◻ **An acquired von Willebrand's disease is observed in what percentage of newly diagnosed Wilms' tumor patients?**

5-10%. All newly diagnosed patients should undergo a coagulation screen with platelet count, bleeding time, prothrombin time, and activated partial thromboplastin time prior to surgery.

☐☐ **What percentage of Wilms' tumors have a tumor diameter greater than 5 cm?**

90%.

☐☐ **How frequently does Wilms' tumor have venous extension into the inferior vena cava?**

4% of patients have tumor thrombus in the vena cava.

☐☐ **What are the common site of metastasis for Wilms' tumor?**

The most common site of distant metastasis is the lungs. Pulmonary metastasis are present at diagnosis in 8% of patients. The other common site of metastasis is the liver.

☐☐ **What microscopic features are seen classically with Wilms' tumor?**

Blastema, stroma, and epithelium. 60% of cases will have a predominant component. Blastema-predominant tumors behave more aggressively with earlier metastasis and more advanced disease at presentation.

☐☐ **What is the most important prognostic indicator in Wilms' tumor?**

Unfavorable histology. The two features now considered unfavorable histology in Wilms' tumor include nuclear anaplasia and concurrent high-grade RCC. Unfavorable histology had the biggest impact when tumor extends beyond the kidney.

☐☐ **T/F: Unfavorable histology is most commonly seen in Wilms' tumors of patients less than 2-years of age.**

False. Unfavorable histology is rare in Wilms' tumors presenting in the first 2 years of life. Anaplastic features are not commonly encountered in infants.

☐☐ **What is the incidence of unfavorable histology among Wilms' tumor patients?**

Unfavorable histology accounts for 10% of Wilms' tumor cases, but is responsible for 50% of Wilms' tumor deaths.

☐☐ **What possible precursor lesions have been implicated in Wilms' tumor?**

Nephrogenic rests. Precursors to Wilms' tumor are found in 25-40% of cases. Presence of precursor lesions in one kidney are highly suggestive of precursor lesions in another kidney and therefore identify patients at risk for tumor in the contralateral kidney.

☐☐ **Differentiate between types of nephrogenic rests.**

Perilobar-more common, smooth, well demarcated, usually multiple, located on the periphery, predominantly blastemal cells, less risk for tumor development.

Intralobar- irregular, usually solitary, random distribution, primarily stromal cells, greater risk of tumor development.

☐☐ **What is nephroblastomatosis?**

Bilateral, symmetrical enlargement of kidneys by diffuse proliferation of immature nephrogenic elements. Usually found in neonates. Differs from Wilms' tumor by absence of stromal elements.

☐☐ **How commonly does preoperative imaging miss evidence of bilateral Wilms' tumors?**

7% of cases. Thus, formal exploration of contralateral kidney is imperative at time of surgery for presumed unilateral disease.

☐☐ What clinical scenarios preclude primary surgical excision for Wilms' tumor?

Most patients with bilateral disease, extensive intravascular tumor extension, tumors that require resection of adjacent organs to complete excision.

☐☐ When should a primary surgical treatment be considered for patients with bilateral Wilms' tumor?

In most instances, patients with bilateral Wilms' tumor should undergo biopsies to establish the correct diagnosis, followed by preoperative therapy. If initial partial nephrectomy or wedge excision can be completed with preservation of two thirds or more of the renal parenchyma on both sides, then a primary surgical treatment should be considered.

☐☐ What effect does tumor spillage at time of surgery have on local abdominal relapse rate?

Tumor spillage results in a six fold increase in local abdominal relapse.

☐☐ Differentiate stage characteristics used by National Wilms' Tumor Study Group.

Stage I-   tumor completely confined to the kidney.
Stage II-   beyond kidney but completely removed: capsule penetration, invasion of renal sinus, previous
            biopsy, local spillage, venous involvement, tumor thrombus
Stage III- residual abdominal disease: nodes involved, diffuse spillage, peritoneal implants, positive
            margin, tumor left behind.
Stage IV-   distant metastasis or distant lymph node involvement.
Stage V-   bilateral disease at diagnosis.

☐☐ T/F: The treatment protocol for patients with unfavorable (focal anaplasia) stage I disease is the same as patients with favorable stage II disease.

True. Both groups of patients should receive 18 weeks of adjuvant actinomycin D and vincristine; no radiotherapy.

☐☐ Do primary Wilms' tumors appear exclusively in the kidneys?

No. Extrarenal Wilms' tumors have been reported in the retroperitoneum, sacrococcyx, cervix, groin, and gonads. The prognosis of patients with extrarenal Wilms' tumors is comparable to patients with intrarenal Wilms' tumors.

☐☐ Do horseshoe or fused kidneys predispose patients for Wilms' tumor?

Wilms' tumor is 2-8 times more common in patients with horseshoe or fused kidneys.

☐☐ T/F: Second malignancies have not occurred in patients with Wilms' tumor.

False. Sarcomas and adenocarcinomas (possibly related to irradiation) have been reported as well as brain tumors and leukemias. The incidence of second malignancies at 15 years post-treatment is 1.6% in the National Wilms Tumor Study Group

☐☐ What factors placed patients at in increased risk for second malignancy?

Prior treatment for relapse, the amount of abdominal radiotherapy, and use of doxorubicin placed patients at increased risk for a second malignancy.

☐☐ Can neuroblastomas arise in the kidney?

Yes.

❑❑ **A 12-year old boy presents with diastolic hypertension and hypokalemia. The patient has a 3.0 cm renal mass on computerized tomography. What laboratory test should be completed?**

A serum renin should be obtained. The suspected diagnosis is a juxtaglomerular tumor and serum renin levels would be elevated.

❑❑ **T/F: By definition, patients with juxtaglomerular tumors have a primary hyperaldosteronism.**

False. Juxtaglomerular tumors secrete renin which causes profound hypertension, and secondary hyperaldosteronism with associated hypokalemia

❑❑ **How do cystic nephromas of childhood differ from adults.**

Pediatric cases more frequently exhibit foci of blastemal cells in the stroma. Boys usually present before four-years of age while girls typically present after four- years of age. Best treated with nephrectomy.

❑❑ **A 16-year old girl with Klippel-Trenaunay syndrome presents with hematuria. What diagnosis should especially be considered?**

Hemangioma. Renal hemangiomas have been reported in the cortex, medulla, or renal pelvis. Most are small, single lesions and 50% are below the limits of radiologic detection. Symptomatic lesions appear more commonly in adults often with hematuria, which may become massive.

❑❑ **A 9-year old girl has microscopic hematuria and a honeycombed peripelvic mass noted on abdominal CT. What is the most likely diagnosis?**

The appearance of a honeycombed mass in a peripelvic location is most consistent with a lymphangioma. About one-third of lymphangiomas have been reported to occur in children.

❑❑ **What tumor is referred to as the bone-metastasizing renal tumor of childhood?**

Clear cell sarcomas. The other tumor to consider is RCC. Patients with either diagnosis should have a bone scan and skeletal survey completed.

❑❑ **How do clear cell sarcomas differ from Wilms' tumors?**

These tumors have a significant component of clear cells, predilection for bone involvement, and very poor prognosis. They represent 5% of pediatric renal tumors and 50% present before two years of life.

❑❑ **T/F: The majority of clear cell sarcomas have bone metastases.**

False. While the eponym has been applied to this tumor, clear cell sarcoma has bone metastasis in only 15-20% of cases.

❑❑ **Have rhabdoid tumors of the kidney been reported in conjunction with brain tumors?**

Yes, rhabdoid tumors have coexisted with medulloblastoma and other intracranial neoplasms and have been known to metastasize to the brain. The other renal tumor with propensity for brain metastasis is clear cell sarcoma. Patients with either diagnosis should have a brain MR completed in the early postoperative period.

❑❑ **A 2-month old boy has a unilateral renal mass. What benign renal tumor is most commonly the cause?**

Congenital mesoblastic nephroma. More common in boys, effectively treated with nephrectomy.

❑❑ **Microscopically, congenital mesoblastic nephroma resembles what other type of tumors?**

Leiomyoma, leiomyosarcoma

❑❑ **What are the typical characteristics of RCC in children?**

RCC accounts for only 3-5% of renal tumors in children. The tumors typically present around 9 years of age more commonly with an abdominal mass. No sex predilectation exists. Survival for RCC in children is worse than Wilms' tumor survival

❐❐ **T/F: All cases of angiomyolipoma reported in children have been associated with tuberous sclerosis.**

False. While angiomyolipma is a very rare tumor in children, cases have been reported without features of tuberous sclerosis.

RENAL/URETERAL STONE SURGERY

Jonathan L. Giddens and Michael Grasso III

☐☐ **What are the most common renal stones in North America?**

Calcium stones (calcium oxalate, calcium phosphate, mixed), account for approximately 70% of stones in the United States while infection stones (struvite, magnesium ammonium phosphate) account for 15-20%. Uric acid stones make up 5-10% and cystine stones 1-5% of stones diagnosed in this country.

☐☐ **Which stones are most dense on plain radiograph?**

Calcium phosphate stones

☐☐ **Which stones are radiolucent on intravenous pyelogram?**

Uric acid, sodium urate, ammonium urate, xanthine stones, 2-8 Dihydroxyadenine (rare) and indinavir stones are all radiolucent on intravenous pyleography, all except one can be visualized with computed tomography.

☐☐ **Which stones are invisible on CT scan?**

Indinavir (Crixivan) stones.

☐☐ **What stone disorder is inherited?**

Cystine stones. Cystine stones result from an inherited disorder of renal tubular reabsorption of Cystine, Ornithine, Lysine, and Arginine. These four amino acids can be remembered by the mnemonic COLA. Of these four, only cystine is relatively insoluble in urine and will precipitate to form stones.

☐☐ **What does ESWL stand for?**

Extracorporeal Shock Wave Lithotripsy.

☐☐ **Which stones are hardest to fragment with ESWL?**

Calcium oxalate monohydrate stones are typically the most difficult stones to fragment with ESWL. Cystine stones are also usually refractory to ESWL therapy.

☐☐ **Which stones are most difficult to fragment with ESWL- proximal, mid, or distal ureteral stones?**

Midureteral calculi, especially those located between the level of the inferior and superior margin of the sacroiliac joint are hardest to approach with ESWL. The patient is positioned prone and the stone may be difficult to visualize / localize against the background of the pelvic bones with current imaging.

☐☐ **What are the two absolute contraindications to ESWL?**

Pregnancy and coagulopathy.

☐☐ **What is "steinstrausse"?**

Steinstrausse, meaning "stone street" in German, refers to a column of stone fragments that may line up in the ureter following ESWL. This may lead to symptoms of obstruction.

❏❏ **What are the three areas of functional narrowing of the ureter?**

The ureteropelvic junction is the proximal site of narrowing, followed by the level at which the ureter traverses the iliac vessels and finally the ureterovesical junction.

❏❏ **What are the two major complications associated with ureteropyeloscopy?**

The two major complications are acute, intraoperative ureteral wall perforation or avulsion and postoperative ureteral stricture.

❏❏ **Where is the most common location for ureteral avulsion and perforations?**

The proximal ureter is the most common site for these complications (the ureteral wall is the thinnest in this location).

❏❏ **Where do ureteral calculi form?**

Ureteral stones form in the kidney and grow in size in the intrarenal collecting system before passing into the ureter. Factors that lead to stone formation in the ureter include congenital anomalies such as ectopic ureters and ureteroceles as well as ureteral strictures, neoplasms and foreign bodies within the upper urinary tract.

❏❏ **What are the indications for hospitalization in a patient with a ureteral calculus?**

The following are indications for hospitalization and/or treatment: Intractable pain requiring parenteral analgesics, severe colic and / or intractable nausea and vomiting with dehydration, fever, leukocytosis, or bacteriuria, a stone in a solitary kidney, complete obstruction of the kidney which is not transient and azotemia.

❏❏ **What are the different types of endoscopic lithotripsy?**

Electrohydraulic, Ultrasonic, Laser, and Ballistic.

❏❏ **Laser lithotripsy of uric acid stones produces which toxin?**

Cyanide.

❏❏ **T/F: Blind basketing of ureteric calculi is an acceptable method of extracting ureteral stones.**

False: With the advent of ureteroscopic lithotripsy, blind basketing has been completely abandoned. Stones extraction with force using this method using this method often results in severe tissue trauma, and a stone could occasionally be engaged within a basket that subsequently could not be safely extracted from the ureter resulting in an adverse situation.

❏❏ **What is the potential consequence of a submucosal stone?**

A stone granuloma may form; this may lead to a ureteral stricture.

❏❏ **What is the incidence of symptomatic urinary calculi in pregnancy?**

The incidence has been estimated at 1 in 1500 pregnancies.

❏❏ **T/F: The incidence of urinary stone formation is higher among pregnant women.**

False. Elevated urinary citrate levels are a protective mechanism correcting for the significant hypercalciuria associated with pregnancy.

☐☐ **What are the indications for urologic intervention of symptomatic ureteral calculi in the pregnant woman?**

Severe intractable pain, urosepsis, prolonged obstruction or a solitary kidney with azotemia are all well established indications for intervention.

☐☐ **What factors affect the success of endoincision for ureteral strictures?**

A stricture length >2cm, associated periureteral fibrosis (ie, secondary to endometrioma, idiopathic retroperitoneal fibrosis, etc.) and a history of prior abdominal radiation are all factors that affect the success of endoincision of ureteral strictures.

☐☐ **What is Dietel's crisis?**

Flank pain that occurs or is exacerbated by increased fluid intake or a diuretic effect from ingestion of fluids such as alcohol. This is often associated with ureteropelvic junction obstruction.

☐☐ **What is a struvite stone?**

A struvite stone is an infectious stone caused by urease splitting bacteria (Proteus, Pseudomonas and Klebsiella are common examples). A struvite stone is comprised of a mixture of magnesium ammonium phosphate and carbonate apatite.

☐☐ **Can struvite stones form in acidic urine?**

No, they cannot. An alkaline urine of pH > 7.0 is necessary.

☐☐ **What is the consequence of an untreated staghorn struvite calculus?**

Over time, an untreated staghorn calculus has a significant chance of causing death due to renal failure or sepsis. As such, the American Urological Association Nephrolithiasis Clinical Guidelines panel recommends that newly diagnosed struvite staghorn calculi be treated actively rather than be followed conservatively and observed.

☐☐ **How are staghorn calculi removed?**

In the past, the standard treatment was a kidney splitting operation called an anatrophic nephrolithotomy. Today, percutaneous stone removal is considered the standard of care. Various combinations of percutaneous surgery, ESWL and ureteroscopic retrograde management are used as alternatives to open surgery.

☐☐ **T/F: Percutaneous nephrostomy tracts should be placed through anterior calyces.**

False. Nephrostomy tracts should be directed through posterior calyces except in special circumstances. This is done to avoid violation of anatomic structures that lie anterior to the kidney, including vasculature and bowel segments.

☐☐ **Why should one avoid placing a percutaneous nephrostomy tube directly into the renal pelvis?**

A direct approach to the renal pelvis may perforate the renal hilar vessels and cause bleeding. Additionally, the renal pelvis is quite fragile and may be associated with greater urinary leakage postoperatively with poor healing.

☐☐ **What is the transfusion rate following percutaneous nephrostomy?**

Approximately 5 % for simple stones and 10 % for complete staghorn therapy.

☐☐ **What are the different methods available to dilate a nephrostomy tract?**

One can use balloon dilatation, Amplatz dilators, or metal telescoping dilators.

☐☐ What are the common causes of delayed bleeding following Percutaneous Nephrolithotomy?

This complication, which occurs in less than 1% of patients, is usually secondary to pseudoaneurysm formation or an arteriovenous fistula.

☐☐ What is the most common postoperative complication following percutaneous nephrolithotomy for a staghorn calculus?

Fever, due extravasation of urine, and / or infection in the urine.

☐☐ Which calculi are the least amenable to chemolysis?

Calcium oxalate stones, the most common of all renal calculi, are the least amenable to chemolysis.

☐☐ Which electrolyte must be monitored closely when using Renacidin chemolysis?

Magnesium levels. Hypermagnesemia , although occurring mainly in those with severe renal impairment, may also occur in those with normal renal function. Mucosal erosions, urinary tract infections, and elevated intrarenal irrigation pressures may contribute to elevated serum magnesium levels.

☐☐ How big is 3 French?

3 French = 1 mm = 0.038 inch.

☐☐ Differentiate between a calyceal diverticulum from a hydrocalyx.

Calyceal diverticulae are considered to be congenital in origin and arise from a fornix of a minor calyx. A hydrocalyx is considered to be an acquired condition secondary to infundibular stenosis caused by various conditions (TB, stones, prior surgery, inflammation). Renal papillae are present within and diagnostic of a hydrocalyx. A calyceal diverticulum will not have a renal papilla inside it but will be lined by transitional epithelium.

TCC OF THE UPPER TRACTS

Thomas W. Jarrett, M.D.

❑❑ What is the most common presenting sign of upper tract urothelial tumors?

Hematuria is seen in 75% of cases followed by flank pain in 30% of cases. Rarely do upper tract tumors remain asymptomatic.

❑❑ Primary urothelial cancers can be located in the bladder and/or upper urinary tracts. What percentage of urothelial tumors are located in the upper urinary tract?

Approximately five to eight percent of all urothelial tumors are located in the ureter and / or renal collecting system.

❑❑ What histology is most commonly found with urothelial tumors of the upper urinary tract?

Transitional cell carcinoma (TCC) accounts for more then 90 % of upper tract urothelial tumors.

❑❑ What are acceptable ways of making the diagnosis of upper urinary tract TCC?

Diagnosis is made by the characteristic radiolucent filling defect of the upper urinary tract as well as cytologic evaluation of the urine. In some cases, sonography or cross sectional imaging may be necessary to rule out a radiolucent stone as the cause of a filling defect. Diagnostic ureteroscopy may be necessary to confirm the diagnosis in equivocal cases.

❑❑ What other histologic patterns are found with upper tract tumors?

Squamous cell carcinoma and adenocarcinoma are less commonly seen and are usually associated with chronic inflammation from kidney stones, obstruction, and / or infection.

❑❑ What is the most common risk factor contributing to the development of upper urinary tract TCC?

Cigarette smoking is the risk factor most strongly associated with transitional cell carcinoma of the bladder and upper urinary tracts. The risk increases three-fold in a patient with a history of significant tobacco abuse when compared to the general population.

❑❑ What is the incidence of a bilateral upper tract involvement (either synchronous or metachronous)?

Approximately two to five percent patients with upper tract TCC will have involvement of the contralateral system at some point in their lives.

❑❑ What percentage of patients who initially present with TCC of the bladder will subsequently develop a tumor of the upper urinary tract?

Upper urinary tract cancer occurs in two to four percent of patients with bladder cancer.

❑❑ What percentage of patients who initially present with TCC of the upper urinary tract will subsequently develop a bladder tumor?

Approximately 50% percent of upper urinary tract TCC patients will develop bladder tumors at some point in their lives. This necessitates vigilant lifetime bladder surveillance in all patients with upper urinary tract tumors.

What are the two most clinically important prognostic variables?

Tumor grade and stage are the most important prognostic indicators. All studies have shown the prognosis significantly worsens with higher grade and stage lesions.

What is the incidence of multifocality with upper tract TCC?

Multifocality is seen in approximately one third of patients and is directly related to tumor grade.

Are tumor grade and stage related?

Tumor grade and stage are matched in the vast majority of cases. It is quite rare for a low-grade lesion to show potential for invasion and / or metastasis. The opposite is true for high-grade lesions.

What is the pattern of spread for upper tract TCC?

TCC of the upper urinary tract can spread by direct extension, lymphatic invasion and/or vascular invasion.

What is the traditional treatment of organ confined TCC of the upper urinary tract?

The propensity of upper tract TCC towards multifocality and ipsilateral recurrence has led to ipsilateral nephroureterectomy with a bladder cuff as the best treatment for reducing the risks of disease recurrence and progression. Exceptions to this rule are patients who may be at risk for renal failure and hemodialysis following removal of a renal unit. Examples include patients with solitary kidneys, bilateral disease, chronic renal insufficiency and / or other risk factors for renal failure. In such cases the risks of long-term hemodialysis may be greater than the risks of the disease itself and an organ sparing approach should be considered.

What surgical approaches may be used for total nephroureterectomy?

Nephroureterectomy requires surgical exposure of the kidney and bladder. This requires either a single midline or thoraco-abdominal incision or a two incision approach, flank and lower abdomen. Laparoscopic techniques have recently been incorporated to reduce the morbidity of the procedure. Both total laparoscopic and laparoscopic assisted procedures have been reported with decreased morbidity and equivalent cancer outcomes.

What organ-sparing alternatives to nephroureterectomy are available in the treatment of localized TCC of the upper urinary tract?

Open local excision and endoscopic resection are established alternatives to nephroureterectomy.

What endoscopic techniques are acceptable for the treatment of upper urinary tract TCC?

Endoscopic therapy can be performed in a retrograde ureteroscopic fashion or an antegrade percutaneous fashion.

Are patients with a normal contralateral kidney candidates for organ sparing therapy?

This is a controversial area of urologic oncology, however, it is generally accepted that patients with low grade and low stage TCC are at low risk for disease progression. Organ-sparing therapy is acceptable provided the patient is compliant and committed to life long follow-up of the ipsilateral collecting system with ureteroscopy.

With patients treated with organ sparing therapy, is there any evidence that ipsilateral recurrence compromises patient survival?

Especially when dealing with low-grade disease, there is little evidence to suggest that survival is compromised by ipsilateral recurrences. Recurrences can be addressed with repeat excision or nephroureterectomy.

❑❑ **What is the benefit of a retrograde ureteroscopic approach over an antegrade percutaneous one?**

The retrograde ureteroscopic approach has two distinct advantages: 1) ureteroscopy can generally be performed on an out-patient basis with minimal risk of complications, 2) ureteroscopic techniques maintain a closed system and thus have a lower theoretical risk of tumor seeding of non-urinary tract surfaces.

❑❑ **What are the limitations of a ureteroscopic approach?**

The ureteroscopic approach works well for low volume and low-grade tumors. Limitations of this approach include: 1) inability to treat a large volume of tumor, 2) limitations of ureteroscopes to reach all portions of the kidney (ie. lower pole system) and 3) limitations of biopsy specimens. Specimens obtained ureteroscopically are generally sufficient to establish tumor grade but are of inadequate depth to establish stage by assessing depth of invasion.

❑❑ **When is a percutaneous approach generally favored?**

The percutaneous approach is generally indicated for larger tumors and / or those that are not easily accessible through a ureteroscopic approach (ie. lower pole lesions). Unlike ureteroscopy, larger caliber instruments can be used for removal of larger tumor burdens. In addition, deep tissue specimens can be obtained for staging purposes.

❑❑ **What is the best follow up study for transitional cell carcinoma of the upper urinary tract treated with conservative management?**

Ureteroscopic evaluation is the most effective way of screening for ipsilateral tumor recurrence. Simple radiographic evaluation is not sufficient, as it has been shown that up to 75% of early tumor recurrences were visible endoscopically and not radiographically.

❑❑ **With endoscopic management, what are the risks of tumor seeding of noninvolved urothelial surfaces or the nephrostomy tract?**

A significant concern of endoscopic therapy has been the theoretical concern of tumor seeding of the normal urothelial surfaces and / or nephrostomy tract. Although there are individual case reports describing such problems, the majority of the literature has not supported this concern.

❑❑ **Topical immuno or chemotherapy has been effective adjuvant therapy for bladder TCC. Have any studies shown significant improvement with regard to tumor recurrence or prevention of disease progression when this therapy is used for the upper urinary tract?**

Adjuvant topical therapy via nephrostomy tubes and ureteral catheters has been described. To date no study has shown a statistically significant benefit with regard to recurrence and disease progression. This may be due to low patient numbers or possibly due to inadequate contact time with the urothelial surfaces of the upper urinary tract.

❑❑ **What systemic chemotherapy regimens are available for the treatment of metastatic upper tract TCC?**

Available chemotherapeutic protocols for TCC of the upper urinary tract are identical to their bladder counterparts. Because of the rarity of the disease, no large studies have been performed to show significant benefit. However, it stands to reason that these tumors are of similar to their bladder counterparts and should respond in the same fashion.

TCC OF THE BLADDER

Howard J. Korman, M.D., F.A.C.S.

❑❑ **What is the most common kind of bladder cancer?**

Transitional cell carcinoma accounts for 85% of all bladder cancers. Squamous cell carcinoma accounts for 10% with adenocarcinoma and metastatic carcinomas uncommon.

❑❑ **Other than smoking, what are the risk factors for bladder cancer?**

Exposure to chemicals in the workplace such as beta-napthalamine, paints, oils, gasoline, zinc and chromium as well as pelvic irradiation, chronic cystitis and treatment with cyclophosphamide.

❑❑ **What is the most common presentation of bladder cancer?**

Gross, painless hematuria. Frequency, urgency and dysuria can be linked to carcinoma in situ (CIS).

❑❑ **Which method of urinary cytology has the best diagnostic yield: voided or bladder wash?**

Bladder washings with normal saline yield a higher number of cells, which are better defined leading to a more accurate diagnosis.

❑❑ **How often do synchronous, upper tract urothelial tumors coexist when a bladder tumor is diagnosed?**

Two to five percent.

❑❑ **What are the most predictive factors of disease progression for superficial TCC of the bladder?**

Tumor grade, stage and the presence of CIS are all significant prognostic factors as are lymphovascular invasion and a sessile / nodular tumor growth pattern.

❑❑ **What are the most predictive factors of lymph node metastasis for invasive TCC of the bladder?**

Tumor grade and depth of tumor invasion.

❑❑ **What is the current TNM staging system for cancer of the urinary bladder?**

Ta - Noninvasive papillary carcinoma.
Tis - Carcinoma in situ.
T1 - Tumor invades lamina propria.
T2 - Tumor invades muscle.
    T2a - Superficial muscle (inner half).
    T2b - Deep muscle (outer half).
T3 - Tumor invades perivesical fat.
    T3a - Microscopic invasion.
    T3b - Macroscopic invasion (extravesical mass).
T4 - Tumor invades adjacent organs.
    T4a - prostate, uterus, or vagina.
    T4b - pelvic or abdominal wall.

❑❑ **What are the main indications for intravesical therapy after transurethral resection of a bladder tumor?**

High grade tumor, tumor size greater than 5 cm, tumor multiplicity, CIS, positive urinary cytology after resection, incomplete tumor resection.

❏❏ **What are the risk factors for systemic side effects from intravesical therapy?**

Anything that increases drug absorption may lead to systemic toxicity. These factors include low molecular weight of the intravesical agent, extensive area of resection and instillation close to the time of the initial resection.

❏❏ **What side effects are common to most forms of intravesical therapy?**

Hematuria, cystitis and irritative voiding symptoms.

❏❏ **Which intravesical agent is most commonly associated with the side effect of myelosuppression?**

Thiotepa, due to its low molecular weight is easily absorbed and can be associated with myelosuppression.

❏❏ **Which intravesical agent is most often associated with the side effect of contact dermatitis?**

Mitomycin C is caustic to the skin when contact is made.

❏❏ **What are common side effects associated with bacillus Calmette-Guerin (BCG)?**

Cystitis, hematuria, fever, sepsis, granulomatous prostatitis, pnemonitis or hepatitis. Deaths have also been reported from systemic BCGosis.

❏❏ **What is the mechanism of action of BCG?**

The bacillus organism binds to the cell surface through fibronectin binding sites which activates the immune system.

❏❏ **What is the effect of anticoagulants on BCG therapy?**

Anti-clotting drugs inhibit the binding of BCG to fibronectin, thus patients should be off anitcoagulants when receiving BCG if at all possible.

❏❏ **What is the treatment for systemic BCGosis?**

Patients with a fever of greater than 103 degrees Fahrenheit should be hospitalized and aggressive therapy implemented. Cycloserine 250mg to 500mg p.o. BID should be started immediately. Patients who are less toxic may be treated with Isoniazid 300 mg and Rifampicin 600 mg a day.

❏❏ **How can the risk of BCG complications be diminished?**

BCG therapy should not be initiated for at least 7 days following transurethral resection of the bladder tumor (TURBT). If gross hematuria is present or catheterization is traumatic, BCG should be withheld.

❏❏ **What are other immunotherapeutic agents that have been used?**

Keyhole Limpett Hemocyanin, oral Bropirimine and interferon have also been studied but are not currently first line therapies.

❏❏ **What is the optimal course of intravesical therapy?**

The optimal duration, dosage and timing of intravesical therapy has yet to be determined and remains under investigation.

❏❏ **What are possible indications for partial cystectomy?**

Tumor in a diverticulum or a small (< 2cm) isolated invasive tumor away from the trigone. Total radical cystectomy remains the treatment of choice for most invasive bladder cancers due to high recurrence rates reported following partial cystectomy patients with muscle invasive disease.

❑❑ What are the indications for radical cystectomy for superficial disease?

Recurrent or persistent high-grade disease / CIS, progression of disease, refractory hematuria from a large volume tumor, and a strong clinical suspicion of understaging.

❑❑ What degree of clinical understaging is associated with T1 disease?

Understaging as high as 30% has been reported.

❑❑ What is the most accepted treatment for muscle invasive bladder cancer?

Radical cystectomy. Bladder preservation with radiation and chemotherapy can be used for select patients but has not been shown to be better than surgical extirpation.

❑❑ What are local recurrence rates after radical cystectomy for invasive bladder cancer?

Ten percent of patients have a local recurrence after radical cystectomy.

❑❑ What are the expected 5-year survival rates for T2, T3 and N1 disease?

Estimated 5-year survival is 65%, 30% and 20%, respectively.

❑❑ What is the urethral recurrence rate following cystoprostatectomy if tumor was present in the prostatic urethra on final pathology?

Urethral recurrence following radical cystoprostatectomy is 30-50% if a concomitant urethrectomy is not performed.

❑❑ In what percentage of patients is incidental adenocarcinoma of the prostate found at the time of radical cystoprostatectomy?

Reports in the literature indicate that approximately 45 to 60% of patients undergoing radical cystoprostatectomy have incidental adenocarcinoma found in the pathological specimen.

❑❑ List the common complications associated with ileal conduit urinary diversions.

Pyelonephritis, stomal stenosis, parastomal hernias, ureterointestinal anastomotic strictures, ureterointestinal anastamotic leaks, metabolic abnormalities and renal stones.

❑❑ List the common complications associated with orthotopic urinary diversions.

Pyelonephritis, stomal stenosis, ureterointestinal anastomotic strictures, metabolic abnormalities, reservoir and renal stones, mucous retention and nocturnal incontinence.

❑❑ What is the cut-off for renal function for performing orthotopic diversions and why?

Patients with a serum creatinine greater than 2.5 mg% are usually excluded due to the high likelihood of metabolic complications.

❑❑ What is the most common metabolic complication associated with orthotopic urinary diversions?

Metabolic acidosis can occur in up to 50% of patients, often requiring life-long oral alkalinization therapy.

❑❑ What is currently the most accepted systemic chemotherapeutic regimen for metastatic bladder cancer?

Methotrexate, vinblastine, adriamycin and cisplatin (MVAC) is the most commonly used chemotherapeutic regimen for metastatic bladder cancer if the patient is healthy enough to tolerate the side effects of treatment with 50-70% response rates reported in the literature. Taxol-based regimens are currently being studied as a means of decreasing toxicity while hopefully maintaining efficacy and are now being evaluated as 2nd line chemotherapy.

❑❑ **What is the most common hematogenous site of bladder cancer metastasis?**

Liver (38%), lung (36%), bone (27%), adrenal (21%) and bowel (13%).

❑❑ **What is the most common site of metastasis overall for bladder cancer.**

Lymph node metastases are the most common (78%), and most frequently involve the obturator lymph nodes (64%).

❑❑ **What is the most common side effect associated with high dose interferon used as intravesical treatment for refractory superficial TCC?**

A flu-like syndrome occurs in up to 20% of patients. Local symptoms are rare. The expense of high dose intravesical interferon has limited its use as a primary therapy. Complete response rates of 25-43% have been reported.

SQUAMOUS CELL CARCINOMA AND ADENOCARCINOMA OF THE BLADDER

Ramon Rodriguez M.D. and Reza Ghavamian M.D.

❑❑ Squamous cell carcinoma of the bladder accounts for what percentage of the bladder neoplasms in the U.S.?

In the U.S. Squamous cell carcinoma accounts for about 3-7% of the total cases of bladder cancer.

❑❑ Why is squamous cell carcinoma of the bladder an important public health problem in Egypt?

In Egypt, where schistosomiasis is endemic, about 80% of squamous cell carcinoma of the bladder are caused by *Schistosoma haematobium*.

❑❑ Is schistosomiasis only associated with squamous cell carcinoma?

No, indeed schistosomiasis also increases the incidence of transitional cell carcinoma of the bladder.

❑❑ Can squamous cell carcinoma co-exist with transitional cell carcinoma?

Yes, transitional epithelium has tremendous metaplastic potential and therefore squamous cell carcinoma elements are also frequently seen with invasive transitional cell carcinoma.

❑❑ What are the cystoscopic and histological characteristics of bilharzial bladder carcinoma?

Bilharzial bladder carcinomas appear as exophytic, nodular, fungating lesions that histologically are well differentiated and have a low incidence of lymph node and distant metastases.

❑❑ What is the proposed etiology of non-bilharzial squamous cell cancers?

Most non-bilharzial bladder cancers are caused by chronic irritation of the bladder mucosa from bladder calculi, long term indwelling Foley catheter, chronic urinary infection or bladder diverticula.

❑❑ What is the proposed carcinogenic mechanism?

This is not completely understood, but could be the result of formation of nitrite and *N*-nitroso compounds that result from parasitic and bacterial metabolism.

❑❑ What other patients are found to have squamous epithelium in their bladder?

Vaginal type non-keratinizing stratified squamous epithelium is commonly found in the trigone of many women and in men receiving estrogen for prostate cancer. These patients should not be diagnosed with squamous metaplasia.

❑❑ What patient populations are at greatest risk for the development of squamous metaplasia?

Eighty percent of paraplegic patients are found to have squamous metaplasia of the bladder.

❑❑ What percentage of paraplegic patients with squamous metaplasia will go on to develop squamous cell carcinoma?

Approximately 5% percent of paraplegics with squamous metaplasia will go on to develop squamous cell carcinoma.

❑❑ What other patient populations are at risk for squamous cell carcinoma of the bladder?

These tumors account for approximately 20% of bladder cancers arising within bladder diverticula, 50% occur in patients with nonfunctioning bladders and also account for 15% of bladder cancers in patients who have had renal transplants.

❑❑ What is the role of cytology in the diagnosis of squamous cell carcinoma of the bladder?

Cytology has a limited role in the diagnosis of squamous cell carcinoma of the bladder. Histologic examination of biopsied tumor more closely correlates with the prognosis of the disease.

❑❑ How does non-bilharzial squamous cell carcinoma differ from bilharzial squamous cell carcinoma of the bladder?

In bilharzial squamous cell carcinoma, the tumors are usually well differentiated with a low incidence of lymph node or distant metastases. In nonbilharzial squamous cell carcinoma of the bladder seen in the U.S. the tumors tend to be poorly differentiated and advanced at diagnosis so the patients tend to have a poorer prognosis.

❑❑ What is the role of chemotherapy in the treatment of squamous cell carcinoma of the bladder?

Chemotherapy has not been very effective in the treatment of squamous cell carcinoma of the bladder. In addition, transurethral resection, partial cystectomy and radiation therapy alone have not been effective.

❑❑ What has been shown to be the most effective treatment against squamous cell carcinoma of the bladder?

The most effective treatment at this time is radical cystectomy with pelvic lymph node dissection. The role of preoperative radiation is not well defined although promising results have been reported.

❑❑ What percentage of patients with squamous cell carcinoma of the bladder are found to have involvement of their urethra?

About 50% of patients are found to have urethral involvement, therefore it has been suggested that urethrectomy should be routinely performed in all patients undergoing a cystectomy.

❑❑ What is the prognosis of squamous cell carcinoma of the bladder?

Stage for stage the prognosis is equivalent to transitional cell carcinoma of the bladder.

❑❑ What percent of primary bladder cancers are adenocarcinomas?

Adenocarcinoma of the bladder accounts for less than 2% of primary bladder cancers.

❑❑ What are the different classifications of bladder adenocarcinoma?

Bladder adenocarcinomas can be classified as primary vesical, urachal, and metastatic.

❑❑ What percentage of bladder neoplasms are adenocarcinomas?

Less than 2% of bladder cancers are adenocarcinomas.

❑❑ What are the different cell types of primary vesical adenocarcinoma?

In one large series vesical adenocarcinomas were mucinous (23.6%), enteric (19.4%), signet-ring cell (16.7%), mixed (12.5%) or not otherwise specified (27.8%).

❏❏ What are the histologic features?

There is a predominantly glandular pattern, but in poorly differentiated tumors, areas of solid growth are evident. The glands resemble intestinal adenocarcinoma of typical or colloid type. The epithelial lining can have a mucinous character. Eight percent of the tumors can have papillary features.

❏❏ What is linitis plastica of the bladder?

This is primary vesical adenocarcinoma of the signet-ring cell type. It accounts for 3-5% of primary adenocarcinomas of the bladder. It can present with a diffusely thickened bladder wall on imaging studies, especially computed tomography or ultrasonography. Sheets of tumor cells, fibrosis and mural thickening typical of linitis plastica of the stomach is characteristic of these tumors and they are generally associated with a worse prognosis.

❏❏ Which patient populations are at increased risk for bladder adenocarcinomas?

Patients with intestinal urinary conduits, augmentations, pouches, and ureterosigmoidostomies are at increased risk. Adenocarcinoma is also the most common type of cancer in bladder extrophy.

❏❏ With what premalignant lesion in the bladder is adenocarcinoma associated?

Adenocarcinomas of the bladder are more often associated with cystitis glandularis.

❏❏ What treatment offers the best chance for cure in patients with adenocarcinoma of the bladder?

Adenocarcinoma is poorly responsive to both radiation and chemotherapy. At this time radical cystectomy with a bilateral pelvic lymph node dissection offers the best chance of cure for localized adenocarcinoma of the bladder.

❏❏ What is the prognosis for bladder adenocarcinomas?

There is no concrete evidence to suggest that adenocarcinoma of the bladder carries a worse prognosis stage for stage than transitional cell carcinoma. However, they are generally thought to be associated with a poor prognosis. Of the different cell types, signet-ring cell carcinoma is more undifferentiated and hence carries the worst prognosis.

❏❏ What is the incidence of urachal carcinoma?

0.35% to 0.7 percent, with predilection for males (72% to 80% of the cases).

❏❏ The majority of urachal tumors are of which cell type?

Urachal tumors are usually adenocarcinomas, however, primary squamous cell carcinoma, transitional cell carcinoma and even rarely sarcomas of the urachus have been described.

❏❏ How do urachal tumors present?

Urachal tumors may present with a bloody or mucoid discharge from the umbilicus. Urachal tumors may also produce a mucocele, which occurs as a midline infraumbilical palpable abdominal mass. Fifteen percent of urachal tumors do not produce mucin.

❏❏ What are the other presenting symptoms?

Tumors invading the bladder lumen can produce mucus in the urine. This happens in only 15-33% of cases. Tumors that complicate extrophy are remarkable primarily for their presence on the anterior abdominal wall. Other symptoms include dysuria and frequency, lower abdominal pain.

❏❏ What is the most common finding on radiography?

Sixty percent of urachal tumors have areas of low attenuation on CT, which is reflective of the tumor's high mucin content.

❏❏ **What is essential in the diagnosis of urachal carcinomas?**

Cystoscopy and transurethral biopsy is essential for tumor location assessment and tissue diagnosis.

❏❏ **What other neoplastic processes can mimic urachal carcinoma?**

Metastatic prostate, colonic, ovarian and endometrial carcinoma all have the potential to locally invade the bladder. Therefore, tissue diagnosis is important.

❏❏ **What is the prognosis of primary urachal adenocarcinomas?**

These tumors usually portend a worse prognosis than primary vesical adenocarcinomas. Patients with predominantly mucin histology have a 79% five-year survival. Patients with papillary, tubular or signet ring cells had a 33 percent five-year survival based on one study.

❏❏ **What is the overall 5-year survival?**

43% to 50 %.

❏❏ **How should urachal tumors be treated?**

Radical cystectomy with an en-bloc excision of the urachus is the treatment of choice in patients with large tumors as histologically these tumors exhibit wider and deeper infiltration of the bladder wall. However, for small localized tumors at the bladder dome, partial cystectomy with complete removal of the urachus is acceptable. Recently, extended partial cystectomy has been shown to be the treatment of choice as survival is related to the stage at presentation rather than extent of surgical resection.

❏❏ **Are urachal tumors sensitive to radiation or chemotherapy therapy?**

Urachal tumors are usually unresponsive to chemotherapy, and radiation therapy is also ineffective.

❏❏ **Where are the common metastatic sites for urachal adenocarcinomas?**

Urachal tumors can metastasize to the iliac and inguinal nodes as well as the omentum, liver, lung, and bones.

❏❏ **What are the more common primary sites for adenocarcinomas metastatic to the bladder?**

Rectum, stomach, endometrium, breast, prostate and ovary.

❏❏ **Are any additional investigations necessary once a diagnosis of adenocarcinoma of the bladder is established?**

Patients should be evaluated for a possible source of a primary adenocarcinoma site. This includes computed tomography of the abdomen and pelvis, barium enema and colonoscopy when the index of suspicion is high and in patients in whom linitis plastica of the bladder is diagnosed, upper endoscopy to rule out a stomach primary is indicated.

URETHRAL LESIONS

Badrinath R. Konety, MD

❑❑ **Describe the different types of epithelia lining the male urethra.**

The prostatic and membranous urethra are lined with transitional epithelium, the bulbar urethra is lined with squamous epithelium and the glanular portion of the urethra is lined by stratified squamous epithelium.

❑❑ **What is the lacuna magna?**

The dorsal expansion of the fossa navicularis in the glans penis is called the lacuna magna.

❑❑ **What portion of the urethra do Cowper's glands and the glands of Littre open into?**

Cowper's glands open into the membranous urethra while the glands of Littre open into the dorsal urethra.

❑❑ **What is the specific feature of male urethral blood supply which is advantageous in planning urethral reconstructive surgery?**

The male urethra has a dual blood supply – proximally from the bulbar artery, a branch of the internal pudendal artery, and distally from the dorsal artery of the penis, which is a terminal branch of the pudendal artery. This fact allows for complete excision of diseased segments of the urethra during urethral reconstruction.

❑❑ **What is commonly believed to be the cause of congenital urethral strictures?**

Incomplete rupture of the cloacal membrane is believed to result in congenital urethral strictures.

❑❑ **What are the most common sites of iatrogenic urethral injury?**

The penoscrotal junction and the external urethral meatus are the most common sites of iatrogenic urethral injury.

❑❑ **What is the incidence of urethral injury following pelvic fractures?**

Approximately 10% of pelvic fractures are accompanied by urethral injury whereas a majority of patients with urethral injury will have pelvic fractures. Approximately 10% of patients with posterior urethral injury will also have an accompanying bladder rupture.

❑❑ **What is the most common cause of external urethral meatal stenosis requiring surgical repair?**

Balanitis xerotica obliterans is the most common cause of meatal stenosis requiring surgical repair.

❑❑ **What other radiologic methods other than a retrograde urethrogram can be employed in evaluating urethral injuries?**

Urethral stricture resulting from urethral trauma can also be evaluated by a sonographic urethrogram. A sonographic urethrogram allows determination of the extent of peri-urethral fibrosis and spongiofibrosis and luminal size. This is important because in the case of most urethral strictures, sub-epithelial spongiofibrosis extends well beyond the grossly identifiable stricture area.

❑❑ **What is the main continence mechanism in men with complete urethral disruption?**

The bladder neck constitutes the main continence mechanism in men with complete urethral disruption.

☐☐ What are the two main principles to be kept in mind during the excision and re-anastomosis of urethral strictures?

Excision and re-anastomosis should be avoided in pendulous urethral strictures since it can result in shortening of the penile urethra and chordee. A similar situation can result if >2 cm of bulbar urethra is excised.

☐☐ What are the most common indications for two stage urethral reconstruction?

The most common indications prompting a two-stage urethral reconstruction are: an extremely long or full-length urethral stricture, multiple strictures, presence of urethro-cutaneous fistula, periurethral inflammation or extensive local scarring.

☐☐ What are the principal advantages and disadvantages of immediate primary urethral re-anastomosis versus delayed primary re-anastomosis?

Immediate primary urethral re-anastomosis results in a low rate of urethral stricture formation but is accompanied by a high rate of complications such as impotence and incontinence. Delayed primary repair results in higher urethral stricture rates but the impotence and incontinence rates are considerably lower. Early endoscopic re-alignment with delayed primary repair combines the two approaches and has been found to yield lower stricture rates while reducing complication rates in small series of patients.

☐☐ Which is the only genitourinary malignancy more common in women?

Urethral carcinoma is the only genito-urinary malignancy more common in women. Squamous cell carcinoma is the most common histologic type in both sexes.

☐☐ What are the most common risk factors for urethral carcinoma in men and women?

The risk factors are: urethral strictures, venereal disease, transitional cell carcinoma of the bladder, human papilloma virus (HPV) subtypes 16 and 18 infections. In women urethral diverticula can also constitute a risk factor for urethral carcinoma.

☐☐ What is the key pathologic feature that determines the need for a urethrectomy along with a radical cystoprostatectomy in patients with transitional cell carcinoma of the bladder?

Presence of transitional cell carcinoma invading the prostatic stroma on urethral biopsy necessitates a urethrectomy along with cystoprostatectomy in cases of transitional cell carcinoma of the bladder. Urethrectomy is not considered mandatory in cases with carcinoma-in-situ of the urethra or tumor invasion into the prostatic ducts and acini without stromal encroachment. In cases where urethrectomy is not deemed necessary, involvement of the prostatic urethral margin dictates the need for urethrectomy which is usually performed within 2-months following the cystoprostatectomy.

☐☐ What are the principles of surgical treatment of urethral carcinoma in men?

Low stage urethral carcinoma especially if located in the anterior urethra is treated with local resection or Nd:Yag laser fulguration while extensive disease requires wider resection. There is no demonstrated benefit to prophylactic lymphadenectomy in these patients.

☐☐ What is the most common site of malignant melanoma in the genitourinary tract?

The urethra is the most common site of malignant melanoma in the urinary tract. It is most often located at the fossa navicularis in men.

☐☐ What is commonly believed to be the site of origin of urethral adenocarcinoma in men?

Cowper's glands are commonly believed to be the site of origin of urethral adenocarcinoma in men.

☐☐ What is the most common histologic type of cancers occurring in a urethral diverticulum in women?

Adenocarcinomas are the most common histologic type of tumor that occur in urethral diverticula in women.

☐☐ What is the Grabstald classification of urethral tumors in women?

According to the Grabstald classification female urethral tumors are classified as involving the anterior (external meatus and distal 1/3) or entire (posterior 2/3 may extend to anterior) urethra. However, survival from urethral carcinoma is only dependent upon stage at diagnosis and tumor size with location having no impact.

☐☐ What are the principles of management of female urethral carcinoma?

Early stage female urethral carcinoma can be managed with laser fulguration or radiation. Invasive tumors require local resection with or without neoadjuvant radiation therapy. Combined external beam and interstitial radiation therapy have been used for palliation.

☐☐ What are the demographic patterns of gonococcal and non-gonococcal urethritis (NGU)?

Gonococcal urethritis caused by the gram negative diplococcus Neisseria gonorrhoeae occurs more commonly in adolescent inner city males with a large incidence in African-Americans. Non-gonococcal urethritis, one of the major causes of which is Chlamydia trachomatis, is commonly found in educated Caucasians of higher socio-economic class including students.

☐☐ Who are the carriers of N. gonorrhoeae?

Both sexes can be asymptomatic carriers of N. gonorrhoeae and symptomatic infections can also occur in both sexes. Humans are the sole host for this organism.

☐☐ What are the criteria for diagnosing NGU?

The presence of inflammatory cells on a urethral smear in the absence of N. gonorrhoeae suggests a diagnosis of NGU. Presence of significant inflammation is indicated by the presence of >4 neutrophils/oil immersion field (400X).

☐☐ What is the optimal means of documenting infection by C. trachomatis?

C. trachomatis infection is best confirmed by culturing the organism from urethral swabs or staining with fluorescin conjugated anti-chlamydial monoclonal antibodies.

☐☐ What associations between gonococcal urethritis and NGU should be considered when evaluating patients with gonococcal urethritis?

45% of patients with gonococcal urethritis will have concomitant infection with C. trachomatis. Hence all such patients should be treated for both infections simultaneously.

☐☐ What are the standard therapeutic antibiotic regimens used to treat gonococcal urethritis and NGU?

Gonococcal urethritis – single dose Ofloxacin (400mg p.o.), Ciprofloxacin (500mg p.o.), Cefixime (400mg p.o.), or Ceftriaxone (250mg i.m.)
NGU – Azithromycin single dose (1g p.o.), Doxycycline 7 days (100mg p.o. b.i.d.), Erythromycin or Tetracycline 7 days (500mg p.o. q.i.d.), Ofloxacin 7 days (300mg p.o. b.i.d.). Ciprofloxacin is not effective in treating C. trachomatis infections. Partners though asymptomatic should be treated since 33% of them will be carriers.

☐☐ What are other organisms commonly implicated in NGU?

Ureaplasma urealyticum, Trichomonas vaginalis, Herpes simplex virus (HSV) types I and II, Human papilloma virus (HPV) are other commonly implicated organisms.

❏❏ What are the best methods to establish infection with HSV and HPV?

HSV infection can be established by viral culture while HPV infection can best be established by testing for the presence of viral DNA.

❏❏ What are the standard therapeutic regimens used in the management of NGU caused by organisms other than C. trachomatis?

Ureaplasma urealyticum responds to treatment with erythromycin and tetracycline (500mg p.o. q.i.d. for 7 days). Trichomonas is treated with metronidazole (250mg p.o. t.i.d. for 7 days). Partners though asymptomatic should also be treated since they could be carriers. HSV infections can respond to topical or oral acyclovir (for primary or recurrent episodes). HPV infections are treated with topical podophyllin, 5-Fluorouracil, cryotherapy, laser fulguration, electrocautery or surgical excision.

❏❏ What are the common complications ensuing from urethritis?

Epididymitis - C. trachomatis is the most common organism responsible for epididymitis in younger men. Urethral strictures can occur as a consequence of both gonococcal urethritis and NGU. Disseminated gonococcal infections with septic arthritis, tenosynovitis occur more commonly in pregnant women. NGU is associated with Reiter's syndrome of uveitis and arthritis. It is the most common cause of peripheral arthritis in young men.

❏❏ Urethral prolapse most frequently occurs in which patient population?

Urethral prolapse occurs almost exclusively in African-American girls between ages 1-9 yrs.

❏❏ What is believed to be the pathophysiology of urethral prolapse?

Urethral prolapse is thought to occur during episodes of increased abdominal pressure in a urethra where there is poor attachment of the smooth muscle layers. The cleavage plane is usually between the inner circular and outer longitudinal muscle layers.

❏❏ What is the standard therapeutic management of urethral prolapse?

Standard therapy for urethral prolapse entails topical application of estrogen cream and sitz baths. Formal surgical excision may be required if the prolapse is persistent.

❏❏ What is the pathophysiologic mechanism resulting in acquired urethral diverticula?

Acquired urethral diverticula result from infected and obstructed peri-urethral glands which rupture into the urethral lumen.

❏❏ What are the tumors which have been found in urethral diverticula?

Urethral adenocarcinoma, transitional cell carcinoma, squamous cell carcinoma and nephrogenic adenoma are the tumors that have been found in urethral diverticula. Of these, adenocarcinoma is the most common.

❏❏ What are the three D's of symptoms which are characteristic of urethral diverticula?

Dysuria, post void Dribbling and Dyspareunia are the symptoms characteristic of urethral diverticula.

❏❏ What is the diagnostic study to demonstrate the presence of a urethral diverticulum?

A retrograde urethrogram with a double balloon catheter best demonstrates a urethral diverticulum.

❏❏ What is circinate balanitis?

Circinate balanitis manifests as a shallow ulcer on the glans penis. It is painless, has gray borders and is typically associated with Reiter's syndrome.

◻◻ What is the difference between senile urethritis and a urethral caruncle?

Both are benign conditions occurring in post-menopausal women, with the former being more common. Senile urethritis results in eversion of the external urethral meatus due to shortening of the vagina. It can be mistaken for a urethral caruncle and responds to estrogen replacement therapy. Urethral caruncle is a red, friable mass located on the posterior lip of the external urethral meatus. It is composed of connective tissue, blood vessels and inflammatory cells. It may require local excision.

DIAGNOSIS AND STAGING OF PROSTATE CANCER

David A. Levy, M.D.

☐☐ **What are the current recommendations for screening for prostate cancer in American men?**

To date there is no consensus on screening for prostate cancer in American men. The American Urological Association currently recommends initiating screening at age 50 for white men with no family history of prostate cancer and age 45 for black men with no family history of the disease. In men with a first degree relative with the disease initiation of screening should begin at age 45 for white men and age 40 for black men.

☐☐ **What is considered a "normal" PSA?**

Normal PSA ranges have been determined to be 0 ng/ml to 4 ng/ml. However, age specific normal reference ranges and acceptable rates of change in the PSA value over time (PSA velocity) have been delineated and may enhance the identification of individuals at risk for the disease.

☐☐ **What are the age specific normal reference ranges for PSA?**

For men aged 40-49 the normal reference range is 0 ng/ml – 2.5 ng/ml.
For men aged 50-59 the normal reference range is 0 ng/ml – 3.5 ng/ml.
For men aged 60-69 the normal reference range is 0 ng/ml – 4-5 ng/ml.
For men aged 70-79 the normal reference range is 0 ng/ml – 6.5 ng/ml.

☐☐ **What is PSA velocity?**

PSA velocity is the rate of change of serum PSA over time. Studies have indicated that the acceptable rate of change in PSA over 12 months is ≤ 0.75 ng/ml. Changes that exceed this rate are considered abnormal and should be carefully considered by the interpreting physician. An individual should have several PSA determinations over time intervals to provide for correct interpretation.

☐☐ **What types of events can adversely affect PSA results?**

A number of factors will affect the accuracy of PSA results. A vigorous digital rectal exam, urinary retention, passage of a Foley catheter, acute prostatitis, recent prostate biopsy and any maneuver that "manipulates" the gland will falsely elevate the PSA. Interpretation of serum PSA results following any of these events should be delayed for 21 days to allow sufficient time for resolution of the false elevation of the PSA.

☐☐ **What is the serum half-life of PSA?**

Published reports have documented the serum half-life of PSA to be 2.2 ± 0.8 days and 3.3 ± 0.1 days, depending upon the testing method used. Based on these data, one should wait at least 21 days following manipulation of the gland to allow for a sufficient number of half-lives to yield a reliable result before drawing a serum PSA.

☐☐ **What is free PSA and what is the significance of free PSA?**

PSA is a glycoprotein produced by the prostatic epithelial cells and once in the serum approximately 40% is bound to alpha-2 macroglobulin and is unmeasureable. The remaining fraction of PSA is bound to alpha 1- antichymotrypsin or circulates free in the serum and both are measurable by commercial techniques. Conclusive studies have indicated that individuals with prostate cancer tend to have a lower percent free

PSA, and cut off limits have been assigned to this value. A free PSA less than 25% is considered to be a prognostic factor for prostate cancer.

❑❏ **Can free PSA be used to assess the relative risk for carcinoma of the prostate in all men?**

No. The utility of free PSA is restricted to men with a total PSA between 4 ng/ml and 10 ng/ml. There have been no definitive studies that indicate an application of free PSA to individuals with a total PSA less than 4 ng/ml. If the total PSA is less than 4.0 ng/ml one may employ the age specific reference ranges for PSA and PSA velocity to better assess an individual's risk for disease.

❑❏ **Can the serum PSA level reliably predict pathological stage?**

No. The serum PSA level alone cannot be used to reliably predict the pathological stage of disease. Approximately 70% to 80% of patients with locally advanced prostate cancer have serum PSA levels >10 ng/ml. The Gleason biopsy score may have more predictive value in predicting the extent of disease.

❑❏ **A 54-year-old man with an enlarged prostate on rectal exam has a serum PSA of 3.6 ng/ml and a free PSA of 45%. There is no family history of prostate cancer. How would you counsel him about his risk for prostate cancer?**

Autopsy studies from 1954 indicate that the overall risk for prostate cancer in 50 year-old men is 30%. This individual has BPH by exam and although his free PSA is over 25%, which is consistent with the diagnosis of BPH, his total PSA is less than 4.0 ng/ml and therefore, the free PSA may not have much bearing. This patient's current risk for indolent disease should parallel the age matched general population. A reasonable course of follow up may consist of serial PSA measurements to track his PSA velocity.

❑❏ **What is the role for digital rectal exam (DRE) in assessing patients at risk for prostate cancer?**

Data reported in the literature indicate that digital rectal exam alone detects less than 1.7% of all diagnosed prostate cancers even when there is a high index of suspicion of glandular abnormalities. However, DRE does provide useful information about the size and potential resectability of the prostate in individuals with prostate pathology.

❑❏ **What is the accuracy of clinical staging based on DRE?**

The accuracy of DRE alone in men with palpable lesions approximates 50%, and of those individuals diagnosed by this modality alone more than 70% will be upstaged at the time of pathological examination.

❑❏ **What is the best role for DRE in assessing patients at risk for prostate cancer?**

Digital rectal exam is utilized best in combination with PSA determination and transrectal ultrasound guided biopsies. This combination provides for the most efficient means of evaluating men at risk for prostate cancer.

❑❏ **What is the expected positive biopsy rate for individuals undergoing prostate biopsy with a normal DRE and an abnormal PSA?**

When performing transectal ultrasound guided needle biopsy of the prostate for men with a clinically benign gland and an abnormal (mildly elevated) PSA, a positive biopsy rate of 30% can be expected.

❑❏ **Can ultrasound reliably diagnose prostate cancer?**

No. Numerous studies have been published that indicate the absence of a pathognomonic appearance of prostate cancer on ultrasound. Although a higher percentage of cancers are hypoechoic, prostate cancer can also be hyperechoic or isoechoic on transrectal ultrasound imaging.

❑❏ **What is the role for ultrasound in diagnosing prostate cancer?**

Ultrasound is a very useful adjunct in diagnosing prostate cancer and has its greatest utility in directing the biopsy needle to particular areas of the prostate gland.

❑❑ **When performing transrectal needle biopsy of the prostate how many biopsies should be done?**

Traditionally, six cores were thought to represent a reasonable sampling of the gland with the cores including left and right sided biopsies from the base, mid and apical portions of the gland. Reports in the literature over the past several years have suggested that six cores may be insufficient and performing additional biopsies will lead to a higher rate of disease detection. Recommendations have been published for as many as 8 and 12 biopsies including transition zone biopsies and far left and right lateral lobe biopsies to maximize detection.

❑❑ **Is the biopsy result indicative of overall disease burden?**

Yes. There have been a number of studies that indicate that the biopsy result has prognositc information about overall disease burden. The Gleason score of the biopsy specimen is the most important prognostic factor for capsular extension of disease. Additionally, the percent of core involved and the number of cores involved can give predictive information for capsular extension and lymph node involvement.

❑❑ **What is the strongest prognostic factor for prostate cancer related death?**

The biopsy Gleason score has consistently been shown to be a significant prognostic factor for cancer related death in individuals diagnosed with the disease. To date there have been no reliable prognostic data reported for preoperative PSA results or free PSA results.

❑❑ **A 64-year-old man with a normal digital rectal exam undergoes a transrectal needle biopsy of the prostate for a PSA of 4.9 ng/ml. One out of eight cores, the left base, is positive for Gleason's 3+3 adenocarcinoma. What is his clinical stage?**

One of the more commonly used staging systems is that outlined by the American Joint Commission on Cancer (AJCC). Based on this staging system, this individual would be classified as having T1c disease, i.e. tumor identified by needle biopsy.

❑❑ **The individual in the previous question underwent a radical retropubic prostatectomy. The pathology report revealed disease involving the entire left side of the gland with no capsular penetration. The lymph nodes were negative. What is his pathologic stage?**

Using AJCC criteria, disease confined by the capsule and involving more than one half of the lobe but not more than one lobe with negative lymph nodes is classified as pT2b, N0, M0 disease.

❑❑ **A 58-year-old man underwent a radical perineal prostatectomy for unilateral Gleason's 3+4 in one out of 8 core biopsies. His PSA was 4.3 ng/ml. The pathology specimen showed disease involving both sides of the gland with capsular penetration at the left apex. What is his stage?**

AJCC criteria support a diagnosis of pT3a, Nx, M0 in this individual. A pelvic lymph node dissection was not done and therefore one cannot assess the status of the lymph nodes.

❑❑ **A 69-year-old man underwent a radical retropubic prostatectomy and the pathology report revealed disease on both sides of the gland with extension through the capsule bilaterally and zero out of 13 lymph nodes involved. What is his pathologic stage?**

Based on the AJCC criteria the correct diagnosis is pT3a, N0, M0 disease.

❑❑ **A 63-year-old man whose father had prostate cancer has a total PSA of 11.8 ng/ml and a free PSA of 11%. A transrectal ultrasound guided needle biopsy of his prostate revealed no evidence of cancer in eight cores. What is a reasonable approach to his management?**

This individual certainly is at high risk for having prostate cancer and probably warrants a repeat biopsy. One could consider doing more extensive biopsies including biopsies of the transitional zone and far lateral peripheral zone biopsies. Mapping biopsies done under anesthesia and often numbering as high as 15 or more cores in which the gland is more thoroughly sampled may be helpful.

❑❑ **A 78-year-old healthy asymptomatic man presents with a PSA of 8 ng/ml and a free PSA of 20%. He has no voiding symptoms, minimal nocturia, and no history of past GU problems. On**

physical exam his prostate is enlarged, asymmetric but not clinically suspicious. What is the next best course of action?

This individual has a minimally elevated PSA when one considers the age specific reference ranges. He is asymptomatic from a GU standpoint. A conservative approach with serial PSA determinations is not unreasonable in this situation.

❏❏ **A 54-year-old man with no comorbid disease underwent a transrectal needle biopsy of the prostate for a PSA of 18 ng/ml and a free PSA of 8%. The pathology showed Gleason 4+5 in all 6 six cores and there was evidence of perineural invasion. What is your next course of action?**

This individual has a very poor chance of being cured of his disease. The overwhelming majority (approximately 80%) of patients with this Gleason pattern will suffer a biochemical failure within 5-years of monotherapeutic intervention. Furthermore, the likelihood of his having positive lymph nodes based on his biopsy results must be considered. Brachytherapy alone would be a poor choice since it does not effectively treat disease in the extracapsular space. Radical prostatectomy for maximal local control of the disease with an option for early adjuvant radiation therapy to sterilize the field may be an option depending upon the lymph node status, but this will likely only extend his time period of biochemical freedom of disease rather than result in cure. A multimodality approach in this young individual with no comorbid disease will be required to maximize his outcome.

❏❏ **A 57-year-old healthy man presents with a PSA of 3.2 ng/ml. His previous PSA 6-months ago was 2.3 ng/ml and six months prior to that his PSA was 1.5 ng/ml. What is your next course of action?**

Although this man has a PSA within the age specific reference range, (0 - 3.5 ng/ml) his PSA velocity is out of the accepted range of normal. He has a sufficient PSA history to make this determination and his most recent findings warrant further investigation. A TRUS guided biopsy of the prostate would not be unreasonable.

❏❏ **A 69-year-old obese insulin dependent diabetic man with a history of hypertension, coronary artery disease, s/p CABG, and a 70-pack year smoking history presents with a PSA of 5.4 ng/ml. What is the next best course of action?**

This individual has significant comorbid disease and his PSA is minimally elevated. He is asymptomatic from a GU standpoint. A careful assessment of his overall condition reveals that he is not a good candidate for anesthesia. One must determine how aggressive they should be in evaluating patients at risk for disease, and whether the risk benefit ratio warrants further evaluation / intervention. Close observation with repeat PSA measurements may not be unreasonable for this individual.

❏❏ **Is there a role for MRI in the routine evaluation for prostate cancer?**

The role of MRI in diagnosing and staging prostate cancer has been studied extensively. Endorectal coil and newer body surface coil MRI of the prostate have shown utility in staging select patients with prostate cancer. However, the lack of sensitivity and specificity of MRI in differentiating benign from malignant prostate tissue preclude the use of MRI as a reliable means to diagnose the disease. Extracapuslar extension and seminal vesicle involvement have been identified with MRI and correlated with pathologic findings, but the associated costs and the availability of the equipment are factors that preclude the use of MRI as a first line imaging modality for patients with prostate cancer. MRI is used by a number of institutions for assessment of metastatic disease and confirmation of bony involvement.

❏❏ **A 64-year-old man presents with a PSA of 52 ng/ml and a free PSA of 8%. He complains of back pain and left hip pain. What is the next best course of action?**

This individual likely has bony metastases from his disease. He requires prompt diagnosis with a prostate biopsy as well as a serum alkaline phosphatase level and a radiologic evaluation of his bones. If he has metastatic disease initiation of hormonal deprivation therapy is reasonable.

❏❏ **What are the risks of starting LHRH therapy alone in a patient with metastatic prostate cancer?**

Initiation of LHRH therapy is associated with a testosterone flare that usually lasts about 14 days, after which castrate levels of testosterone are achieved. During the flare period individuals can suffer from exacerbation of obstructive voiding symptoms, increased bone pain and if there is vertebral involvement with bony metastases they can develop spinal cord compromise or even paralysis. Additionally, compression fractures of the spine or any other involved bone may occur during the flare period depending upon the degree of bony involvement. Therefore, it is wise to begin antiandrogen therapy at the time of initiation of LHRH therapy in an effort to minimize potential morbidity in these select patients. The duration of antiandrogen administration should be a minimum of 2-weeks.

❒❒ **A thin 52-year-old man is referred by his internist with complaints of obstructive voiding symptoms, pelvic pain and bilateral lower extremity weakness and swelling. On physical exam he has palpable non-tender periaortic masses and his prostate is consistent with TIIIc disease. He also has 2+ pitting edema of the lower extremities. A phone call to the internist reveals a PSA was drawn and the result is 914 ng/ml. How would you proceed?**

This patient requires urgent intervention. A CT scan of the abdomen and pelvis reveals massive retroperitoneal adenopathy with compression of the vena cava. There are large iliac lymph nodes identified on the CT scan. There is no evidence of vertebral bony involvement with disease or cord compression. His findings are consistent with advanced prostate cancer as well as vascular compromise from metastatic disease. An urgent orchiectomy should be performed since initiation of LHRH therapy will not result in castrate levels of testosterone for approximately 14 days. Additionally, one should consider CT guided needle biopsy of the retroperitoneal lymph nodes to confirm the absence of a second primary such as lymphoma.

❒❒ **Should all patients with prostate cancer have a bone scan as part of the staging evaluation?**

No. Bone scans are often employed to evaluate patients at risk for metastatic prostate cancer. Studies have indicated that the likelihood of a positive bone scan in an individual with a PSA less than 10 ng/ml in the absence of symptoms of bone pain is less than 1%. However, poorly differentiated cancers are known to have diminished PSA production, therefore, PSA can be misleading in patients with poorly differentiated prostate cancer. If an individual has symptoms of bone pain and / or an elevated alkaline phosphatase a bone scan is a reasonable staging examination.

❒❒ **Which is more sensitive for the detection of bone metastases, bone scans or plain radiographs?**

Bone scintigraphy is much more sensitive than plain radiography for detection of bony metastases. Plain radiography generally requires a 50% change in the cortical bone density to diagnose a bony metastasis, while bone scintigraphy can detect disease with as little as 10% change in the cortical bone density. Ninety-five percent of bone lesions due to prostate cancer are osteoblastic while five percent are osteolytic.

❒❒ **A 73-year-old man presents with a PSA of 23 ng/ml 10 years following 64 Gy external beam radiation therapy for prostate cancer. He has significant bladder outlet obstructive symptoms and a clinical TIIIb prostate. There are no other pertinent findings on history and physical. What is your next course of action?**

This individual should be evaluated with a TRUS biopsy of the prostate to establish the diagnosis of recurrent disease. If the diagnosis of locally recurrent disease is made LHRH therapy can be initiated cognizant of the fact that he may develop urinary retention due to the testosterone flare. To address his bladder outlet obstruction one might consider a "channel" TUR of the prostate, but the associated risk of incontinence in a previously radiated patient is as high as 30% in some series. LHRH therapy will not have impact on his voiding function for several months, and alpha blockers are not always effective with a high tumor burden in the prostate. Finally, a metastatic evaluation would be predicated upon abnormal findings on physical exam or blood work, which are not present in this individual.

❒❒ **Is there a role for computed tomography (CT) in the routine staging of prostate cancer?**

No. CT scanning lacks sufficient sensitivity and specificity to reliably increase the accuracy of clinical staging for patients with prostate cancer. Numerous studies have been published that report accuracy rates ranging between 15% and 65% for staging individuals with disease. In the absence of bulky disease, CT lacks the resolution necessary to delineate extracapsular extension, and CT cannot differentiate benign from pathologic tissue within the prostate.

❑❑ **Is there a role for CT scanning in assessing the status of the pelvic lymph nodes?**

CT scanning cannot differentiate a suspicious (> 1 cm) from an abnormal lymph node (> 1.5 cm) with regards to a benign inflammatory condition versus a pathologic process. However, in select individuals with prognostic factors suggestive of lymph node involvement, i.e. significantly elevated PSA, high Gleason score (> 7) or bulky clinical disease CT scanning may have a role in staging the patient.

❑❑ **Is there a role for radioimmunoimaging in staging patients with prostate cancer?**

Yes. Radiolabled immunoconjugates have been studied for the assessment of the pelvic lymph nodes in individuals diagnosed with prostate cancer. These agents have been employed by a number of institutions in an effort to enhance the preoperative predictability of pelvic lymph node involvement as well as the presence of occult soft tissue metastasis. The sensitivity of studies reported in the literature for detection of lymph node involvement is in the 62% range with a specificity approximating 72% and the positive predictive values are in the low 60% range. Limiting factors to the reliability of the immunoconjugates are the proximity of large blood vessels to the areas of interest. These studies when combined with other predictive factors of lymph node involvement such as Gleason score and PSA levels are helpful in predicting lymph node and occult soft tissue disease status for individuals with prostate cancer who are at high risk for metastatic disease.

RADIATION THERAPY FOR PROSTATE CANCER

Richard K. Valicenti, M.D.

☐☐ List the most important clinical prognostic factors predicting disease free survival for prostate cancer?

T stage.
Biopsy Gleason score.
Pretreatment PSA.

☐☐ Describe the most important clinical prognostic factors predicting disease free survival for prostate cancer?

The above three factors have been the most extensively studied. They also appear to provide reproducible outcomes among prostate cancer patients treated with radiation therapy alone. Several investigators (Pisansky) have used a combination of these factors to stratify disease free survival according to low, intermediate, and high-risk groups. Such a strategy is helpful in order to select patients who may stand the greatest benefit from adjuvant therapy.

☐☐ Which of these factors is the strongest predictor of death from prostate cancer?

Biopsy Gleason score is the clinical prognostic factor that has been consistently shown to predict death from prostate cancer. Interestingly, no investigator has been able to demonstrate that pretreatment PSA reliably predicts death from prostate cancer.

☐☐ How would this affect treatment recommendations for radiation therapy?

In recommending radiation therapy for prostate cancer, careful consideration should be given to the Gleason score over any other factor. Several studies now purport that an improved effect to using higher radiation dose is restricted to patients with Gleason scores 8 to 10. In addition, the RTOG has shown in two prospective randomized trials that patients with high Gleason score tumors have a survival benefit from the use of long duration adjuvant hormonal therapy.

☐☐ A 65 year-old man was recently diagnosed with a Gleason score 4 T1aNxM0 carcinoma of the prostate. His most recent PSA was 30 ng/ml. His prostate gland size is 40 cc. What is the significance of PSA in this stage of disease?

Despite his PSA being 30 ng/ml, he has a low risk (<5%) of having prostate cancer extending outside the prostate. Because he has a transition zone cancer, his PSA is not necessarily indicative of the prostate cancer volume, which strongly correlates with the presence of extracapsular disease.

☐☐ What is your recommendation for treatment for the above mentioned patient?

One may argue that based on his Gleason score and T stage that this patient may be suitable for watchful waiting, but his age may point you in another direction. Despite his PSA having little prognostic significance, his PSA may be too anxiety provoking not to recommend any definitive treatment. Of course, one may consider watchful waiting if he has multiple comorbid conditions that may lead to death in the immediate future. In any event, recommendations should include monotherapy with radiation therapy or surgery since these treatments appear to be equally efficacious for this stage of disease. The use of hormonal therapy is less clear and probably is not necessary for this patient.

❏❏ **A 50 year-old has a PSA of 15.0 ng/ml, Gleason 8, and clinical stage T1cNxM0 prostate cancer. How does the PSA influence your treatment decision?**

Whether the patient has monotherapy with standard dose (66 to 70 Gy) radiation therapy or surgery his chances of freedom of biochemical failure at 5 years is under 25%. This most likely translates into a 15 year overall survival of 50%. His PSA of 15.0 ng/ml puts him at a greater risk. In this situation most oncologists would recommend combined modality therapy with long duration (> 2 years) hormonal therapy and standard dose radiation therapy. Other therapies that look promising include combined surgery and adjuvant radiation therapy or dose escalated radiation therapy if lymph nodes are confirmed as pathologically uninvolved.

❏❏ **A 61 year-old man undergoes hormonal downsizing (3-months) and has a radical prostatectomy. Pathologically, he is found to have extensive capsular penetration and positive surgical margins. His surgical Gleason score can not be classified by his pathologist. His postoperative PSA at 10 days is .4 ng/ml (Chiron assay). What are your recommendations?**

In this situation, one should recommend that the patient return in one week for repeat measurement of his PSA. This recommendation is justified since the biological half-life after a radical prostatectomy is probably no less than 2.2 days. In actuality, his PSA was less than 0.2 ng/ml on repeat measurement a week later.

❏❏ **Same patient as the previous question and tumor characteristics but the PSA is undetectable. What are your recommendations?**

Because of the high preoperative PSA value and the presence of capsular penetration and surgical margin positivity, his risk of biochemical failure at 5 years is greater than 50%. The use of neoadjuvant hormonal therapy (up to 3 months) has little effect on biochemical outcome after a radical prostatectomy. Salvage radiation therapy for a delayed biochemical failure has about 20% chance of long-term biochemical control (PSA< 0.2 ng/ml). Early adjuvant radiation therapy may provide an 84% reduced risk of biochemical failure and perhaps a long-term survival benefit.

❏❏ **What radiation dose range is effective adjuvant postoperative radiation therapy and why?**

Radiation doses from 63 Gy - 66.6 Gy in 1.8 Gy fractions to a radiation portal 8x8 to 10x10 appears effective. Similar to other postoperative situations where radiation therapy is used adjuvantly, this dose range appears effective and safe. In addition, there has been a recent publication on a radiation dose response for patients after radical prostatectomy. A radiation dose > 61.2Gy appeared to be more effective than lower doses (Valicenti).

❏❏ **What are the clinical benefits from adjuvant radiation therapy?**

Early adjuvant postprostatectomy radiation therapy appears to reduce the risk of biochemical failure and local progression, but a reduction in the risk of dying from prostate cancer is less clear.

❏❏ **Would an isolated local recurrence after a radical prostatectomy require higher radiation doses for biochemical control?**

Larger tumor volumes require more radiation dose than smaller tumors for the same probability of local control. Several authors have reported on radiation dose response for patients with rising PSA after radical prostatectomy and have found that doses higher than 64 Gy are necessary (Valicenti).

❏❏ **What are the important predictors of response to salvage radiation therapy for patients with a rising PSA after a radical prostatectomy?**

The magnitude of PSA elevation, surgical Gleason score, and seminal vesicle invasion are the most significant prognostic factors. Rate of rise and time of rise (early vs. late) have not been consistently reported to predict response.

❏❏ **Which factor is perhaps the strongest predictor?**

The magnitude of the PSA elevation. Generally, patients with postoperative PSA > 2.0 ng/ml do not have a durable long-term response to salvage radiation therapy.

❑❑ What would combined modality treatment provide over monotherapy for an isolated biochemical failure after a radical prostatectomy?

There has been no completed prospective trial of combined modality therapy for patients with an isolated biochemical failure after a radical prostatectomy. Decisions regarding management thus depend on clinical judgement. Since the majority of patients fail after salvage radiation therapy, either insufficient radiation therapy is delivered or subclinical distant metastases are already present. If there is still androgen sensitive prostate cancer clones, there may be a benefit to use hormonal therapy to both potentiate radiation therapy locally and to eradicate disseminated disease.

❑❑ A 70 year-old man has a T1cNxM0 Gleason 8 prostate cancer in 5% of one of six cores. His prebiopsy PSA level was 0.9 ng/ml. Prostate gland size of 30 cc. Would you expect this patient to have a large tumor burden?

The patient has findings suggestive of having low volume prostate cancer. A single core biopsy containing 5% or less cancer correlates with low volume of disease and a low risk of capsular penetration.

❑❑ What is his risk of having lymph nodal metastases?

He has less than 15% risk of having lymph nodal involvement. Since the risk is relatively low, evaluation of the pelvic lymph nodes with either ProstaScint or pelvic lymph node dissection probably would not provide useful information for guiding therapy.

❑❑ What are your recommendations and why?

External beam radiation therapy alone (>70.2 Gy) to the prostate alone. It is not clear whether hormonal therapy would enhance the effect of radiation therapy for this patient.

❑❑ A 55 year-old man is diagnosed with T3bN1M0 Gleason 6 prostate cancer, PSA of 29 ng/ml. What is his prognosis with radiation therapy alone?

His expected survival at 10 years is less than 20% although there appears to be a wide range of estimates made in the literature.

❑❑ What is his prognosis with combined hormonal therapy and radiation therapy?

Several retrospective and prospective studies purport 70% to 80% expected survival at 5-years.

❑❑ Which patients with clinically localized disease are most suitable for prostate seed implantation alone?

The patient most suited for an implant alone as monotherapy has a tumor with a clinical stage T1 –T2a, biopsy Gleason score < 7, and / or PSA < 10 ng/ml.

❑❑ What is the incidence of potency after external beam radiation therapy for prostate cancer?

Depending on patient age, comorbid conditions, use of beta blockers, patients undergoing external beam radiation therapy for prostate cancer have 40% to 60% chance of remaining potent after treatment.

❑❑ What is the incidence of potency after prostate seed implantation?

There are few studies on this subject. The incidence is probably comparable to external beam radiation therapy.

❑❑ Which form of radiation treatment may lead to higher incidence of urinary incontinence?

Prostate seed implantation. The incidence can be as high as 50% if the patient had a prior TURP. External beam radiation therapy causes urinary incontinence in less than 5% of the patients.

SURGICAL THERAPY FOR PROSTATE CANCER

Daniel M. Hoffman, M.D.

☐☐ What are the treatments for prostate cancer?

There are four general categories of treatment for prostate cancer:

1. The monitoring of the patient without any aggressive therapy. This is sometimes called watchful waiting and consists of a physical exam with serial PSA determinations.
2. Radiation therapy. This can be administered in two ways: external beam radiation therapy and interstitial brachytherapy.
3. Radical prostatectomy either by a retropubic or perineal approach.
4. Hormonal manipulation.

☐☐ How effective is orchiectomy?

Orchiectomy results in a reduction of circulating androgens by approximately 97%. Castrate levels of testosterone are achieved within 24 - hours of orchiectomy. The hormonal deprivation results in remission of the hormone dependent prostate tumor growth. Depending upon the Gleason's grade of the cancer, the duration of the remission varies, and biochemical failure / hormone independent tumor growth can develop.

☐☐ Why are there are two ways of administering radiation therapy?

The efficacy of external beam radiation therapy was established in the 1960s and prior to the implementation of PSA external beam radiation therapy was as effective as surgical removal of the prostate for control of localized prostate cancer. Brachytherapy utilizing radioactive Iodine or Palladium seeds placed directly into the prostate gland to achieve a higher radiation dose to the prostate while minimizing radiation dose to the surrounding organs and tissues is considered a less morbid means of achieving higher doses of radiation to the prostate.

☐☐ What are the complications of radiation therapy?

The complications are primarily intestinal with radiation proctitis which leads to diarrhea. Patients also experience urinary frequency and urgency. This is usually transient, but may become debilitating in some cases and may involve urinary incontinence. New onset of impotence occurs in approximately 10% of the patients treated with external beam radiation therapy.

☐☐ How is brachytherapy performed?

Brachytherapy is performed under real time transrectal ultrasound guidance. The patient undergoes a pretreatment mapping of the prostate and iodine or palladium implants are placed transperineally directly into the prostate under general anesthesia with the patient in the dorsal lithotomy position.

☐☐ How do the results of brachytherapy compare with surgical therapy?

In a recent report comparing brachytherapy and radial retropubic prostatectomy in patients matched for similar pretreatment clinical pathological characteristics, the results showed a mean seven-year disease free survival rate of 84% for surgical extirpation versus 79% for the iodine brachytherapy series. Although there was a proportionately higher probability of nonprogression for brachytherapy this was not statistically significant. In other studies, brachytherapy has compared favorably to radical prostatectomy in biopsy-confirmed patients post treatment.

❏❏ **What are the complications of brachytherapy for prostate cancer?**

Patients transiently experience urinary frequency and urgency and may need catheter placement for management of severe symptoms. Impotence has been reported. Other complications include rectal ulcers and urethral sloughing. Although rare these complications are severe.

❏❏ **What are the surgical approaches to the prostate?**

Radical prostatectomy can be performed two different ways with similar results. A radical retropubic prostatectomy allows for a wider margin around the gland as well as simultaneous lymphadenectomy through the same incision. The perineal prostatectomy was first reported by Hugh Hamptom Young, M.D. in 1905 and was modified by Dr. Belt in 1939. Radical perineal prostatectomy has its advantages in avoidance of the plexus of Santorini and is generally associated with less discomfort postoperatively.

❏❏ **How are the lymph nodes assessed for metastatic disease?**

Although CT scan may be used to evaluate for lymphadenopathy, one cannot differentiate pathologic from non pathologic nodes if they are < 1.5 cm in size. Thus, computed tomography is both nonspecific and non sensitive. To adequately rule out metastatic disease of the lymph nodes, a lymphadenectomy is required.

❏❏ **What are the options for pelvic lymphadenectomy?**

If the patient is undergoing radical retropubic prostatectomy, a lymphadenectomy may be performed simultaneously and the lymph nodes can be sent for frozen section analysis to rule out micrometastases. Alternatively, a laparoscopic pelvic lymph node dissection can be performed or a mini-lap lymph node dissection may be performed.

❏❏ **How is a laparoscopic lymph node dissection performed?**

Laparoscopic lymph node dissection can be performed transperitoneally or through a preperitoneal approach. A standard pelvic lymphnode dissection is carried out and the tissue is sent for analysis.

❏❏ **What are the boundaries for lymph node dissection?**

The distal limit of the dissection is the node of Cloquet located in the femoral canal. The proximal limit of the dissection is the bifrication of the iliac vessels. The superior limit of the dissection is the external iliac artery, the lateral limit is the pelvic side wall and the inferior limit is the obturator vessels. Thus, all the lymph nodes are dissected off of the external iliac vein, the pelvic side wall laterally, and the obturator nerve and vessels.

❏❏ **What are the complications of pelvic lymph node dissection?**

The most common complication is lymphocele formation. Lymphocele formation can be minimized by clipping or tying feeding lymphatics as coagulation of lymphatics commonly results in postoperative leakage. Damage to the external iliac vein, obturator vessels and obturator nerve can also occur during pelvic lymphadenectomy. Additionally, injury of the genitofemoral nerve from tractor blades has been reported.

❏❏ **What is meant by a mini-lap lymph node dissection?**

A mini-lap lymph node dissection is performed using a 4 cm to 6 cm midline incision. It is an extra-peritoneal lymph node dissection performed using the standard anatomic limits for dissection.

❏❏ **How is the patient prepared for radical prostatectomy?**

The patient should have adequate cardiac and pulmonary function. If there are any risk factors of cardiopulmonary disease, the patient should be optimized prior to surgery. Screening tests for coagulopathy are mandatory. Preoperative determination should be made of the patient's hemoglobin, hematocrit and electrolytes. Although the risk of rectal injury is low, patients should undergo a bowel prep prior to surgery.

❏❏ Should the patient donate autologous blood?

This depends on the surgeon's experience. If the surgeon historically loses more than 500 cc of blood during a radial prostatectomy, it is reasonable to offer the patient the option of donating autologous blood. The blood is commonly donated within the month before surgery. This bears substantial cost, but decreases the risk of a transfusion reaction or a transfusion-associated morbidity.

❏❏ Are antiembolism precautions necessary for radical prostatectomy / pelvic lymphnode dissection?

Many of the risk factors for deep vein thrombosis and pelvic thrombosis are present: general anesthesia, blood loss, pelvic surgery, and possibly a hypercoagulable state. However, utilization of some sort of anti-embolic protection remains controversial. Lower extremity sequential compression devices and anti-embolism stockings are commonly employed to help minimize pooling of blood in the deep veins of the legs. This may be used with or without some sort of medical anticoagulation such as subcutaneous heparin.

❏❏ What is the positioning for the radical retropubic prostatectomy?

The radical retropubic prostatectomy is performed through a midline infraumbilical incision extending from the umbilicus to the pubic symphysis. The patient is placed supine or in a low lithotomy position with the kidney rest or a rolled towel just above the sacrum with the table slightly hyperextended. During the procedure, reverse Trendelenburg may be helpful in visualizing the apex of the prostate. A Bookwalter or other self-retaining retractor is useful for adequate exposure.

❏❏ Describe the approach to the prostate in a retropubic prostatectomy.

The radical retropubic prostatectomy is an extra-peritoneal procedure. The rectus muscles are split in the midline and the space of Retzius is developed. The bladder is freed from the posterior surface of the pubic symphysis and cleared from the lateral pelvic sidewall. At this time, if so indicated, a bilateral lymph node dissection is performed. After the lymph node dissection is complete and the pathological results obtained, incisions are made in the endopelvic fascia, lateral to the apex of the prostate, to gain exposure to the apex of the prostate. If the apex of the prostate is not easily visualized, the puboprostatic ligaments are divided.

❏❏ Are puboprostatic ligaments vascular structures?

These are fibrous bands that connect the prostate to the underside of the pubic symphysis. They may be incised using Metzenbaum scissors without causing excessive bleeding.

❏❏ What is the structure that is most likely to cause significant bleeding?

Santorini's plexus, which is a continuation of the dorsal vein of the penis. This is the structure found in the midline that drains between the puboprostatic ligaments and forms the dorsal venous complex which is superior and anterior to the urethra at the apex of the prostate gland.

❏❏ How is bleeding prevented from the dorsal venous complex?

A variety of techniques for controlling the dorsal venous complex have been described. In the radical retropubic prostatectomy, the dorsal venous complex must be transected in order to visualize the apex of the prostate. Bunching sutures paced deeply into the dorsal surface of the prostate from the level of the bladder neck and continuing distally to the apex of the gland are exceedingly helpful in controlling back bleeding. The doral venous complex must be dissected off of the anterior surface of the urethra. A right angle clamp is passed between the dorsal vein complex and the anterior surface of the urethra and the dorsal vein complex is tented up. Some surgeons prefer to transect the dorsal vein complex at this point and oversew the free ends of the dorsal vein complex. Other authors feel it is best to suture ligate or doubly ligate the dorsal vein complex before transection.

❏❏ What if these measures do not control bleeding from the dorsal venous complex.

Direct visualization suture ligation of the transected veins under the pubic symphysis is the best means of stopping the bleeding. Rarely, temporary compression of and possibly suture ligation of the deep dorsal vein of the penis below the level of the pubic symphysis may be helpful in gaining control of bleeding from the dorsal venous complex. Suture ligation will require dissection of the veins at the base of the penis at the dorsal vein.

❑❑ Aside from the dorsal vein complex, what other important structures are located at the level of the apex of the prostate?

The external sphincter is located distal to the apex of the prostate. Injury to this sphincter can cause permanent urinary incontinence. The neurovascular bundles which supply the erectile function run laterally along the apex of the prostate from 3 o'clock and 9 o'clock at the level of the external urinary sphincter and 5 and 7 o'clock at the base of the gland. If both neurovascular bundles are transected, impotence results.

❑❑ What is the major blood supply to the prostate?

The main blood supply to the prostate is from the inferior vesical artery which is a branch of the hypogastric artery. This penetrates the substance of the prostate at the prostatovesical junction at 8 o'clock and 4 o'clock posteriorly.

❑❑ Describe the technique for avoiding injury to the external sphincter and the neurovascular bundles.

The anterior urethra is incised under direct vision. The Foley catheter is delivered through the urethrotomy and transected while maintaining the fluid in the balloon. The posterior urethra is carefully dissected off of the rectum and is divided. The rectourethralis muscle is divided at apex of the gland in the midline and then the mid-portion of the dorsal surface of the prostate or Denonvilliers' fascia can be freed in the midline from the rectal surface. Dissection is then carried out along the prostate sharply freeing it off of the neurovascular bundles. When vascular branches are identified, they are controlled with fine ligatures or clips. Cautery should be avoided to prevent injury to the neurovascular bundles. As the base of the prostate is encountered, the main prostatic pedicle is encountered. The prostatic pedicle at this point should also be secured with ligatures or clips. The prostate is then carefully dissected at the level of the prostatovesical junction, starting anteriorly and progressing posteriorly.

❑❑ What structures are important to preserve at the base of the prostate?

The bladder neck should be preserved when possible to improve continence. Posteriorly, the trigone can easily be encroached upon during the dissection of the posterior aspect of the base of the prostate and trigonal injury can occur.

❑❑ What can one do to prevent damage to the ureteral orifices?

Bladder neck preservation surgery is the safest way to preserve the ureteral orifices. Indigo carmine or methylene blue may be administered intravenously to identify the ureteral orifices. Alternatively, ureteral catheters can be placed under direct vision to delineate the ureteral orifices. If there is any question subsequently whether the ureteral orifices have been violated, placement of ureteral stents prior to the urethrovesical anastamosis should be entertained.

❑❑ After freeing up the apex of the prostate, the prostatic pedicles and the prostatovesical junction, what structures remain to be dissected free to allow the prostate to be removed?

The seminal vesicles and ductus differentia. The ductus differentia are identified in the midline. They are transected and ligated using clips or absorbable suture. These are then used to delineate the medial side of the seminal vesicles. The seminal vesicles are dissected free from the surrounding tissue and the apical artery identified, controlled and divided.

❑❑ What is the blood supply to the seminal vesicle?

The artery to the seminal vesicle is also a division of the hypogastric artery. It penetrates the seminal vesicle at its superior end. These need to be secured before removing the seminal vesicle. After the seminal vesicles and the ductus differentia are freed, the prostate specimen may be removed.

❑❑ How is continuity of the urinary tract restored?

The urethrovesical anastomosis is performed in two steps:

1. The bladder neck is reconstructed so that the opening is approximately 1.2 cm to 1.5 cm an appropriately sized catheter or sound can help one approximate the size. Typically this is accomplished by closing the bladder neck in a tennis racquet manner anteriorly and / or posteriorly, with care taken to avoid damage to the ureteral orifices. The mucosa is everted using 4-0 absorbable suture to "stomatize" the bladder neck.

2. Sutures are then placed in the urethral stump. This may be done earlier, as the urethra is transected from the prostate or at the time of bladder neck reconstruction. Often a Van Buren sound placed per urethral meatus may help delineate the urethral stump. Once 4 to 6 sutures are placed in the urethra they are sewn through the bladder neck. After all sutures have been placed, a Foley catheter is passed per urethra and directed into the bladder. The sutures are then tied down individually with gentle traction on the Foley catheter to bring the bladder down to the urethra.

❑❑ What sort of drains are necessary for this surgery?

The two potential areas of drainage from radical retropubic prostatectomy are urinary drainage from the urethrovesical anastomosis and lymphatic drainage if a lymphadenectomy was performed. Drains (suction or non-suction) are placed in the left and right side of the pelvis, respectively. The incision is then closed in the midline in the usual fashion.

❑❑ What is the positioning for perineal prostatectomy?

The patient is placed in the extreme dorsal lithotomy position with a rolled towel or sheet under the sacrum so that the perineum is parallel to the floor. Allen stirrups are used to stabilize the patient's legs.

❑❑ What incision is used for perineal prostatectomy?

The incision is made in a convex curvilinear fashion between the ischial tuberosities, anterior to the anus. Prior to the incision a curved Lowsley tractor is placed per urethra into the bladder.

❑❑ What are the layers to be divided between the skin and the prostate?

Scarpa's fascia, the central tendon or perineal body and the rectourethralis muscule are all divided during the dissection. The levator ani muscles which meet in the midline posterior to the rectourethralis muscle are also encountered. These are retracted laterally.

❑❑ What are the "pearly gates?"

The "pearly gates" are also known as Denonvilliers' fascia. This indicates that the base of the prostate is in view. The rectum is then dissected off of the posterior surface of the prostate by dividing Denonvilliers' fascia using sharp and blunt dissection.

❑❑ Is there any retractor that can be used to facilitate this prostatectomy?

There are several devices that can be used to retract the levator ani and the padded rectum out of the operative field. It is at this point in the operation that these self-retaining retractors are generally employed.

❑❑ Describe the apical dissection in a perineal prostatectomy.

The prostatourethral junction is visualized from the posterior surface in the perineal exposure. A right angle clamp is gently passed around the urethra, between the dorsal venous complex and the anterior surface of the urethra. This dissects the underside of the dorsal vein complex off of the anterior surface of the urethra. The posterior aspect of the urethra is then transected, and the curved Lowsley tractor is removed. A straight Lowsley tractor is placed into the bladder through the urethrotomy and the wings expanded. The anterior surface of the urethra is then divided.

❑❑ Can the neurovascular bundles be seen and / or preserved in the perineal prostatectomy?

If the Denonvilliers' fascia is divided in the midline towards the apex of the prostate, then a right angle can used to follow the prostatic contour more closely and preserve the neurovascular bundles laterally at the level of the apex of the prostate. Care must be taken subsequently to continue to dissect the neurovascular bundles off of the prostate throughout their course.

❑❑ How is the anterior prostate dissected?

The anterior prostate is visualized by pushing downward posteriorly on the Lowsley tractor. A plane of dissection is developed between the anterior surface of the prostae and the endopelvic fascia. This plane is actually below the dorsal venous complex / Santorini's plexus. With this approach to the prostate, Santorini's plexus is rarely encountered or injured during the perineal prostatectomy. Once the wings of the Lowsley can be palpated, this indicates that the dissection has carried to the prostatovesical junction.

❑❑ How is the prostatovesical junction delineated?

The prostatovesical junction can be delineated by rotating the wings of the Lowsley in a circumferential manner. Once the junction is well defined, the detrussorotomy is made in the anterior midline at the level of the prostatovesical junction. The wings of the Lowsley tractor can be delivered through this detrussorotomy and dissection is carried circumferentially around the bladder neck using the Lowsley tractor for retraction.

❑❑ Is there any option to using the Lowsley tractor?

The Lowsley tractor may be removed and a right-angle clamp passed through the apex of the prostate and used to deliver an 18-French red rubber catheter. This allows some pliability and some flexibility.

❑❑ How is the blood supply to the prostate controlled?

As large vessels are encountered, they may be suture ligated or clipped prior to dividing the apex. The prostate may be rotated anteriorly and the posterior pedicles at the base of the prostate can be visualized and suture ligated before apical dissection.

❑❑ Are there any pitfalls to the dissection of the ureters or the trigone in the perineal approach?

The perineal prostatectomy and the radial retropublic prostatectomy are analogous at this point in that either Indigo carmine or methylene blue may be administered intravenously to delineate the ureteral orifices. Alternatively, if there is concern, ureteral stents may be placed.

❑❑ Are the seminal vesicle dissections analogous too?

The seminal vesicle dissection is somewhat more problematic with a perineal prostatectomy than a retropubic prostatectomy. Again, the vasa deferentia and ductus deferens are identified in the midline and clipped. Though the dissection down to the apex of the seminal vesicle may sometimes be awkward, with patience, the artery to the seminal vesicle may be ligated at the tip of the seminal vesicle and the prostate gland removed.

❑❑ How is the urethrovesical anastomosis performed in a radical perineal prostatectomy?

One of the advantages of the perineal prostatectomy compared with the retropubic prostatectomy is that urethrovesical anastomosis is often easier to perform. The bladder neck is tailored to 1.2 cm to 1.5 cm in diameter, using a tennis racquet approach to avoid damage to the ureteral orifice. The bladder mucosa is everted at the surgeon's discretion. Interrupted sutures are used to re-anastomose the bladder neck to the urethra, starting in the anterior midline and extending laterally. However, once three-quarters of the anastomosis has been performed, a Foley catheter is placed per urethra and directed into the bladder and the remainder of the anastomosis is performed.

❑❑ How is the perineal prostatectomy drained?

A separate perineal stab incision is made and a Penrose drain is placed at the level of the urethrovesical anastomosis. The wound is closed in layers with absorbable suture. The patient is treated with routine post-operative care. Post-operative care is consistent between retropubic prostatectomy and perineal prostatectomy.

❑❑ How long does the patient stay in the hospital?

Patients stay in the hospital until they are tolerating a diet and drainage has tapered off sufficiently and they are hemodynamically stable. Patients are discharged with their Foley.

❑❑ How long does the Foley catheter remain?

The Foley catheter remains in place for two to three weeks, then it is removed in the office.

❑❑ Do any confirmatory tests need to be performed before the Foley catheter is removed?

Traditionally, a gravity cystogram was performed before removal of the catheter. Due to refinement in technique, this has not been considered necessary by most surgeons. Although if there is any question of urinary leak, a cystogram should be performed prior to removal of the Foley catheter.

❑❑ If there is excessive drainage from the wound or drainage sites, how can one tell the origin of the fluid?

The fluid should be sent for creatinine determination. If the creatinine is equivalent to the serum creatinine, a urine leak is ruled out. The drains should be managed conservatively and left in place until the fluid accumulation has subsided. If the drainage persists without evidence of improvement a lymphatic source is more likely. The patient should be placed on broad spectrum oral antibiotics and the drains gradually advanced and removed. The lymphatic leak should subside with time, but a lymphocele may accumulate and require internal drainage.

If the fluid has a markedly elevated creatinine a urine leak is confirmed. Similarly, the patient should be placed on broad spectrum oral antibiotics and the drains should be taken off of suction and advanced gradually until they are removed. The Foley catheter should be maintained. With adequate drainage, urinary leakage should subside.

❑❑ What are the intraoperative complications from radical prostatectomy?

1. Hemorrhage.
2. Rectal injury.
3. Ureteral injury.

❑❑ How is hemorrhage handled?

The source must be identified. Generally, this is from the dorsal vein complex or from the prostatic pedicle. The most important step in controlling hemorrhage is to first make sure the patient remains hemodynamically stable. Communication with anesthesia is of major importance. Initially, pressure may be placed on the bleeding area so that anesthesia can maintain or reestablish hemodynamic stability. Dorsal vein complex bleeding was previously described. If the prostatic pedicles are bleeding, then they must be suture ligated. Mass ligatures or widespread electrocautery should not be used because it may damage the surrounding structures. If the urine is grossly bloody in the post-operative period, gentle traction on the Foley catheter can be utilized for short periods of time.

❑❑ How does rectal injury occur and how is it managed?

The incidence of rectal injury for patients undergoing a radical perineal prostatectomy is 10%. Injury usually occurs during takedown of the rectum and rectourethralis musculature. In some patients, the rectum is densely adherent to the posterior surface of the prostate, and an enterotomy occurs. If an enterotomy occurs at this stage, it is safe to continue with the dissection of the posterior surface of the prostate unless there is fecal soilage. If feces contaminate the wound the area should be thoroughly irrigated and the operation ended after formation of a diverting colostomy.

If the patient has had a good antibiotic and mechanical bowel prep the prostatectomy may be continued. The rectum should be closed in two layers. Some Urologists favor the input of a general surgeon. Assuming that the patient has had a preoperative bowel prep, a primary repair should be safe. In addition, a manual dilation or defunctionalization of the anal sphincter should be performed following closure of the incision, and the patient should be kept on a low residue diet for one to two weeks post-operatively.

Rectal injuries are less common with radical retropubic prostatectomy with an incidence of 5% to 7%. Generally, this occurs during apical dissection in the midline. Again, the rectal injury should be closed in two layers, and following closure of the incision the anus should be manually dilated and the patient kept on a low residue diet.

▢▢ What if the patient has fecal drainage from his wound or his drain post-operatively.

Provided the patient is clinically stable and fit for anesthesia, a diverting colostomy is indicated. The only way to heal a rectal fistula is by complete diversion.

The risk of a rectal injury during a perineal prostatectomy can be minimized by placing a gloved finger in the rectum during the dissection so that the rectum is clearly identifiable throughout the dissection.

▢▢ How is ureteral injury handled?

Ureteral injury, which may occur during lymph node dissection or less likely during dissection of the prostatovesical junction if one got into the wrong plane, is best handled by ureteral re-implantation in the standard fashion.

▢▢ What are the post-operative complications of radical prostatectomy?

As with any major pelvic surgery for cancer, deep vein thrombosis of the lower extremity and femoral veins is always a possibility. As mentioned before, TED hose and sequential compression devices can be useful intraoperatively. If deep vein thrombosis is clinically suspected, a Doppler ultrasound of the lower extremities and pelvic veins should be ordered immediately.

▢▢ What are the complications of a DVT?

The catastrophic complication of DVTs is pulmonary embolus, which is life threatening. Pulmonary embolus causes circulatory collapse and should be suspected when a patient has shortness of breath, tachypnea, tachycardia and unexplained fever. A confirmatory study is a pulmonary arteriogram. Pulmonary embolism is an emergent situation that should be treated initially with anticoagulation and urgent cardiac or general surgery consultation.

▢▢ What if the Foley catheter is removed accidentally or falls out?

If the catheter falls out, a coudé catheter may be gently passed. If it does not pass easily on the first gentle attempt, the patient should be taken to the cystoscopy suite and under direct visualization a guide wire is placed in the bladder and a Council-tipped catheter can be placed into the bladder. This prevents any disruption of the vesicourethral anastomosis.

▢▢ What if the patient does not void after removal of the Foley catheter?

If the patient does not void or is uncomfortable, a catheter can be gently passed per urethra. If this does not pass easily, a suprapubic tube can be placed into the patient's bladder, and trials of voiding can be carried out at a later date. Edema at the site of the urethrovesical anastamosis is usually the etiology of failure to void in this situation.

▢▢ What if there is drainage through the incision after a perineal prostatectomy?

Urinary drainage will usually subside. Depending upon the severity of leakage, a Foley catheter can be placed or the patient can be managed conservatively.

▢▢ What if the patient develops urinary retention three months after operation?

A bladder neck contracture is a likely etiology. The urethra may be gradually dilated with filiforms and followers. Alternatively, a direct vision internal urethrotomy should be performed.

❑❑ What is the complication of a direct vision internal urethrotomy or bladder neck contracture after radical prostatectomy?

Urinary incontinence. The urethrovesical anastomosis is very close to the external urinary sphincter and in incising an anastomotic stricture, the sphincter may be damaged leading to urinary incontinence.

❑❑ What if the stricture occurs three years after surgery?

Cystoscopy should be performed to evaluate the stricture. It should be handled with care to avoid incontinence. The surgeon should also be cognizant that this may represent a local recurrence of disease and a PSA should be checked to evaluate this possibility and a biopsy of the stricture may be considered.

❑❑ What is the incidence of urinary incontinence following radical prostatectomy?

Depending on the study, continence rates have been reported between 100% and 45% with most studies describing full continence in 85 to 90% of the patients treated with radical prostatectomy. Certainly it takes a while to establish continence, and surgeons feel that some stress incontinence between the first catheter removal and six months post-surgery is not worrisome or negatively prognostic in terms of the patient's overall continence rate postoperatively.

❑❑ How is incontinence managed?

For the first year postoperatively, anticholinergics or alpha-agonists can be used to try to minimize the incontinence. If the incontinence persists, management with artificial urinary sphincter or a trial of submucosal collagen injections at the bladder neck may be indicated.

❑❑ What is the incidence of impotence following radical prostatectomy?

Reported potency results following radical prostatectomy vary widely between 75% potent and 10% potent.

❑❑ Is there an advantage in terms of potency to radical retropubic prostatectomy over radical perineal prostatectomy?

Certainly radical retropubic prostatectomy allows improved visualization and preservation of the neurovascular complexes that run along the lateral surface of the prostate gland. Certainly, if the neurovascular bundles are included in the specimen, there is unlikely preservation of potency even during radical retropubic prostatectomy.

❑❑ Is potency possible after radical perineal prostatectomy?

Yes. Several techniques have been described that allow for an apical dissection that will preserve the neurovascular bundles and in younger men with excellent preoperative potency has been maintained during a perineal approach. Preservation of potency is related to the patient's preoperative erectile status. Potency will be covered more completely in another chapter in this book.

TREATMENT OF LOCALLY RECURRENT PROSTATE CANCER

Badar Mian, M.D. and Louis L. Pisters, M.D.

❏❏ **What is the current incidence of clinical stage T3 prostate cancer?**

15 to 20% of patients in modern series present with extracapsular disease.

❏❏ **What is the incidence of pathological T3 disease in patients who are initially diagnosed with organ-confined disease?**

25 to 50% of these patients may have extracapsular disease, depending on the Gleason score and the prostate-specific antigen (PSA) concentration.

❏❏ **Does PSA level reliably predict pathological stage?**

70 to 80% of patients with locally advanced prostate cancer have a serum PSA level of >10 ng/ml, but serum PSA level alone cannot reliably predict pathological stage.

❏❏ **What is the incidence of seminal vesicle invasion (SVI) in patients with clinical T3a disease?**

Approximately 15 to 20% of patients will have SVI after radical prostatectomy.

❏❏ **What are the pitfalls of seminal vesicle biopsies to assess local tumor extent in patients with locally advanced prostate cancer?**

A significant number of *false negative* biopsy results can occur due to sampling error in the presence of focal SVI. Even when SVI is suspected clinically and biopsies are performed, only 50% of patients will have positive biopsy results. *False positive* results can occur because of a drag-through artifact where the needle goes through the base of the prostate. Lipofuscin staining can identify seminal vesicle tissue and help minimize the *false positive* results.

❏❏ **What is the extent of clinical staging error for locally advanced prostate cancer?**

Overstaging occurs in 20 to 25% of patients who are found to have organ confined disease. Understaging has been reported in 20 to 40% of patients who are found to have T4 lesions or nodal metastases.

❏❏ **What percentage of patients with locally advanced prostate cancer will require surgical or medical intervention for disease progression if initially placed on watchful waiting?**

Approximately 70% will require some form of intervention secondary to local or distant disease progression. Most patients are treated with hormonal ablation therapy. Up to 50% of patients may need a transurethral resection of the prostate (TURP) or nephrostomy tube placement for urinary obstruction.

❏❏ **What are the long-term results following radical prostatectomy for clinical T3 disease without adjuvant therapy?**

At 5 years, approximately 70% of such patients will have a biochemical (PSA) relapse, while 85% will have rising PSA levels if lymph nodes were positive. At 10 years, 70% are expected to have clinical progression and more than 50% of patient deaths are due to prostate cancer.

❑❑ **What effect does local failure have on quality of life after external beam radiation therapy (EBRT)?**

A significant decrease in quality of life is noted secondary to pelvic pain, hematuria, bladder outlet obstruction, and ureteral obstruction requiring nephrostomy tube placement. There is a significantly higher incidence of metastatic progression with bone pain and pathological progression.

❑❑ **What percentage of patients with local disease progression following EBRT may require surgical procedures?**

Depending upon the length of follow-up, up to 80% of such patients can require surgical intervention such as TURP, salvage radical prostatectomy, or nephrostomy tube placement. Also, 30 to 50% of patients undergoing TURP in this situation become incontinent.

❑❑ **What strategies have been used to improve local control and the disease-free survival rate following EBRT?**

EBRT has been used in combination with neoadjuvant / adjuvant hormonal deprivation therapy and with brachytherapy. Also, dose escalation and conformal techniques have been utilized to deliver a larger dose to the target area.

❑❑ **What are the results of cryotherapy for patients with clinical stage T3 prostate cancer?**

At 6 months follow-up, up to 75% of patients may have negative prostate biopsies and 50% may have an undetectable PSA level. However, only 15% continue to have an undetectable PSA level after 1 year.

❑❑ **What are the more common sites for T3 disease recurrence following cryotherapy?**

Residual tumor is found more commonly in the seminal vesicle biopsies and apical biopsies. These sites may be inadequately treated secondary to technical difficulties.

❑❑ **What are the most common complications following cryotherapy?**

Common complications include voiding symptoms such as frequency, urgency, and urinary retention related to local edema and urethral sloughing. Up to 30% of patients have reportedly required transurethral resection of necrotic debris. The risk of urinary incontinence is significantly higher in patients who have received radiation therapy in the past (up to 60 to 70% incidence). With improvements in technology and better ability to monitor urethral and intraprostatic temperature, these complications may decrease over time.

❑❑ **A patient presents with a high-grade Gleason combined score 9, clinical stage T2b N0M0 adenocarcinoma. After a lengthy discussion of treatment options, the patient decides to pursue initial observation. What are the disease- specific and metastasis-free survival rates at 10 years for patients with high- grade, clinically localized prostate cancer that has been observed?**

Reports in the literature indicate that patients with clinically localized (clinical stage ≤ T2) high grade prostate cancer who are treated conservatively, will have a disease-specific survival rate of only 34% at 10 years, and only 26% of these patients will be free of metastasis at 10 years. Patients with high-grade prostate cancers are over six times more likely to die of prostate cancer than are patients with lower-grade tumors.

❑❑ **A patient with initial clinical stage T3 prostate cancer undergoes external beam radiation therapy and is noted to have a rising PSA level. The patient elects to be initially observed for his rising PSA. What is the time interval from the rise in the PSA level to development of clinically detectable prostate cancer (change in rectal examination or radiographic bone metastasis)?**

A rising PSA level after initial radiation therapy precedes clinically detectable disease relapse by 3 to 5 years on average. In the absence of salvage therapy, at least three quarters of men will have clinical evidence of recurrent disease 5 years after PSA elevation is detected.

❏❏ **A 55-year-old man with Gleason combined score 7, clinical stage T2a prostate cancer elects to receive initial external beam radiation therapy. His pretreatment PSA value is 7.5 ng/ml and falls to a nadir level of 1.2 ng/ml. It then rises to 5.5 ng/ml. The patient is now 60 years old. What staging studies should be considered prior to salvage radical prostatectomy?**

Restaging for patients with rising PSA levels after radiation therapy should include a bone scan and possibly a computerized tomography of the abdomen and pelvis to rule out metastatic disease. Although it is well established that bone scans rarely detect metastasis in untreated patients with a PSA value below 20 ng/ml, this has not been established for patients with rising PSA levels after radiation therapy. In surgical candidates, cystoscopic examination is helpful to rule out bladder neck involvement.

❏❏ **For the patient described above, what is the role for prostate biopsies and what is the likelihood that prostate biopsies will be positive in this clinical setting?**

A biopsy is indicated only in those patients who are considering further aggressive local therapy, namely salvage prostatectomy, cryotherapy, or radiation therapy. Performing a prostate biopsy under transrectal ultrasound (TRUS) guidance is important, as up to 80% of patients with a rising PSA after initial radiation therapy will have positive biopsies.

❏❏ **The above-described patient elects to undergo a salvage radical prostatectomy. Given that his presalvage serum PSA concentration is <10 ng/ml, what are his chances of having an undetectable serum PSA 5 years later?**

The 5-year biochemical disease-free survival rate is 70% for patients undergoing salvage prostatectomy with a presalvage PSA <10 ng/ml compared with 47% for patients with a presalvage PSA >10 ng/ml.

❏❏ **In salvage prostatectomy series performed in the PSA era, what are the rates of capsular penetration, positive margins, and seminal vesicle involvement?**

Many patients with recurrent prostate cancer after radiation therapy have larger cancers with more advanced pathological stage than anticipated from the preoperative clinical staging. Adverse pathologic features are commonly present. Series that include patients diagnosed in the PSA era have shown a 26% to 43% rate of capsular penetration, a 32 to 36% rate of positive surgical margins, and a 28 to 49% rate of seminal vesicle involvement.

❏❏ **A patient undergoes a salvage radical prostatectomy following radiation therapy. The final pathologic evaluation shows Gleason combined score 9 adenocarcinoma with extracapsular extension and a positive surgical margin. The seminal vesicles and lymph nodes are negative. Is a positive surgical margin in a patient undergoing salvage radical prostatectomy biologically significant?**

A positive surgical margin in a previously irradiated patient is biologically significant, and patients with positive margins have a worse cancer-specific survival rate than do those with negative surgical margins. In previously irradiated patients, there are no curative treatments to fall back on should the surgery fail to remove all the cancer.

❏❏ **What is the risk of urinary incontinence following salvage radical prostatectomy?**

Incontinence in recent salvage prostatectomy series remains high at 50 to 65%, despite improvements in operative technique.

❏❏ **A patient with recurrent prostate cancer after radiation therapy does not want to undergo salvage radical prostatectomy but does desire further local therapy. Other than salvage radical prostatectomy, what other salvage local therapies are available? What are the biochemical disease-free survival rates and complications of these alternate salvage local therapies?**

Salvage cryotherapy and salvage brachytherapy are alternate salvage local therapies. Approximately 40% of patients undergoing salvage cryotherapy will have a durable biochemical response. The main patient-reported complications of salvage cryotherapy are urinary incontinence (72%), obstructive symptoms (66%), impotence (85%), and severe perineal pain (44%). The 5-year biochemical disease-free survival rate following salvage brachytherapy is only 34%, which appears lower than the biochemical disease-free survival rates reported for salvage prostatectomy or cryotherapy. There is a 37% incidence of serious gastrointestinal or genitourinary complications following salvage brachytherapy. Obstructive symptoms are common, and up to 14% of patients undergo a transurethral resection for relief of obstructive symptoms following salvage brachytherapy. Four percent of patients develop significant rectal ulceration, and there are reports of patients undergoing colostomy for rectal bleeding.

❐❐ **Pathological features have been shown to be extremely important in establishing risk for local versus distant recurrence after radical prostatectomy. For patients with a rising PSA level after radical prostatectomy, which pathological features of the radical prostatectomy specimen support the presence of distant metastasis?**

Patients with a radical prostatectomy specimen Gleason score of ≥8, seminal vesicle invasion, or positive pelvic lymph nodes are at higher risk for distant metastasis. Patients with a specimen Gleason score ≤7, no seminal vesicle invasion, and negative pelvic lymph nodes are at higher risk for local recurrence.

❐❐ **Does the presence of negative surgical margins in a radical prostatectomy specimen preclude the development of a local recurrence?**

Reports indicate that patients with negative surgical margins still have a substantial risk of local recurrence. Of patients with an elevated PSA level and negative bone scan following radical prostatectomy the chances of a biopsy proven local recurrence have been reported to be as high as 34%. These data objectively demonstrate that a significant subset of patients with negative surgical margins may develop local recurrences. Patients with negative surgical margins should, therefore, not be excluded from salvage radiation therapy.

❐❐ **What are the PSA features of local versus distant disease recurrence following radical prostatectomy? Is the timing of the PSA recurrence important?**

Many studies have shown that a short interval from surgery to detectable PSA is often indicative of distant metastasis. The development of a detectable PSA ≤1 year following radical prostatectomy, a PSA velocity of ≥0.75 ng/ml per year following radical prostatectomy, and a PSA doubling time of ≤6 months have all been associated with significant risk for distant metastasis in patients with a rising PSA level after radical prostatectomy. By comparison, patients who develop a detectable PSA >1 year following radical prostatectomy, or having a PSA velocity <0.75 ng/ml per year, or having a PSA doubling time of >6 months are at higher risk of local recurrence.

❐❐ **A 70-year-old man develops a rising PSA value after radical prostatectomy. This patient elects to undergo observation. What is the median actuarial time from postsurgical PSA elevation to the development of clinically evident metastasis?**

Eight years.

❐❐ **A 60-year-old patient has a rising PSA value after radical prostatectomy. Four years after radical prostatectomy, his serum PSA concentration is 1.2 ng/ml. The patient is concerned about the possibility of metastasis, and staging studies including a bone scan and CT scan are ordered. What is the likelihood that a bone scan or CT scan will be positive in this patient?**

Although bone scans and CT scans of the pelvis are often recommended for patients with a rising PSA value after surgery, results of these studies are initially negative in the majority of patients, particularly in those with low PSA values (<30 ng/ml). There have been anecdotal cases of patients who had positive bone scans but undetectable PSA levels, although this is extremely rare. The literature supports the low likelihood of a positive bone scan (<5%) in this setting until the PSA increased to 40 to 45 ng/ml. Bone scans have limited usefulness until the PSA increases above 30 ng/ml. In general, there is no need to obtain a bone scan if systemic therapy is planned. Furthermore, CT scans of the pelvis are often inaccurate for assessing lymph node metastasis. The decision to obtain a bone scan or a CT study in a patient with rising PSA after surgery should therefore be individualized.

❐❐ **A 60-year-old nervous lawyer develops a rising PSA 5 years after radical prostatectomy. He is well informed and requests an indium-111 capromab pendetide (ProstaScint®) scan. What is the usefulness of this type of scan in patients with a rising PSA value after radical prostatectomy? What are the positive and negative predictive values of the scan?**

The indium-111 capromab pendetide scan is associated with a low negative predictive value of 70%, suggesting that the technique may be falsely negative in up to 30% of cases. False-positive scans may occur as a result of inflammation or vascular abnormalities following surgery. Therefore, owing to its inaccuracy, indium-111 capromab pendetide imaging has limited value in evaluating patients with elevated PSA values after surgery.

❑❑ **What proportion of patients with a detectable PSA level after radical prostatectomy will experience a fall or decrease in their PSA level with salvage radiation therapy?**

Most patients (approximately 80 to 85%) who receive postoperative radiation therapy to the prostatic bed experience a decrease in their serum PSA following the initiation of radiation therapy. This fact objectively demonstrates that at least some cancer cells persisted in the local field after radical prostatectomy.

❑❑ **In what proportion of patients who undergo salvage radiation therapy for a detectable PSA level does the PSA level become undetectable and stay undetectable?**

The PSA becomes undetectable and stays undetectable in approximately 10 to 59% of patients following salvage radiation therapy. This widely divergent outcome in terms of a persistently undetectable PSA level is almost certainly related to substantial differences in patient selection, dose of radiation, and timing of radiation therapy.

❑❑ **A patient has a PSA value of 0.8 ng/ml 5 years after radical prostatectomy. What is his likelihood of having a durable biochemical response to salvage radiation? What would his chance of having a durable biochemical response be if his PSA value was 3.5 ng/ml?**

The preradiation PSA value has a profound effect on outcome following salvage radiation therapy. It is clear that the lower the preradiation PSA value, the greater the likelihood of achieving a durable biochemical response. If the preradiation PSA is <2 ng/ml, then 83% of such patients will be disease-free at 4 years compared with only 33% of patients with a PSA >2 ng/ml. For this reason, patients who have a rising PSA value after surgery and who have pathologic features favorable for salvage radiation therapy should have this radiation therapy administered early, while the PSA is well below 2 ng/ml. Observing these patients and letting the PSA rise above 2 ng/ml may significantly compromise their chances for a cure.

❑❑ **What pathologic features of radical prostatectomy specimens have been shown to have prognostic value for patients undergoing salvage radiation therapy?**

Several studies have shown that patients with pathological evidence of seminal vesicle or lymph node involvement are unlikely to have a durable response to salvage radiation therapy. The risk of treatment failure is 5.6 times higher if patients have pathological evidence of lymph node or seminal vesicle involvement. In patients with no evidence of seminal vesicle or lymph node involvement, 82% and 38% of patients with PSA values of ≤2 ng/ml and >2 ng/ml, respectively, were disease free at 4 years (Forman, J Urol 158:1436, 1997). Some reports have shown that patients with higher-grade cancer (Gleason score of 8 to 10) in the radical prostatectomy specimen are at much higher risk for biochemical failure following salvage radiation therapy.

❑❑ **What are the complications of salvage radiation therapy for a detectable PSA level following radical prostatectomy? If a patient has good continence, is he likely to develop incontinence?**

In general, salvage radiation therapy is extremely well tolerated with few serious side effects. The most common side effects are related to radiation-induced cystitis and proctitis, which may cause irritative voiding symptoms and diarrhea. The irritative voiding symptoms and diarrhea typically resolve within 3 months of therapy. A worsening of incontinence has been noted in approximately 4% to 8% of patients undergoing salvage radiation therapy. In general, however, most patients who have good urinary control following radical prostatectomy continue to have good urinary control after salvage radiation therapy. The effect of salvage radiation therapy on potency has not been well studied.

❑❑ **What is the biochemical disease-free survival rate for patients with clinical stage T3-4 prostate cancer who undergo external beam radiation therapy alone?**

Studies have indicated a 10-year biochemical disease-free survival rate of only 18% in patients with clinical stage T3-4 disease who were treated with external beam monotherapy. Because the results of external beam radiation therapy alone for locally advanced prostate cancer have been disappointing, there has been a dramatic shift toward treating patients with combined hormonal therapy and radiation therapy.

❏❏ **Is there convincing evidence to indicate that the combined use of hormonal therapy along with radiation therapy is superior to radiation therapy alone?**

There have been at least four randomized prospective studies that demonstrate improvement in disease-free survival rates for patients treated with combined hormonal treatment with radiation therapy compared with radiation therapy alone. Only one study demonstrated an improvement in the overall survival rate for patients treated with combined hormonal therapy and radiation therapy, compared with radiation alone.

❏❏ **Is there any randomized prospective evidence to indicate that the combined use of hormonal therapy and radiation therapy is superior to the use of hormonal treatment alone?**

A randomized prospective study including three treatment groups: an orchiectomy-only group, a radiation therapy-only group, and a combined orchiectomy plus radiation therapy group indicated no statistical difference between the orchiectomy-only and combined therapy treatment groups with regard to distant disease progression and overall survival rate.

❏❏ **A 60-year-old man presents with palpable extracapsular extension with Gleason combined score 7 adenocarcinoma and a PSA value of 15 ng/ml. He is considering 3 months of neoadjuvant hormonal therapy prior to radical prostatectomy. Is there any evidence that neoadjuvant hormonal therapy results in downstaging of clinical stage T3 prostate cancer?**

There have been many studies of neoadjuvant hormonal therapy in patients with clinical stage T3 disease. These studies showed a drop in PSA level in more than 90% of cases, with a 30 to 50% decrease in prostate volume after neoadjuvant hormonal therapy. However, only about 21% of these patients had organ-confined disease, which is not substantially different from the frequency of organ-confined disease noted in patients undergoing surgery without neoadjuvant hormonal therapy for stage T3 disease. Thus, there is no evidence whatsoever that neoadjuvant hormonal therapy results in downstaging of T3 prostate cancer.

❏❏ **The use of neoadjuvant hormonal therapy prior to radical prostatectomy has been shown to reduce the risk of positive surgical margins in which patients?**

The observed reduction in the rate of positive margins has been limited to patients with clinical stage T2 disease, and a reduced rate has not been seen in patients with clinical stage T3 disease.

❏❏ **Is there any proven reduction in the rate of biochemical failure for patients treated with 3 months of neoadjuvant hormonal therapy prior to surgery?**

Several recent randomized prospective series comparing the use of neoadjuvant hormonal therapy before surgery with the use of surgery alone for clinical stage T1-T3 prostate cancer found no difference in the rate of subsequent biochemical failure between the two treatment groups. Thus, there does not appear to be any improvement in biochemical outcome following 3 months of neoadjuvant hormonal therapy given before surgery.

TESTICULAR AND PARATESTICULAR TUMORS

John D. Seigne, M.B.

❑❑ **A 26-year old man complains of a right testicular mass. He noticed the mass after falling 3-weeks ago. Physical examination is remarkable only for a mildly tender 3 cm lower pole testicular swelling. Laboratory studies and tumor markers are negative. Ultrasound demonstrates a well circumscribed heterogeneous mass in the lower pole of the right testicle. What is the next step in management?**

Many patients with testicular tumors report a recent history of mild testicular trauma. The ultrasound shows a solid mass classical for a testicular tumor. Therefore right inguinal exploration and orchiectomy is the appropriate management.

❑❑ **A 38-year old man presents with a left testicular mass. Tumor markers are normal. He undergoes a left inguinal orchiectomy. What is the likely histology? If the patient's BHCG was 25 would this change your prediction?**

Seminoma is the most common histology found in men over the age of 35. However, if BHCG is elevated, this is more likely to be a non seminomatous germ cell tumor, despite the patients age and the fact that 10-25% of men with seminoma have an elevated BHCG prior to orchiectomy.

❑❑ **A 22-year old man recently had a left orchiectomy for a seminoma. He has low risk metastatic seminoma to the lungs and is due to start BEP chemotherapy. Sperm banking is not covered by his insurance company. He wants to know if the expense is justifiable.**

Between 40% and 60% of patients with testicular cancer are hypofertile at diagnosis with sperm counts returning to normal in 75% of patients following orchiectomy. With newer reproductive technologies fertility is likely to be possible for more than 80% of patients. However, sperm banking is a sensible precaution as the sperm can be discarded after 2-3 years if the patient remains disease free and the sperm count reverts to normal.

❑❑ **A 30-year old man presents with a left testicular mass. He undergoes a left orchiectomy. Pathology shows a 4 cm embryonal cancer invading the tunica albuginea. Vascular invasion is noted. Metastatic work up consists of an abdominal CT scan, which shows a 7 cm left paraaortic mass. Chest CT shows five 0.5 cm to 2 cm lung nodules. LDH is 3 times normal. BHCG is 3000. AFP is 1500. What stage is the patient according to the 1997 American Joint Commission on Cancer TNM staging system.**

The patient has a T2N3S2M1a, Stage IIIA tumor.

❑❑ **A 27-year old man has a right orchiectomy for a mixed germ cell tumor (70% embryonal, 30% yolk sac). Tumor markers are negative. CBC and complete metabolic profile are normal. CT scan of the abdomen and pelvis is normal. Chest X-ray is normal. The patients referring doctor asks you if he should order a CT scan of the chest for the patient to bring with him to your appointment. Would this study be helpful?**

A chest CT is not necessary. In the absence of abdominal disease chest x-ray has been reported to have up to a 100% sensitivity in the detection of lung metastasis. Chest CT scan has a false positive rate of 5-7% leading to unnecessary further evaluation.

❑❑ A 22-year old has a left orchiectomy for a mixed germ cell tumor of the testis. Preoperative AFP is 80. Assuming that this is the only site of disease. How long would it take the AFP to return to normal (<5).

The half-life of AFP is 5-6 days therefore it would take 20-24 days to return to normal.

❑❑ A 36-year old has a left orchiectomy for a pure Seminoma BHCG. Preoperative BHCG is 25. Assuming that this is the only site of disease. How long would it take the BHCG to return to normal (<2).

The half-life of BHCG is 12-24 hours therefore it would take 48-120 hours to return to normal.

❑❑ A 29-year old has a left orchiectomy for a mixed germ cell tumor (70% embryonal, 30% yolk sac). Tumor markers are negative. Lab tests and Chest X-ray are normal. CT scan of the abdomen and pelvis is shown (Fig 1). What is the likelihood that the patient will be found to have metastatic germ cell tumor at the time of RPLND?

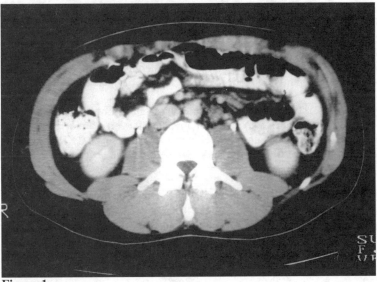

Figure 1

The CT scan shows a 1.5 cm node in the primary landing site of the left testicle. The likelihood that this contains tumor is approximately 75%.

❑❑ A 28-year old has a right orchiectomy for a testicular tumor. Final pathology shows a mixed germ cell tumor with 85% embryonal, 10% teratoma and 5% yolk sac. Vascular invasion is present. Metastatic work up including tumor markers, Chest X-ray and CT scan of the abdomen and pelvis are normal. What is the likelihood that the patient will be found to have metastatic germ cell tumor at the time of RPLND?

Vascular invasion and the percentage of embryonal cell carcinoma have been shown to reflect the risk of finding disease in the draining lymphatics. This patient falls into a high risk group and has an 80% chance of having disease at the time of RPLND.

❑❑ A 28-year old has a right orchiectomy for a mixed germ cell tumor (10% embryonal 30% teratoma and 40% seminoma). There is no vascular invasion. Metastatic work up including tumor markers, Chest x-ray and CT scan of the abdomen and pelvis are normal. What is the likelihood that the patient will be found to have germ cell tumor at the time of RPLND?

Vascular invasion and the percentage of embryonal cell carcinoma have been shown to reflect the risk of finding disease in the draining lymphatics. This patient falls into a low risk group and has a 10% chance of disease at the time of RPLND.

❑❏ **A 28-year old man with an embryonal carcinoma of the left testicle, normal tumor markers and negative metastatic evaluation undergoes a modified left nerve sparing RPLND. Final pathology demonstrates microscopic foci of embryonal cell carcinoma in 2 of 10 left para aortic nodes. If the patient elects observation what is the chance that the tumor will recur and what follow-up would you recommend?**

The risk of recurrence of the testicular cancer is between 8 and 48% in patients with pathological Stage II disease. The average likelihood of relapse is approximately 35% for patients with less than 5 nodes all less than 2 cm in diameter (as in this example). The most likely site of recurrence is the lungs. Recommended follow up is a physical exam, chest x-ray and tumor markers every 2 months for the 1st year, every 3 months for the 2nd year, every 4 months for the 3rd and 4th years and every 6 months for the 5th year. An abdominal CT scan should be performed at six months.

❑❏ **A 27-year old man has a right orchiectomy for a mixed germ cell tumor. Prior to orchiectomy his AFP was 25 and BHCG was <2.0. Final pathology shows a mixed germ cell tumor with 40% embryonal 20% yolk sac and 40% seminoma. There is no vascular invasion. Metastatic work up including chest x-ray and CT scan of the Abdomen and Pelvis are normal. One month after orchiectomy AFP is 12. What is the next step in management?**

Patients with persistently elevated tumor markers without evidence of disease on chest X-ray and abdominal CT scan are generally considered to have systemic disease and have a high relapse rate after RPLND. Reported data indicate that this patient should receive 3 cycles of Bleomycin, Etoposide and Cis-Platinium chemotherapy or 4 cycles of Etopiside and Cis-Platinium.

❑❏ **A 32-year old man undergoes a right orchiectomy for a mixed germ cell tumor of the testis (25% embryonal, 25% yolk sac and 50% seminoma. No vascular invasion is seen). Prior to orchiectomy AFP was 25 and BHCG was <2.0. He is now 3 weeks post orchiectomy. CXR is normal, CT of the abdomen and pelvis are normal as are tumor markers. He wants to be observed. What would you recommend as follow-up?**

A definitive protocol for follow up of patients on surveillance does not exist. The risk of recurrence is greatest in the first year, less in the second and then rapidly decreases. Therefore, patients require the most intensive monitoring during the first and second years, and decreasing frequency of visits during the following years.

❑❏ **A 36-year old homeless alcoholic undergoes a left orchiectomy for a pathological stage T1 non seminomatous germ cell tumor (20% embryonal, 40% seminoma, 40% yolk sac). Tumor markers prior to orchiectomy were BHCG 30 and AFP 45. An abdominal CT scan and chest x-ray show no evidence of disease. He is lost to follow up. Five-years later he returns to your office and wants follow-up. He has recently married and is currently working. He has no complaints, physical examination is normal. Tumor markers are notable for an AFP of 20 (nl. < 5). BHCG is normal. Chest X-ray and abdominal CT scans are normal. What is the cause of his AFP and what further management is necessary?**

Elevated AFP can be seen in patients with hepatocellular, pancreatic, gastric and lung carcinomas as well as benign conditions such as cirrhosis and hepatitis. This patient had a low risk tumor at diagnosis (T1, low percentage of embryonal cell) and has a negative evaluation 5-years after diagnosis. He is unlikely to have recurrent testicular cancer and should be evaluated for liver disease due to his history of alcohol abuse.

❑❏ **A 25-year old receives 4 cycles of chemotherapy for a Stage III nonseminomatous germ cell tumor. At diagnosis both BHCG and AFP were markedly elevated. He is now 1 month after completing chemotherapy and his BHCG has been stable for 2 months but slightly elevated at 6 (normal < 2). He has no complaints. Physical examination is notable only for an absent right testicle and a small soft left testicle. An extensive radiologic evaluation demonstrates a complete response. What is the next set in this patient's management?**

Occasionally some older assays for HCG can cross react with LH leading to a false positive elevation of BHCG. The patient has a small soft residual testicle suggesting he has hypogonadism. An intramuscular injection of 200mg of testosterone will suppress LH production and if BHCG is measured 48-hours later a true elevation of BHCG can be distinguished from cross reactivity in the assay.

❏❏ **A 25-year old man is undergoing a right modified template RPLND for a clinical stage I testis cancer. On abdominal exploration you note he has a 4 cm healthy appendix. Should an appendectomy be performed at the time of RPLND?**

An incidental appendectomy performed at the time of RPLND increases the risk of an infectious complication from 2% to approximately 10%. Therefore, incidental appendectomy at the time of RPLND is not recommended.

❏❏ **A 28-year old man with an embryonal carcinoma of the left testicle, normal tumor markers and negative metastatic evaluation undergoes a modified left nerve sparing RPLND. What are the boundaries of dissection?**

The boundaries of dissection are superiorly the renal artery and vein, inferiorly the bifurcation of the common iliac artery, laterally the ureter and medially the medial boarder of the aorta to the level of the inferior epigastric artery. Below the inferior epigastric artery the boundaries are the lateral aspect of the aorta and the common iliac artery. Additional inter aortocaval nodes should be removed below the right renal artery.

❏❏ **A 25-year old man with an embryonal carcinoma of the right testicle, normal tumor markers and negative metastatic evaluation undergoes a modified right nerve sparing RPLND. What are the boundaries of dissection?**

The boundaries of dissection are superiorly the right renal artery and vein, inferiorly the bifurcation of the common iliac artery, laterally the ureter and medially the mid-point of the aorta to the level of the inferior epigastric artery. Below the inferior epigastric artery the boundaries are the lateral aspect of the aorta and the common iliac artery.

❏❏ **A 25-year old man with an embryonal carcinoma of the left testicle, normal tumor markers and negative metastatic evaluation undergoes a modified left nerve sparing RPLND. At the time of RPLND gross nodal disease is unexpectedly discovered in the interaortocaval area. What is the appropriate course of action?**

The surgeon should abandon the plan to perform a modified nerve sparing operation and proceed with a full bilateral node dissection

❏❏ **A 28-year old man with an embryonal carcinoma of the left testicle, normal tumor markers and negative metastatic evaluation undergoes a modified template RPLND. What are the chances that he will have normal antegrade ejaculation? If the surgeon prospectively preserves the symphathetic nerves at the time of the template RPLND how much will that improve the rate of antegrade ejaculation?**

A template RPLND will result in approximately 75% of patients ejaculating normally. If prospective nerve sparing is performed this will increase to 98%.

❏❏ **A 25-year old man with an embryonal carcinoma of the left testicle, normal tumor markers and negative metastatic evaluation undergoes a modified left nerve sparing RPLND. At the time of RPLND gross nodal disease is unexpectedly discovered in the interaortocaval area. The surgeon performs a bilateral non nerve sparing dissection. How likely is the patient to ejaculate normally?**

Reports indicate that 18% of patients undergoing a bilateral infra hilar node dissection had antegrade ejaculation. If an extended suprahilar dissection was performed the rate decreases to 9%.

❏❏ **A 27-year old undergoes a right modified RPLND for a mixed germ cell tumor of the right testicle. Final pathology shows 3 interaortocaval nodes involved by tumor. The patient receives two cycles of adjuvant BEP chemotherapy. What are his chances of recurrence and survival?**

In a large randomized trial comparing observation to adjuvant chemotherapy in patients found to have stage II testis cancer at RPLND the relapse rate was reported as 6% after adjuvant chemotherapy. Overall survival was 97%.

❑❑ **A 30-year old with a clinical stage I nonseminomatous germ cell tumor is considering having an RPLND and asks that aside from ejaculatory problems what are the most common short and long term complications of the procedure. What would you tell him?**

In a report from the Testicular Inter Group Study, 3.4% of patients undergoing RPLND had a prolonged ileus for greater than 7 days, 3.3% developed pneumonia and 2% a UTI. Long-term complications included a 2.3% incidence of small bowel obstruction for an overall significant complication rate was 13.8%. Rarer complications included intraoperative hemorrhage, enterotomy, unplanned nephrectomy, thromboembolism, chylous fistula, lymphocoele and pancreatitis.

❑❑ **A 35-year old had a right orchiectomy for a stage I non seminomatous germ cell tumor of the right testis. Metastatic work up and tumor markers were negative. A right modified template RPLND showed no evidence of malignancy in 18/18 lymph nodes removed. What is the chance of relapse and where are the most common sites of relapse?**

Reports indicate that following RPLND 8% of Stage I patients relapsed within 2 years. 76% of these patients relapsed in the lungs and 14% of patients developing a marker only recurrence. Relapse in the retroperitoneum is rare after a properly performed RPLND.

❑❑ **A 32-year old undergoes a right orchiectomy for a Stage I non seminomatous germ cell tumor and enters a surveillance protocol. At the end of one year he is asymptomatic, all radiologic and laboratory studies are negative. He asks you what are his chances of recurrence.**

90% of recurrences occur within the first year. If he has no evidence of disease at five-years the likelihood of relapse is less than 3%.

❑❑ **A 27-year old man undergoes a left orchiectomy. Pathology shows a T1 non seminomatous germ cell tumor (50% teratoma, 40% embryonal cell carcinoma and 10% seminoma. Vascular invasion is noted). Within the teratomatous component foci of dedifferentiation to squamous cell carcinoma are noted. Metastatic evaluation including chest x-ray, abdominal CT scan and tumor markers are all normal. How does the presence of the squamous cell carcinoma effect the management of this patient?**

The presence of de-differentiation into another malignant tumor type within a teratoma is found in approximately 2% of patients. If the patient has Stage I disease the current recommendation is to treat these patients as you would a patient with a standard NSGCT. Thus, the recommendation would be for the patient to undergo a modified left template nerve sparing RPLND. In the presence of metastatic disease most patients do not respond to primary cisplatin based chemotherapy. In these cases the treatment needs to be tailored to the stage and histologic sub-type of the tumor.

❑❑ **A 32-year old is referred to you after under going a trans-scrotal exploration followed by an inguinal orchiectomy for an unsuspected non seminomatous germ cell tumor. After orchiectomy his tumor markers remain persistently elevated and he receives 3 cycles of BEP chemotherapy. Clinical, laboratory and radiological examination show no evidence of disease 1 month after completion of his chemotherapy. He is referred to you for hemiscrotectomy. What is your recommendation?**

Reports indicate that scrotal violation at the time of orchiectomy demonstrated no evidence of local recurrence in those patients who had received subsequent chemotherapy. Therefore, no surgery is indicated and the patient should be observed.

❑❑ **An 18-year old present with acute right testicular pain and a tender right testicle that is elevated in the scrotum without any obvious masses. The left testicle is normal. The patient is brought to the operating room and explored trans-scrotally for a diagnosis of testicular torsion. At exploration the testicle is not twisted and a definite firm mass is palpated in the upper pole of the testicle. The epididymis is normal. What is the next step in management?**

10% of patients with testicular tumor present with acute testicular pain. The presence of a firm testicular mass in an otherwise normal testis is highly likely to be a tumor and a radical orchiectomy is indicated. The site of the prior scrotal exploration should be excised by performing a hemiscotectomy. A biopsy of the testicle should not be performed through the scrotal incision as this will lead to definite wound contamination as the testis is transposed into the inguinal area for orchiectomy. If substantial doubt still exists a biopsy can be performed after the testicle is delivered into the inguinal incision, the cord is clamped and the field isolated. If doubt exists it is better to perform an orchiectomy than replace a malignant tumor in the scrotum

❑❑ **A pediatrician's 1-year old son has an orchipexy for an inguinal cryptorchid testis. The pediatrician wants to know what is his son's chance of developing testicular cancer.**

Patients with crytorchidism have a 3 to 14 times increased risk of developing testicular cancer. The lifetime probability of developing testis cancer is therefore between 0.6 and 2.8%

❑❑ **A 32-year old undergoes a right orchiectomy for a Stage I non seminomatous germ cell tumor and enters a surveillance protocol. At the end of one year he is asymptomatic, all radiologic and laboratory studies are negative. He asks you what are his chances of developing a tumor in the opposite testicle?**

Approximately 2-4% of patients develop a contralateral germ cell tumor which is a 20-40 fold increased risk compared to the general population. Therefore, it is important to teach patients with testicular tumors to perform regular contralateral testicular self-examination.

❑❑ **A 28-year old man, four years post orchiectomy and adjuvant chemotherapy (3 cycles of BEP) for a left Stage II nonseminomatous germ cell tumor, presents with a 2 cm right lower pole testicular mass. Tumor markers are negative. An ultrasound demonstrates a solid mass. What is the likely histology and why did the systemic chemotherapy not prevent the formation of this tumor?**

Patients less than 30-years of age, who are diagnosed with germ cell tumors are at higher risk of developing recurrent tumors. If the tumor is diagnosed within 5- years of the prior tumor it is more likely to be of similar histology. There is some controversy as to whether prior chemotherapy is protective in preventing subsequent germ cell tumor formation. The likely reason for the absence of full protection is poor diffusion of chemotherapy across the blood testis barrier. Additionally 5% of patients with unilateral testis cancer have contralateral CIS and studies have shown that the cumulative incidence of recurrent CIS after chemotherapy in this subgroup is approximately 40%

❑❑ **A 28-year old man has a testicular ultrasound for chronic left testicular pain. The study is normal except for a cluster of small calcifications or an area of microlithisasis in the right testicle. (Fig 2) The patient has never had a problem with this the right testicle and it is normal on examination. What further steps should be taken?**

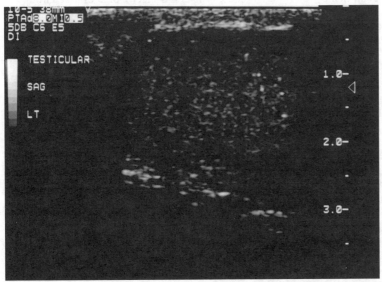

Figure 2

Testicular microlithiasis is an uncommon and usually incidental finding on ultrasound. It is probably of no significance. However, microlithiasis has been found in association with testicular tumors in up to 40% of cases. In this patient it is in all likelihood an incidental finding. The patient should be taught testicular self-examination and should have a follow up ultrasound in six months to a year.

❑❑ **A 36-year old man undergoing evaluation for infertility is found to have small testicles bilaterally. No masses are appreciated. Semen analysis demonstrates severe oligospermia. As part of his infertility evaluation he has bilateral testicular biopsies. Biopsy of the right testicle demonstrates Intratubular Germ Cell Neoplasia (Carcinoma In–Situ). Left testicular biopsy shows incomplete spermatogenesis but no evidence of CIS. Bilateral testicular ultrasound and tumor markers are normal. What is this patient's risk of developing a germ cell neoplasm and what is the recommended management?**

The identification of CIS reliably identifies patients at high risk of developing testis cancer. Approximately 50% of patients diagnosed with CIS will develop a germ cell tumor within the next 5-years. The recommended management in this patient would be a right radical orchiectomy. Patients with bilateral CIS can be treated with low dose radiation approximately 20Gy. Low dose radiation will allow preservation of testicular endocrine function but will almost certainly cause infertility.

❑❑ **A 28-year old status post left radical orchiectomy with adjuvant chemotherapy for a left Stage II nonseminomatous germ cell tumor presents with a 2 cm right lower pole testicular mass. Tumor markers are negative. An ultrasound demonstrates a solid mass located on the anterior surface of the lower pole of the right testis. The remainder of the testis is normal. The patient is recently married and is interested in having children in the future. What are the management options?**

There are three management options: 1. Radical orchiectomy which is associated with endocrine abnormalities and sterility but assures local control. 2. Partial orchiectomy followed by low dose radiation (20Gy) which is associated with sterility but preserves endocrine function and is associated with a low incidence of local recurrence. 3. Partial orchiectomy alone which preserves endocrine function, may preserve fertility and is associated with a higher risk of local failure. As this patient has a favorably located tumor. Partial orchiectomy with negative margins and preceded by sperm banking would be a good therapeutic choice.

❑❑ **A 27-year old man has a right orchiectomy for a nonseminatous germ cell tumor. Metastatic work up reveals a 4 cm inter aortocaval mass and four 1 cm pulmonary nodules. HCG is 250, AFP is 80 and LDH is at the upper limit of normal. How should this patient be treated and what is his chance of a complete response?**

The patient would be stratified as good risk by the International Germ Cell Cancer Collaborative Group (LDH < 1.5x normal, HCG < 5000, AFP < 1000, No non pulmonary metastasis). This group makes up about 50% of all patients diagnosed with metastatic germ cell tumor. He should receive either 3 courses of Bleomycin Etopiside and Platinum or 4 cycles of Etopiside and Platinum. His chances of a complete response are 95%.

❑❑ **A 32-year old man has a left orchiectomy for a nonseminatous germ cell tumor. Metastatic work up reveals a 10 cm left para aortic mass, multiple small pulmonary and liver nodules. HCG is 30,500, AFP is 880 and LDH is 12 x normal. How should this patient be treated and what is his chance of long-term survival?**

The patient would be stratified as poor risk by the International Germ Cell Cancer Collaborative Group (LDH >10 x normal, HCG >50,000, AFP 10,000 and evidence of non pulmonary metastasis). This group makes up about 15% of all patients diagnosed with metastatic germ cell tumor. There is controversy about the best management but most centers would suggest either 4 cycles of Bleomycin, Etopiside and Platinum or inclusion in a clinical trial with high dose chemotherapy followed by autologous bone marrow transplant. Four cycles of BEP is likely to give a response rate of approximately 60% with a long-term cure rate of between 40 and 50%.

❑❑ **A 32-year old man has a left orchiectomy for a seminoma. Metastatic work up reveals a 10 cm left para aortic mass, multiple 1cm pulmonary and liver nodules. HCG is 300, AFP is 5 and LDH is 12 x normal. How should this patient be treated and what is his chance of long-term survival?**

The patient would be stratified as intermediate risk by the International Germ Cell Cancer Collaborative Group (No patients with Seminoma are considered poor risk). This group makes up about 10% of all

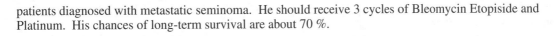

patients diagnosed with metastatic seminoma. He should receive 3 cycles of Bleomycin Etopiside and Platinum. His chances of long-term survival are about 70 %.

❏❏ A 26-year old man has a right orchiectomy for a nonseminomatous germ cell tumor. Metastatic work up reveals a 10 cm inter aotocaval mass, multiple 1 cm pulmonary nodules. HCG is 25,000, AFP is 2000 and LDH is 6 x normal. How should this patient be treated and what is his chance of long-term survival?

The patient would be stratified as intermediate risk by the International Germ Cell Cancer Collaborative Group (LDH >1.5x normal and < 10x normal, HCG >5000 and < 50,000, AFP>1000 and < 10,000, No non pulmonary metastasis). This group makes up about 28% of all patients diagnosed with metastatic germ cell tumor. He should receive 4 courses of Bleomycin, Etopiside and Platinum. His 5 year overall survival is 80%.

❏❏ A 26-year old man has a right orchiectomy for a nonseminomatous germ cell tumor. Metastatic work up reveals a 10 cm inter aotocaval mass, multiple 1 cm pulmonary nodules. HCG is 25,000, AFP is 2000 and LDH is 6x normal. He receives 4 cycles of BEP with shrinkage of pulmonary metastasis and retroperitoneal mass. However, the HCG which had been falling at the appropriate rate is now noted to be increasing significantly. How should this patient be treated and what is his chance of complete response?

The patient is showing signs of progression upon completion of chemotherapy. Treatment options would be inclusion in a clinical trial of high dose therapy with autologous bone marrow transplantation or regimens such as Vinblastine, Ifosfamide and Cisplatin. Such regimens have reported complete response rates of 30-50%.

❏❏ A patient with intermediate risk nonseminomatous germ cell tumor is about to start BEP chemotherapy. He requests that you inform him of the major long-term risks of this treatment.

There are five major long-term risks:

1. Infertility. Combination chemotherapy for testis cancer is toxic to spermatogenesis. Almost all patients become azoospermic during chemotherapy. The toxicity is usually reversible with approximately 50% of patients having normal sperm counts at 2 years. About 25% of patients have persistent azoospermia.
2. Nephrotoxicicty. Most patients have an irreversible decline in renal function after cisplatin chemotherapy. However, in general this is subclinical.
3. Cardiovascular toxicity. The major risk is Raynaud's phenomen which occurs in 20-50% of patients following Cisplatin and Bleomycin chemotherapy.
4. Neurotoxicity. Clinically relevant peripheral neuropathy occurs in 10 - 40% of patients. Injury to the 8th cranial nerve from cisplatin causes tinitus in up to 30% of patients. However, major hearing loss is rare.
5. Pulmonary toxicity. Bleomycin induced pulmonary fibrosis occurs when the dose exceeds 450-500 units (4 cycles of standard BEP contains 360 units of bleomycin). Bleomycin pulmonary toxicity is fatal in 1-2% of patients and clinically significant fibrosis occurs in an additional 2-3%.

❏❏ A patient has an RPLND for a nonseminomatous germ cell tumor. At RPLND he is found to have 4 / 12 nodes containing 1 cm^3 of tumor each. Two cycles of BEP chemotherapy are recommended to the patient. He is reluctant to undergo the treatment as he has heard that chemotherapy can give you cancer. What information can you give him to support or refute this assertion?

Large databases have suggested that patients treated for testicular cancer incur little increased risk of for secondary malignancies. Etoposide treatment is associated with an increased risk of developing a secondary leukemia. However, the rate is less than 0.5% and would probably not occur unless additional cycles of etoposide based chemotherapy are required.

❏❏ A 28-year old newly married patient is diagnosed with low risk metastatic non seminomatous germ cell tumor. He has fathered a child in a previous relationship. His wife wants to know what are his chances of future fertility and how long will it take his sperm count to recover from

chemotherapy. She also wants to know if future children will be at increased risk of developing congenital abnormalities?

Combination chemotherapy for testis cancer is toxic to both spermatogenesis and Leydig cell function. Almost all patients become azoospermic during chemotherapy. The toxicity is usually reversible with approximately 50% of patients having normal sperm counts at 2 years. About 25% of patients have persistent azoospermia. Children conceived after patients have been treated for testis cancer do not appear to be at increased risk of congenital malformations.

❑❑ **A 29-year old undergoes biopsy of a neck mass. Pathology demonstrates a poorly differentiated tumor consistent with embryonal carcinoma. Further examination reveals a 3 cm nodule in the left testis and an ultrasound shows a solid mass. Metastatic workup reveals a Stage III tumor and he receives 4 cycles of BEP. Now tumor markers are normal and an extensive evaluation reveals that the patient has had a complete response. Testicular examination is now normal and an ultrasound shows only a 5 mm scar. What further treatment if any does this patient need?**

The patient should have a left orchiectomy. Studies indicate that 30% of patients have residual teratoma and 25% have active germ cell tumor in the testicle. Orchiectomy is recommended even in patients with a partial and complete response.

❑❑ **A 26-year old man has a right orchiectomy for a nonseminomatous germ cell tumor. Metastatic work-up reveals a 10 cm inter aortocaval mass (Fig 3), multiple 1 cm pulmonary nodules. HCG is 5,000, AFP is 100 and LDH is 3x normal. He receives 4 cycles of BEP with regression of the pulmonary nodules and normalization of tumor markers. A representative section of his post chemotherapy CT scan is shown. (Fig 4) An RPLND is recommended. Is this the correct treatment recommendation? If an RPLND is performed what is the expected histology?**

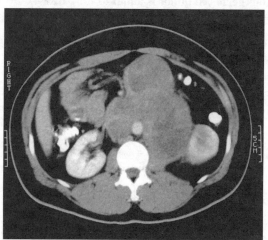
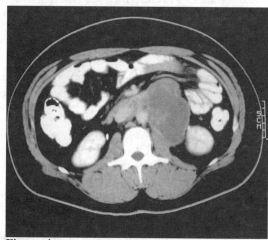

Figure 3   **Figure 4**

This patient has a moderate residual mass after chemotherapy. Approximately 40% of patients will be found to have mature teratoma, 40% necrosis and 20% viable germ cell tumor. A RPLND is recommended as it is important to identify active tumor and resection of teratoma can prevent the growing teratoma syndrome or malignant degeneration within a teratoma.

❑❑ **A 28-year old has a left orchiectomy for a non-seminomatous germ cell tumor (60% embryonal, 30% Yolk sac and 10% Seminoma). He has a 3 cm paraaortic node at diagnosis with negative chest CT and negative tumor markers. He receives 3 cycles of BEP. Tumor markers and CXR are normal. A representative image of the CT Scan is shown. (Fig 5) What is the next step in management?**

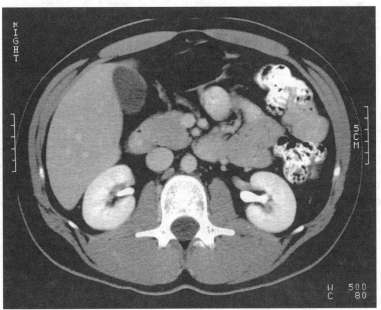

Figure 5

The patient has had a complete response in the retroperitoneum. In these circumstances an RPLND rarely provides important diagnostic or therapeutic value. Therefore the patient should be observed.

❑❑ **A 25-year old has a left orchiectomy for a non-seminomatous germ cell tumor (60% embryonal, 30% Yolk sac and 10% Seminoma). He has an 8 cm paraaortic node at diagnosis with multiple nodules on chest CT (largest 4 cm). He receives 3 cycles of BEP. Evaluation demonstrates resolution of all disease except a 4 cm left paraaortic mass and a 3 cm right lower lobe pulmonary nodule. (Fig 6) Tumor markers are negative. What is the next step in management and why?**

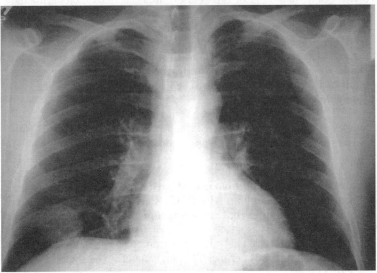

Figure 6

Initially, the patient should have resection of the retroperitoneal mass since this is more likely to show active tumor than the chest. Additionally, the pathology in the retroperitoneum is more predictive of the pathology in the chest than vice-versa. If there is no active tumor in the retroperitoneum, resection of the lower lobe lung mass should be carried out. Surgery can be done simultaneously but is generally only performed at the same time if both lesions can be excised through the same incision.

❑❑ **A 32-year old has a right orchiectomy for a non-seminomatous germ cell tumor (60% embryonal, 30% Teratoma , 10% Seminoma). He has an 8 cm intra aortocaval node at diagnosis with multiple nodules on chest CT (largest 4 cm). He receives 3 cycles of BEP. The chest nodules** resolve. The patient still has a 5 cm aortocaval lymph node. AFP is normal but BHCG is still elevated at 30. He is referred to you by the medical oncologist for RPLND. What do you recommend?

The persistent elevation of the BHCG after chemotherapy is indicative of active disease. Therefore the patient should undergo salvage chemotherapy prior to tumor resection.

❏❐ A 28-year old has a right orchiectomy for a non-seminomatous germ cell tumor (60% embryonal, 30% Teratoma, 10% yolk sac). He has a 10 cm inter aortocaval node at diagnosis with multiple nodules on chest CT (largest 2 cm). He receives 3 cycles of BEP. The chest nodules resolve. The patient still has a 4 cm inter aortocaval lymph node. BHCG is normal but the AFP is still elevated at 100. He receives 4 cycles of VIP salvage chemotherapy. The AFP is now 25 (nl < 5) and a repeat CT scan shows a residual stable 4 cm mass in the inter aortocaval area and an extensive evaluation reveals no other disease. What do you recommend?

Despite the continued marker elevation the patient has few treatment options left. He should undergo resection of the mass or so called "desperation RPLND" as complete resection can result in prolonged survival in 20-33% of patients.

❏❐ A 22-year old is scheduled for a post chemotherapy retroperitoneal node dissection. On reviewing the records it is apparent that he has received a total of 550 units of Bleomycin over the course of his chemotherapy. He reports that he noticed a dry cough during the last cycle of chemotherapy but currently has no respiratory symptoms. What perioperative testing and precautions may aid in management of this patient?

A series of 5 deaths after Bleomycin chemotherapy in the 1970's drew attention to the problem of post-operative pulmonary problems. The causes of Bleomycin pulmonary toxicity are not entirely clear but an increased incidence occurs once the cumulative dose is greater than 400 - 450 units. Pre operative pulmonary function tests (CO diffusion and forced vital capacity) maybe useful in identifying patients at higher risk. Careful management (restriction) of perioperative fluids and transfusions as well as minimizing operative time are important interventions that may decrease the risk of this complication. More recent studies have questioned the need to maintain low levels of inspired (28%) oxygen during the perioperative period.

❏❐ A 28-year old man with a stage III Non seminomatous germ cell tumor has 4 cycles of BEP chemotherapy. The patient's tumor markers are now negative and the only residual disease is a 6 cm inter aortocaval mass. An RPLND and resection of the mass is performed. Final pathology demonstrates 95% necrosis with small foci of residual active germ cell tumor. All margins are negative. What further teatment if any do you recommend?

The patient should receive 2 further cycles of BEP chemotherapy. Studies indicate that 100% of patients with this clinical scenario who do not receive adjuvant therapy relapse compared to less than 70% receiving chemotherapy.

❏❐ A 32-year old undergoes a left orchiectomy for a pathological stage T2 pure seminoma. Preoperative markers are notable for a BHCG of 25 and an AFP of 15. Post-operative markers are normal. Abdominal CT and Chest X-ray are normal. What is the appropriate treatment?

The patient with a pure seminoma after careful histological analysis of the entire testis and elevated tumor markers should be treated as if he has a non-seminomatous germ cell tumor. Therefore he should be recommended to have a RPLND for the pT2 tumor.

❏❐ A 28-year old newly married man presents with a right testis mass. He has a history of a right orchidopexy for a cryptorchid testis at the age of 8. Tumor markers are negative. A right radical orchiectomy is performed and pathological analysis reveals a T1 pure seminoma. Metastatic work up including a Chest X-ray and abdominal CT scan are negative. His referring urologist has recommended radiation. Do you agree? If he is, to undergo radiation what fields and dosage would you recommend. What is his likelihood of long-term survival?

The recommended treatment for Stage I Seminoma is 25cGy in 15-20 fractions of high energy X-rays (> 6 Mev) to the retroperitoneum. Standard fields include the periaortic and ipsilateral pelvic nodes in a so-called "hockey stick" fashion. Exact field boundaries are decided at CT guided planning. There is controversy about whether the inguinal lymph nodes and / or scrotum need to be treated in patients who have had a prior orchidopexy or scrotal violation at the time of surgery. However, the incidence of contralateral inguinal or pelvic relapse is so low even in this group of patients that it is unlikely to be of benefit and may compromise future fertility. Overall survival in patients with Stage I seminoma treated with radiation is between 93-100%.

❏❏ **A 56-year old man undergoes a left orchiectomy for a stage T1 Spermatocytic Seminoma. Tumor markers are negative. Abdominal CT scan and chest X-ray are normal. What treatment do you recommend?**

Spermatocytic seminoma has a very low metastatic potential. In several literature reviews, no documented cases of metastasis have been observed. Therefore, observation is recommended as opposed to classic seminoma where the recommendation is for retroperitoneal radiation.

❏❏ **A 32-year old man undergoes a right orchiectomy for a pathological stage T2 anaplastic Seminoma. Tumor markers are notable for a BHCG of 25 that returns to normal within 2-weeks of orchiectomy and a normal abdominal CT scan and chest X-ray. What therapy do you recommend?**

Anaplastic seminomas make up 5-10% of all seminomas. They tend to present with more locally advanced tumors and have a higher incidence of associated BHCG elevations. However, stage for stage prognosis is the same as that of classical seminoma. Therefore, this patient should receive 25 cGy of radiation to the retroperitoneum.

❏❏ **A 40-year old man presents with a centrally located 2 cm right testicular mass. At the age of 32 he had a left orchiectomy and 25cGy of radiation to the retroperitoneum for a stage I seminoma. A right orchiectomy is performed and pathological analysis reveals a stage T1 seminoma. Tumor markers are normal and metastatic evaluation is negative. What is the likelihood that this patient has retroperitoneal metastasis and what treatment option would you recommend?**

There is little prospective data to guide treatment of bilateral seminomas. However, we know from surveillance series that the risk of retroperitoneal relapse is between 13% and 19%. Treatment alternatives include 1: Retroperitoneal radiation. This would not be a good option considering the patients prior history of radiation (despite the relatively low doses), 2: Chemotherapy. Several small phase II studies have examined the efficacy of short course chemotherapy (one or 2 cycles of single agent cisplatin or carboplatin) and shown that the risk of relapse can be decreased to less than 5%. 3: Surveillance. The recommended treatment for this patient given that he has a low risk tumor (< 3 cm and no vascular invasion) and that an excellent survival rate of as high as 99% is seen in surveillance protocols despite any retroperitoneal recurrences.

❏❏ **A 40-year old man has a left orchiectomy for a T1 pure seminoma. Tumor markers are negative. Chest X-ray is normal. An abdominal CT scan shows a 4 cm preaortic mass. Provide treatment recommendations, risk of recurrence and risk of long-term adverse effects?**

The patient has low volume retroperitoneal disease. Standard therapy is 35-40 cGy of > 6 MEv x-ray treatment to the retroperitoneum and ipsilateral pelvic region through PA and AP fields with appropriate testicular shielding. A CT based planning system should guide the treatment to ensure adequate coverage of all nodal areas as marginal recurrences are well documented. The risk of recurrence is from 10-15% with overall survival of >95%. The primary long-term adverse events are a 6% incidence of dyspepsia and a 3% incidence of frank peptic ulceration. Bowel obstruction is a rare complication occurring <1% of the time. There is a 2 fold increased incidence of solid tumors developing within the radiation field as well as a small increase in the risk of long term cardiac disease (the risk is substantial in patients receiving posterior mediastinal irradiation). Appropriate testicular shielding should minimize radiation to the remaining testicle and maximize the chances for future fertility.

❏❏ **A 42-year man has a right orchiectomy for a pathological stage T2 pure Seminoma of the testis. Tumor markers are negative. An Abdominal CT scan shows an 8 cm retroperitoneal mass surrounding the aorta and vena cava. A chest CT scan is normal. What are the treatment options and which do you recommend?**

The patient has bulky stage II seminoma. Treatment is controversial and the options are retroperitoneal irradiation (35-40 cGy) or chemotherapy (3 cycles BEP or 4 cycles EP). Results with retroperitoneal irradiation are variable with recurrence free survival rates ranging between 45 and 100%. Most patients who fail radiation are salvaged with subsequent chemotherapy. Initial chemotherapy in patients with bulky (>5 cm) disease avoids the necessity for dual treatment in 20-50% of patients.

❏❏ **A 37-year old has a left orchiectomy for a T2 pure seminoma. BHCG and LDH are elevated. AFP is normal. An abdominal CT shows a 10 cm retroperitoneal mass surrounding the great vessels. Chest CT shows multiple pulmonary nodules. He receives 3 cycles of BEP chemotherapy with normalization of markers and resolution of his pulmonary nodules. A representative section of his post chemotherapy abdominal CT scan is shown. (Fig 7) What are the treatment options and what do you recommend?**

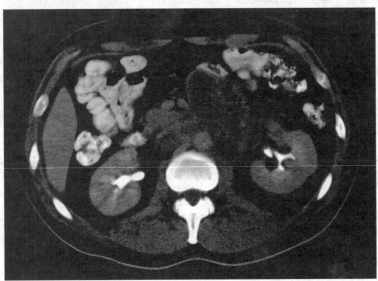

Figure 7

Treatment of a residual retroperitoneal mass (>3 cm) after chemotherapy in patients with Seminoma is controversial. There are three options including observation, radiation and surgery. Unlike nonseminomatous germ cell tumors, only two pathological entities occur in patients with seminoma follwoing chemotherapy, active tumor and / or necrosis. Post chemotherapy surgery in patients with seminoma is usually very difficult due to the intense fibrotic reaction that occurs, and complete resection is rare due to the obliteration of tissue planes.

❏❏ **A 40-year old man presents with a mediastinal mass and pulmonary nodules. BHCG is 125 and AFP is 430. Testicular examination and testicular ultrasound is normal. CT guided biopsy is consistent with embryonal carcinoma. What is the diagnosis and what does this mean from a prognostic perspective?**

The diagnosis is extragonadal germ cell tumor. These tumors make up about 3% of all germ cell tumors. The most common site is the mediastinum followed by the sacrum and pineal gland. These tumors are thought to arise from either aberrant migration of primitive germ cells during embryogenesis or from pluripotent stem cells located in the somatic rests. Patients with extragonadal germ cell tumors have a significantly worse prognosis, stage for stage, than tumors of testicular origin. This patients' 5-year survival is approximately 40%.

❏❏ **A 50-year old man with a 3-year history of gynecomastia discovers a left testicular mass. A radical orchiectomy is performed. On bisecting the testicle a 2 cm homogeneous brown tumor seen in the upper pole. Pathology shows closely packed uniform cells with eosinophilic cytoplasm and Reinke crystals. What is the diagnosis and malignant potential of this tumor?**

The patient has a Leydig cell tumor. Approximately 10% of Leydig cell tumors are malignant. The malignant potential of these tumors is difficult to predict based on histology. However, in the absence of a histological suspicion of malignancy (no hemorrhage, uniform cells, few mitosis) observation is the preferred form of management.

❏❏ **Your 8-year-old labrador retriever develops a left testicular mass. What is the most likely diagnosis and how common is this tumor in humans?**

The likely diagnosis is sertoli cell tumor. Sertoli cell tumors make up less than 1% of human testicular tumors. Approximately 90% are benign and most are successfully managed by radical orchiectomy

❏❏ **A 60-year old man presents with a 2-month history of bilateral testicular masses. Physical examination is otherwise normal and the patient has no complaints. Testicular ultrasound shows diffuse enlargement of both testis. What is the likely diagnosis and prognosis?**

The most common cause of testicular masses in men over the age of 50 is lymphoma. Approximately 10% of men have bilateral disease at presentation. Patients presenting with bilateral disease tend to have a worse prognosis than men presenting with a secondary or unilateral primary testicular lymphoma.

❏❏ **A 30-year old man is referred to you by his family doctor for a 1.5 cm epididymal mass. The patient has no complaints and did not notice anything unusual himself. Physical examination reveals a 1.5 cm mass in the epididymis that does not transilluminate. Ultrasound confirms a 1.5 cm homogeneous solid intraepipdidymal mass. What is the likely and differential diagnosis?**

The likely diagnosis is an adenomatoid tumor. The differential diagnosis is paratesticular sarcoma, atypical spermatocoele or epididymal cyst. The mass is probably growing very slowly as the patient has not noticed a change. Therefore, it is likely a benign process and transscrotal excision is appropriate. If there is any suspicion of malignancy an inguinal exploration is indicated.

❏❏ **A 40-year old man notices a mass in his right groin that has doubled in size in the last 2 months. He otherwise feels well. A radical orchiectomy is performed. Final pathology demonstrates a rhabdomyosarcoma. What are the major determinants of prognosis in patients with sarcomas?**

The main prognostic determinants of sarcomas are tumor grade, tumor size (greater or less than 5 cm) and the presence of metastasis. Complete surgical resection with wide margins holds the best prospect for cure.

❏❏ **A 40-year old molecular biologist has a diagnosis of seminoma. He asks you are there any genetic markers specific for testicular cancer?**

An isochromosme of the short arm of chromosome 12, i (12p), is a relatively frequent finding in germ cell tumors. Tumors not containing i (12p) generally have additional genetic material located on the short arm of chromosome 12. Isochromosome 12p is found in up to 80% of germ cell tumors and can be identified in lesions as early as CIS.

PENILE CANCER

John W. Davis, M.D. and Donald F. Lynch, M.D.

☐☐ **T/F: Bowenoid Papulosis of the penis is a premalignant condition with the natural history of progression to invasive disease.**

False. Bowenoid Papulosis has the histologic criteria of carcinoma in situ, but has a benign course.

☐☐ **What is the best palliative treatment for a patient with AIDS and Kaposi's sarcoma of the glans penis causing obstruction?**

Radiation therapy.

☐☐ **Which form of Kaposi's sarcoma (KS) is associated with acquired immunodeficiency syndrome?**

Classic KS
Immunosuppressive treatment-related KS
African KS
Epidemic KS

☐☐ **T/F: Verrucous carcinoma is a well-differentiated variant of squamous cell carcinoma with similar metastatic potential.**

False. Verrucous carcinoma of the penis invades locally and can cause local tissue destruction; metastasis does not occur unless invasive SCC co-exists.

☐☐ **T/F.: Both Verrucous carcinoma and condyloma acuminatum remain superficial lesions.**

False. Verrucous carcinoma can invade locally causing unrestrained local growth.

☐☐ **Which of the following local treatments is not recommended for Verrucous carcinoma: partial penectomy, radiation therapy, topical podophyllin or 5-flourouracil, Nd:YAG laser.**

Radiation therapy has been associated with malignant degeneration and is ineffective. Partial or total penectomy is standard therapy.

☐☐ **What differentiates condyloma accuminata from Buschke-Lowenstein tumors?**

Condyloma never invades adjacent normal tissues and always remains superficial. Buschke-Lowenstein tumors displace and invade adjacent tissues, destroying them by comparison.

☐☐ **What terms are used for carcinoma in situ?**

CIS is also known as erythroplasia of Queyrat when it involves the glans penis or prepuce, and Bowen's disease if it involves the penile shaft.

☐☐ **A 55-year-old uncircumcised male presents with a 0.5 cm reddish, well defined, barely raised plaque on the glans. The biopsy diagnosis is erythroplasia of Queyrat (CIS). What is the chance of progression to invasive disease and how is the lesion best managed?**

The relative risks of progression to an invasive lesion and develeopment of metastases is 10%, and 2%, respectively. Superficial premalignant lesions may be treated with local excision, topical 5-fourouracil, or laser therapy. Sexual partners should be counseled and examined for CIS.

❑❑ **Diagnosis of erythroplasia of Queyrat requires biopsy. For the lesion described in the previous question, what is the clinical differential diagnosis?**

Chronic circumscribed balanitis, inflammatory process, drug eruption, psoriasis, and lichen planus among others.

❑❑ **What is the importance in differentiating Bowenoid Papulosis from Bowen's Disease in the clinical setting?**

Bowenoid Papulosis is a dysplastic lesion of the epithelium involving the penile shaft in younger men. The histopathologic appearance may be similar to other forms of CIS. The lesions are light brown to gray papules that may coalesce to form plaques. These lesions have an indolent course, respond well to excision or podophyllin, may spontaneously regress, and do not progress to invasive cancer. Bowenoid papulosis is similar to multifocal vulvovaginal dysplasia in young women.

❑❑ **How does the incidence squamous cell carcinoma of the penis (SCC) differ in the United States and Europe versus some African and South American countries?**

In the U.S. and Europe, SCC of the penis accounts for only 0.4-0.6% of all male malignancies. In some African and South American countries, SCC accounts for up to 10% of all diagnosed malignancies in men.

❑❑ **Describe the relationship between penile cancer and circumcision.**

Chronic exposure to smegma in the prepubertal period is thought to contribute to the development of penile cancer. Phimosis may accentuate this effect, as it is a finding in up to 50% of cases of penile cancer. Neonatal circumcision virtually eliminates the risk of penile cancer whereas adolescent or adult circumcision has no protective effect.

❑❑ **T/F: In populations that practice good hygiene but are uncircumcised, the incidence of penile carcinoma is similar to that of circumcised populations.**

True.

❑❑ **Other than smegma, what other etiologic factor is associated with penile cancer?**

Sexually transmitted human papillomavirus (HPV).

❑❑ **What is human papillomavirus (HPV), approximately how many HPV subtypes are known, and which are well know to be benign versus malignant?**

HPV is a double-stranded, supercoiled DNA virus with more than 65 sub-types identified. "Low risk" strands HPV-6 and HPV-11 are associated with benign condylomata of the anogenital area. "High risk" types such as HPV-16, 18, 31, 33, 35, and 39 are associated with premalignant lesions of the cervix and penis, and have been demonstrated in 50% of penile SCC.

❑❑ **How are penile cancer and cervical cancer related?**

Both cancers have HPV as a potential etiology. In some studies, female sexual partners of men with SCC of the penis have a 3-fold increased risk of invasive cervical carcinoma. However, there are key differences as cervical carcinoma is much more common and affects younger women whereas penile cancer is rare and affects older men.

❑❑ **Describe the lymphatic spread of penile cancer.**

Lymphatics from the glans and shaft drain to the superficial inguinal, deep inguinal, and pelvic lymph nodes. Drainage is bilateral, and crossover may occur.

❑❑ **What is the natural history of untreated penile cancer.**

Untreated penile cancer progresses to death in the majority of patients within 2 years. Local and regional nodal enlargement and complications predominate over distant metastases to lung, liver, bone or brain.

Death may occur by erosion into the femoral vessels with subsequent hemorrhage. Spontaneous remission has not been reported.

❏❏ **List the sites of the primary tumor in penile cancer in order of frequency.**

Glans (48%), prepuce (21%), glans and prepuce (9%), coronal sulcus (6%), and shaft (<2%).

❏❏ **What precautions should be taken to prevent dissemination of tumor during biopsy of a penile lesion?**

None—tumor dissemination due to biopsy has not been reported.

❏❏ **What factor is most predictive of survival in penile cancer?**

While histologic grading may be predictive, the presence or absence of nodal metastases is the strongest predictive factor for survival.

❏❏ **How does the appearance of well-differentiated (grade 1) SCC differ from poorly-differentiated (grade 3)?**

Grade 1 SCC shows downward finger-like projections of atypical squamous cells from the papillomatous epidermis. Keratin pearls are present, and there is limited cellular atypia and mitotic figures. Grade 3 SCC shows little to no keratin pearls and marked cellular nuclear pleomorphism, mitoses, necrosis, and deep invasion.

❏❏ **Compare the 5-year survival for the following groups of patients with SCC of the penis: all patients, negative nodes, positive inguinal nodes, and positive pelvic nodes.**

All patients=50%, negative lymph nodes=66%, positive inguinal nodes=27%, positive pelvic lymph nodes = rare.

❏❏ **What radiologic studies have proven useful in staging penile cancer?**

Lymphangiography has been replaced by CT and MRI due to their technical ease and ability to image the hypogastric and presacral nodes. Ultrasound and MRI can stage the depth of invasion of the primary lesion. Ultrasound and CT can image the inguinal nodal regions where physical exam is hindered by obesity or prior surgery.

❏❏ **Assessment of the primary tumor is important in deciding whether to perform inguinal lymph node dissections. List the TNM staging system for penile cancer (UICC, 1994).**

Primary tumor:
    Tx=primary tumor not assessed.
    T0=no primary tumor.
    Tis=carcinoma in situ.
    Ta=verrucous carcinoma.
    T1=tumor invades subepithelial connective tissue.
    T2=tumor invades corpus spongiosum or cavernosum.
    T3= tumor invades urethra or prostate.
    T4=tumor invades other adjacent structures.

Regional lymph nodes:
    Nx=nodes not assessed.
    N0=no regional nodes.
    N1= metastasis in a single, superficial inguinal lymph node.
    N2= metastasis in multiple or bilateral superficial nodes.
    N3= metastasis in deep inguinal or pelvic lymph nodes, unilateral or bilateral.

Distant Metastases:
    MX= distant metastasis not assessed.
    M0= no distant metastases.

M1= Distant metastases.

❑❑ **Review the Jackson staging and how it equates to the TNM system above. What is the disadvantage of the Jackson staging system?**

Jackson staging system:
    Stage I = limited to the glans or prepuce
    Stage II = involving the shaft
    Stage III = palpable nodes
    Stage IV = invades adjacent structures, or distant metastases.

The Jackson system roughly equates to TNM as follows:
    Stage 0 = Tis-Ta N0M0.
    Stage I = T1N0M0.
    Stage II = T1-2N1M0 or T2N0M0.
    Stage III = T1-3N2M0 or T3N0-1M0.
    Stage IV = T4anyNM0 or AnyTN3M0 or AnyTAnyNM1

The Jackson system has the disadvantage of conveying less information about the tumor and makes interpretation of studies using different staging systems difficult.

❑❑ **What is the gold standard treatment for the primary tumor in penile cancer?**

The gold standard is resection of the primary tumor with a 2-centimeter margin to ensure complete resection of microscopic finger-like projections of tumor that may extend from the grossly evident tumor. This goal can be accomplished with a partial penectomy if the residual stump is serviceable for upright voiding and/or sexual function. Otherwise, total penectomy is indicated.

❑❑ **When is circumcision appropriate treatment for penile cancer and what are the risks/benefits?**

Circumcision is less disfiguring than partial penectomy and may be appropriate for small lesions of the prepuce. However recurrence rates are as high as 50%. Close patient follow-up and low threshold for biopsy and additional surgery is necessary for this approach to the primary tumor.

❑❑ **What is the best management for a primary tumor located on the proximal penile shaft?**

In rare circumstances when the tumor invades only the epidermis, excision of skin only is appropriate. In cases of a deeply invasive tumor of the shaft where a 2-cm margin is not possible, or if the residual stump would not allow upright voiding, then total penectomy with perineal urethrostomy is the best management.

❑❑ **A 70-year-old male underwent a partial penectomy one year ago for a T1 N0M0 grade I SCC of the glans penis. He presents with increasing lower urinary tract symptoms. What operative complications apply to this scenario?**

Stricture of the neo-meatus is a common complication of partial penectomy and can be avoided by widely spatulating the urethra, performing a tension free anastamosis, and adequate vascularization of the urethral stump. Strictures are initially managed by dilation or meatotomy. Recurrent local disease must be ruled out.

❑❑ **What are the risks and benefits of Mohs Micrographic Surgery (MMS) for penile cancer?**

MMS for small, distal lesions in the hands of an experienced Mohs surgeon can provide cure rates equivalent to partial penectomy with a decrease in the amount of tissue that is sacrificed. MMS is less successful for larger (>3cm) lesions since large resections can create defects in the glans that are difficult to reconstruct. Excessive resections can create significant glans defects and meatal stenosis that is difficult to reconstruct.

❑❑ **What are the risks and benefits of radiation therapy for penile cancer?**

Many patients undergoing radiation therapy (external beam or brachytherapy) refused surgery. Organ preservation is accomplished with cancer control rates for minimally invasive T1-2 lesions that are comparable to conventional surgery. Radiation therapy for larger lesions is less successful and carries higher morbidity. Potential complications include: urethral fistula, stricture, penile necrosis requiring penectomy, lengthy treatment schedule, and difficulty distinguishing post-irradiation scar from tumor recurrence.

❏❏ **What are the indications for lasers in penile cancer?**

Both CO_2 and Nd:YAG lasers are effective in treating CIS. Select patients with low stage invasive SCC can be treated as long as they are followed carefully for local recurrence.

❏❏ **What is the major drawback to laser surgery for small squamous cell carcinomas of the penis?**

No histologic specimen to assess stage and grade.

❏❏ **A 40-year-old healthy man presents with a large fungating lesion of the glans penis with erosion into the penile shaft and extensive fungating bilateral inguinal lymphadenopathy. The patient delayed seeing a doctor for a considerable amount of time but now requests maximal therapy. Describe the treatment options.**

In such extreme cases, the anatomy will dictate treatment possibilities. Fixed lymph nodes may require neoadjuvant chemotherapy followed by treatment of the primary lesion and lymphadenectomy. Aggressive approaches for these extreme cases include total emasculation, scrotectomy, resection of the lower abdominal wall and pubic symphysis, and hemipelvectomy.

❏❏ **What is the most common reconstructive option for a patient following partial or total penectomy?**

Free flap reconstruction of the penis with a radical forearm flap is the procedure of choice at many centers. Subsequently, a prosthesis can be placed for erectile function.

❏❏ **What is the efficacy of inguinal lymphadenectomy in terms of cure and palliation?**

Inguinal lymphadenectomy is curative in about 50-80% of cases and palliates possible complications of inguinal disease such as ulceration, infection, and vascular compromise.

❏❏ **At the time of diagnosis of an invasive penile cancer, a patient has palpable inguinal lymph nodes. Following 4-6 weeks of oral antibiotics therapy the lymphadenopathy persists. What is the likelihood that the lymph nodes are pathologic?**

Initially—50%; after 4-6 weeks of antibiotics—70-85%.

❏❏ **What are the disadvantages of routine inguinal lymphadenectomy?**

Early complications include phlebitis, pulmonary embolism, wound infection, and flap necrosis. Long term complications include of severe lymphedema from the scrotum to the lower extremities.

❏❏ **Define the terms "early" or "immediate" inguinal lymphadenectomy (LND), and "delayed" LND as they relate to the management of cancer of the penis.**

Early/immediate LND is carried out following 4-6 weeks of antibiotic therapy even though the inguinal nodes are not palpably abnormal. Delayed LND is performed when an abnormal inguinal node exam demonstrates lymphadenopathy some time after penectomy is performed.

❏❏ **T/F: Penectomy and lymphadenectomy should be performed concurrently to maximize staging information.**

False. Mortality from sepsis can occurr when a combined procedure is performed. Additionally, the histology of the nodes is often difficult to assess in the presence of severe inflammation.

❑❑ What is the incidence of subclinical metastasis (negative groin examinations) and what factors increase the likelihood of metastatic nodal disease?

The reported incidence of subclinical metastasis ranges from 2% -25% in most reports. Primary tumor stage (tumor invading the basement membrane of the penile skin) and higher tumor grade increase the likelihood of nodal disease.

❑❑ What is the major drawback to the sentinel node concept of penile cancer metastasis?

Some series have shown metastatic spread to the inguinal nodes without involvement of the sentinel node. Hence sentinel node biopsy alone can miss the diagnosis of inguinal metastasis.

❑❑ What is the key advantage of prophylactic groin dissections of clinically negative nodes versus delayed dissection if they become palpable?

Recent studies have pooled results and indicate a potential survival advantage for patients with positive inguinal nodes who underwent prophylactic versus delayed groin dissection. The survival benefit of prophylactic LND if the nodes are positive, must be weighed against risk of morbidity in the 75% of patients who will have negative dissections.

❑❑ What are the key elements of the modified inguinal lymph node dissection?

Shorter skin incision, skin flaps elevated deep to Scarpa's fascia, narrower field of dissection—exclude dissection lateral to the femoral artery and caudal to the fossa ovalis, preservation of the saphanous vein, and elimination of sartorius muscle transposition (unless subsequent deep nodes dissected).

❑❑ When and why is sartorius muscle transposition performed?

When standard inguinal lymphadenectomy is performed, the deep nodes and fascia lata over the femoral vessels are resected. In the event of erosion from wound infection or major flap necrosis, a sartorius muscle transposition protects the femoral vessels.

❑❑ What are the boundaries of the femoral (Scarpa's) triangle?

Base - inguinal ligament; laterally - sartorius muscle, medially - adductor longus muscle; floor - (lateral to medial) the iliacus, psoas major, pectineus and adductor brevis muscles; roof - fascia lata with small opening (fossa ovalis) through which the greater saphanous vein enters the underlying femoral vein.

❑❑ What 3 small branches of the femoral artery and vein are usually encountered in inguinal lymph node dissection?

Circumflex iliac, superficial epigastric, and superficial external pudendal.

❑❑ A 65-year-old male with SCC of the penis s/p penectomy has bulky eroded groin metastases that would necessitate excision of a large portion of overlying skin. What are treatment approaches?

Palliative or neoadjuvant chemo/radiation therapy may be given for inoperable nodes. Lymph node dissection is preferred and with the assistance of a reconstructive surgeon to rotate a myocutaneous skin flap such as the tensor fascia lata, gracilis, or rectus abdominis flap, the large defect can be covered.

❑❑ A 60-year-old male presents with a biopsy proven SCC of the glans penis and is found to have T1 grade I SCC at partial penectomy. Clinical examination reveals palpable lymphadenopathy on the right and a negative left groin. Describe the management of the lymph nodes.

Following treatment of the primary tumor, 4-6 weeks of oral antibiotics should be administered. If the unilateral lymphadenopathy resolves, then the patient can be carefully followed for recurrence. If the unilateral adenopathy does not resolve, then bilateral superficial inguinal LND should be performed as anatomic crossover of penile lymphatics is well established. If either superficial dissection is positive for malignancy, then a deep inguinal dissection is performed. If any deep dissection is positive, then complete ileoinguinal/pelvic lymph node dissections may be indicated.

❏❏ **How does pelvic lymphadenectomy for penile cancer differ from prostate and bladder cancer?**

Pelvic lymphadenectomy for penile cancer should extend more distally removing all lymph nodes tissue between the deep inguinal node group and the iliac group.

❏❏ **A patient with clinically negative inguinal nodes undergoes resection of a TI Grade III penile tumor. During follow up he develops unilateral inguinal adenopathy. What is the appropriate management?**

In this setting, unilateral dissection of the palpable lymph nodes is appropriate. The elapsed time has increased the likelihood that the clinically negative side is free is metastasis.

❏❏ **Describe the optimal strategy for surveillance of low stage SCC of the penis and clinically negative inguinal nodes.**

Most inguinal metastases occur within 2-3 years of the diagnosis of the primary tumor. Patients must be closely examined during these 2-3 years at 2-3 month intervals, as well as taught self-examination. Follow-up should continue indefinitely.

❏❏ **A 60-year-old male undergoes partial penectomy for a T2 Grade II glanular SCC (corporeal tissue invasion); inguinal nodes are non-palpable. Appropriate management of the lymph nodes includes.**

T2-3, N0M0 patients have a higher incidence of metastases and should undergo 6-weeks of oral antibiotics followed by bilateral inguinal lymph node dissection even if the nodes remain negative. The extent of dissection varies, but it is common to start with a superficial dissection and only perform a deep dissection if positive nodes are encountered; "skip" metastases are rare.

❏❏ **What is the current status of chemotherapy for advanced SCC of the penis?**

Multi-agent chemotherapy with cisplatin, bleomycin, and methotrexate has shown low response rates of only a few months duration. The rarity of the disease in the U.S. makes clinical trials difficult.

❏❏ **What percentage of patients with metastatic penile cancer exhibit hypercalcemia, and what is the mechanism?**

Approximately 20%. The cause is unknown, but systemic release of paraneoplastic hormonal substances is suspected.

❏❏ **How does the incidence of SCC compare with other types of penile cancer?**

SCC accounts for more than 95% of penile cancers. The remaining cancers are rare and include sarcomas, melanomas, basal cell carcinomas, and metastases.

❏❏ **How does malignant melanoma of the penis differ from SCC?**

Malignant melanoma of the penis is rare with <100 cases reported. The glans and prepuce are most common sites. The Breslow thickness scale provides important prognostic information. Most cases of penile melanoma present at an advanced stage with early metastases and poor survival. Hematogenous metastases are more common than lymphatic spread.

❏❏ **How does sarcoma of the penis differ from SCC?**

Sarcomas of the penis are usually locally invasive, low grade, and respond well to local excision. Local recurrence is characteristic, but metastases are rare.

❏❏ **Where do penile metastatic lesions usually originate?**

While rare, metastases to the penis may come from the bladder, prostate, and rectum. The primary disease is usually very advanced when the penis is involved and survival is <1 year.

❏❏ **What is the most common presenting sign of involvement of the penis with metastatic tumor?**

Priapism.

PEDIATRIC ONCOLOGY

Bruce W. Lindgren, M.D.

❏❏ **The Wilms' tumor suppressor gene WT-1 is located on which chromosome?**

The Wilms' tumor suppressor gene (WT-1) is located on the distal portion of the short arm of chromosome 11, in the 11p13 location.

❏❏ **What congenital anomalies are associated with Wilms' tumor?**

Congenital anomalies are seen in about 15% of patients with Wilms' tumor. These include:
- Aniridia
- WAGR syndrome (Wilms', Aniridia, Genitourinary anomalies & Retardation)
- Hemihypertrophy
- Beckwith-Wiedemann syndrome (macroglossia, gigantism, organomegaly)
- Denys-Drash syndrome (Wilms', pseudohermaphroditism, glomerulopathy, retardation)
- Trisomy 18

❏❏ **The histologic picture of Wilms' tumor is described as "triphasic." What are these three components?**

The classic microscopic appearance of Wilms' tumor includes blastemal, epithelial and stromal components.

❏❏ **A patient with Wilms' tumor undergoes nephrectomy. The tumor penetrates the surface of the capsule. At the time of nephrectomy there is tumor spillage, which is confined to the flank. Lymph nodes are negative. Contralateral kidney is negative. Chest X-Ray is negative. What stage is this tumor?**

This is a Stage II Wilms' tumor. The staging system is as follows:

Stage I: Tumor limited to the kidney and completely excised. Renal capsule intact. No tumor rupture.
Stage II: Tumor extends beyond the surface of the renal capsule but is completely removed. Regional extension of the tumor, including perirenal soft tissue, tumor thrombus, or local spillage from tumor rupture. No apparent residual tumor at or beyond the margins of excision.
Stage III: Residual nonhematogenous tumor confined to the abdomen (e.g. positive lymph nodes, diffuse peritoneal contamination from spillage or tumor penetration through the peritoneum, tumor extends beyond the margins of resection, tumor not completely resectable because of local infiltration into vital structures).
Stage IV: Hematogenous metastases (lung, liver, bone, brain)
Stage V: Bilateral involvement at diagnosis.

❏❏ **What is the most important factor in the prognosis of patients with Wilms' tumor?**

The most important aspect of Wilms' tumor is the histology. Unfavorable histology (anaplasia) at any stage is associated with a worse prognosis. The relapse rate is four times higher and the death rate is nine times higher in patients with anaplasia than those without anaplasia.

❏❏ **What are the chemotherapeutic agents used to treat patients with Wilms' tumor?**

Most patients receive Dactinomycin and Vincristine. Patients with higher stage disease and / or anaplasia may also receive Doxorubicin, Etoposide and / or Cyclophosphamide.

❏❏ **What is the most common extracranial solid tumor of childhood?**

Neuroblastoma is the most common extracranial solid tumor in children. It accounts for 6 – 8% of all childhood malignancies.

❑❑ **An 18-month-old male presents with malaise, weight loss and diffuse pain. An abdominal mass is palpable. What is the most likely diagnosis?**

Neuroblastoma. At the time of presentation of neuroblastoma approximately 50% of patients have disseminated disease versus less than 10 – 15% with Wilms'. Patients with Wilms' tumor generally appear in good health, in contrast to patients with neuroblastoma in whom the tumor may be widespread at presentation, and systemic symptoms are very often present.

❑❑ **When does the peak incidence of neuroblastoma occur?**

The peak incidence of neuroblastoma is seen in the first year of life. The incidence decreases progressively with age, and is rarely diagnosed in patients older than 6 to 7 years old.

❑❑ **Neuroblastoma is a malignant neuroendocrine tumor. There is a spectrum from this to benign tumors. What are these other tumors, and what are their characteristics?**

Ganglioneuroma is the benign counterpart to neuroblastoma. It does not metastasize, but can envelop adjacent structures and even extend into intervertebral foramina. Histologically, they contain mature ganglion cells in a collagen-rich background.

Ganglioneuroblastoma is intermediate between neuroblastoma and ganglioneuroma. There is a histologic spectrum between these; the outcome for ganglioneuroblastoma is varied.

❑❑ **What is the most common site of occurrence of neuroblastomas?**

More than half originate in the abdomen (retroperitoneum), and two-thirds of these are in the adrenal gland.

❑❑ **T/F: Metastases are uncommon at the time of diagnosis of neuroblastoma.**

False. Up to 70% of patients have disseminated metastases at the time of diagnosis. This is one of the factors which accounts for the fact that children with neuroblastoma often appear quite ill at the time of presentation, in contrast to patients with Wilms' tumor.

❑❑ **When is a bone marrow aspirate and / or biopsy indicated in the evaluation of patients with confirmed or suspected neuroblastoma?**

All patients with neuroblastoma should undergo bone marrow aspirate and/ or biopsy. As many as 70% of bone marrow aspirates have been reported to be positive in patients with neuroblastoma. The timing of this is variable. In patients with suspected "favorable" disease, bone marrow sampling may be delayed until the time of surgical excision so that it may be done under anesthesia. In patients with suspected "unfavorable" disease, a bone marrow sample which is diagnostic for neuroblastoma may obviate the need for open surgical biopsy, thus should be done early in the evaluation.

❑❑ **What molecular markers have been shown to carry prognostic significance in patients with neuroblastoma?**

The copy number of N-myc has been shown to be consistent throughout the course in a given patient. There is a trend that a lower number of copies of N-myc is associated with a better prognosis.

Hyperdiploid tumors (those that contain more than the normal amount of DNA material found in somatic cells) have demonstrated a favorable outcome.

Transketolase (TRK) gene product quantity may have prognostic significance, especially in combination with N-myc copy number.

❑❑ **What are the characteristics of Stage IV-S neuroblastoma?**

The definition of Stage IV-S is: patients who would otherwise be classified with stage I (tumor confined to the organ of origin) or stage II (tumor extending in continuity beyond the organ of origin, but not crossing the midline; ipsilateral regional nodes may be involved) but who have remote spread of tumor confined to one or more of the following: liver, skin, or bone marrow (without evidence of bony involvement). This stage disease is limited to patients less than 1 year of age.

❏❏ **What is the treatment for Stage IV-S neuroblastoma?**

Although local growth may occur, it rarely causes a serious problem. These tumors generally regress spontaneously without treatment. These infants with Stage IV-S disease have an excellent prognosis.

❏❏ **What are the histologic types of rhabdomyosarcoma, and which is most common in childhood?**

The types of rhabdomyosarcoma are embryonal, alveolar and pleomorphic. Mixed rhabdomyosarcomas also occur, and in about 10 – 20% of cases the tumor is so undifferentiated that it does not fit into the standard classification.

Embryonal rhabdomyosarcoma is the most common type seen in childhood, accounting for 2/3 of GU rhabdomyosarcomas, and 50 – 70% of all rhabdomyosarcomas in children.

Sarcoma botryoides is a descriptive term for an exophytic embryonal tumor that looks grossly like a cluster of grapes. It tends to arise in hollow organs (bladder, vagina).

Another histologic variant of the embryonal type is the "spindle cell sarcoma." It often arises in a paratesticular location and is associated with an especially favorable outcome.

❏❏ **Besides histologic type, what are some adverse prognostic factors in patients with rhabdomyosarcoma?**

Tumors arising in the prostate, children under 1 year of age, and tumors in adults generally have a poorer prognosis.

❏❏ **A 4-year-old male has a rhabdomyosarcoma of the bladder. At the time of surgery the tumor appears grossly removed, however pathological analysis reveals positive margins. Lymph nodes are negative. What stage disease is this (International Rhabdomyosarcoma Study (IRS) staging system)?**

This patient is in Group IIA. The staging system is as follows:

Group I: Localized disease, completely removed, regional nodes not involved. Confined to muscle or organ of origin. Contiguous involvement with infiltration outside the muscle or organ or origin, as through fascial planes; this includes tumors where the gross impression of complete removal is confirmed microscopically

Group II: Grossly removed tumor with microscopic residual disease; no gross residual tumor; no regional nodal involvement Regional disease, completely removed (regional nodes involved, and / or extension to adjacent organ; no microscopic residual disease). Regional disease with involved nodes, grossly removed, but with microscopic residual disease

Group III: Incomplete removal or biopsy with gross residual disease.

Group IV: Distant metastatic disease present at onset.

❏❏ **What is the primary mode of therapy for patients with stage T2a rhabdomyosarcoma of the bladder?**

Multiagent chemotherapy is the primary mode of treatment for patients with rhabdomyosarcoma. The combination of agents is often determined based on randomized trials (e.g. RMS-IV currently), but often includes one or more of the following: vincristine, actinomycin D, ifosfamide, etoposide and / or cyclophosphamide. Radiation therapy may be added, and patients who do not have complete response to these treatments undergo surgical excision. The current trend, however, is toward organ preservation.

❏❏ **What is the most common testicular tumor in a prepubertal boy?**

Yolk sac tumors are the most prevalent in prepubertal boys, accounting for nearly half of all testicular tumors in this age group.

❏❏ **What is the histologic hallmark of a testicular teratoma?**

Teratomas contain elements derived from more than one of the three germ tissues: ectoderm, endoderm, and mesoderm.

❐❐ **A 14-month-old male presents with a testicular mass. Tumor markers are negative. Radical orchiectomy is performed, and the pathology reveals a teratoma. What is the next step in management of this patient?**

Observation. Teratomas in prepubertal boys are consistently benign. Either orchiectomy or enucleation of the tumor with preservation of the remaining testicular tissue is curative. An older, post-pubertal patient with teratocarcinoma, however, is managed the same as an adult with a nonseminomatous germ cell tumor.

❐❐ **What testicular tumor must be ruled out in boys who present with precocious puberty?**

Leydig cell tumors can produce high levels of testosterone resulting in increased somatic growth, deepening of the voice, phallic growth and secondary sexual characteristics. Serum levels of testosterone and gonadotropins must be checked, along with testicular ultrasonography.

❐❐ **What disease can mimic a Leydig cell tumor?**

Congenital adrenal hyperplasia (non-salt-wasting) can present similar to a Leydig cell tumor. This is particularly true if a hypertrophic adrenal rest is present in the scrotum. These patients will exhibit elevated 17-ketosteroids as well as testosterone; gonadotropin levels will be low. Treatment with corticosteroids usually results in prompt resolution of the scrotal mass (adrenal rest).

❐❐ **What condition or conditions are associated with the development of gonadoblastoma?**

Gonadoblastoma is a tumor that contains both germ cells and germinal stromal cells (although often the germ cells predominate and the tumor resembles a seminoma). This tumor develops almost exclusively in patients with abnormal gonads. The karyotype of these children contains either a Y chromosome or a translocation, which includes a portion of the Y chromosome, most commonly 46XY or 45XO / 46XY. All of these children have genital / sexual abnormalities. Eighty percent are phenotypic females with intraabdominal testes (or streak gonads); 20% occur in patients with predominantly male phenotype, often with ambiguity. The risk of tumor development increases at puberty, and the preferred treatment is gonadectomy prior to tumor development.

❐❐ **T/F: The younger the patient is at the time of diagnosis of a sacrococcygeal teratoma the worse the prognosis.**

False. The prognosis for malignant sacrococcygeal teratomas is much worse than that for benign lesions. Malignancy is seen in 7% of girls and 10% of boys diagnosed at less than 2-months of age. In contrast, malignancy was seen in 48% of girls and 67% of boys diagnosed after 2-months of age.

❐❐ **What structure must be excised along with a sacrococcygeal teratoma?**

Resection of the coccyx is an extremely important part of the surgical management of sacrococcygeal teratoma. Failure to resect the coccyx has been associated with a recurrence rate of up to 35%.

❐❐ **What is the primary mode of treatment for a sacrococcygeal teratoma?**

Surgical excision is the mainstay in the management of patients with sacrococcygeal teratoma. Patients with benign tumors need to be followed with imaging to detect any recurrence. Patients with malignant tumors have a poor long-term prognosis despite the multiagent chemotherapy that is required following surgical resection.

RADIOLOGY-CT/ULTRASOUND

Carlin A Ridpath, M.D.

❑❑ **What are posterior urethral valves?**

In the male urethra, there are three types of posterior urethral valves, which may develop. Depending on the extent of the valves predicts the severity of the urethral stricture. Type I valve, the most common, occur distal to the verumontanum. In this instance, several folds are present which encircle a portion of the membranous urethra. However, when these folds fuse anteriorly, they form a stricture of the urethra. This may lead to bladder outlet obstruction. Findings of posterior urethral valves on a VCUG include dilatation of the prostatic urethra, bladder trabeculation and potentially vesicoureteral reflux.

The type II valve extends from the verumontanum and inserts at the bladder neck. This type is nonobstructing.

Type III valves create a membrane below the verumontanum.

❑❑ **What findings constitute prune-belly syndrome?**

Eagle-Barrett or prune-belly syndrome consists of absent abdominal musculature, cryptorchidism and urinary tract abnormalities.

❑❑ **An infant's renal ultrasound shows the right kidney to have multiple cysts of varying sizes, which do not communicate. A right renal pelvis is not identified. What is the diagnosis?**

Multicystic dysplastic kidney (MCDK) is the result of atresia of the renal pelvis. If the disorder is bilateral, it is incompatible with life. MCDK is associated with contralateral renal abnormalities, most commonly, ureteropelvic junction obstruction and vesicoureteral reflux.

❑❑ **What is nephroblastomosis and what is its significance?**

Nephroblastomosis are persistent embryonal remnants (metanephric blastema) in the kidney. Although not malignant itself, nephroblastomosis is associated as a precursor to Wilms' tumor. The involved kidney is enlarged with a lobulated contour. Lesions are hypovascular, with little to no enhancement on contrasted CT.

❑❑ **What is the typical age range for diagnosing Wilms' tumor?**

Wilms' tumor is diagnosed between the first and fifth years of life. They are uncommon in the first year of life.

❑❑ **Describe the typical imaging findings of a Wilms' tumor.**

A large (mean 12cm) mass arising from the renal cortex, displacing and distorting the pelvocalyceal system, with less contrast enhancement than the surrounding parenchyma. Uncommonly Wilms' tumors may have calcifications and may invade the adjacent vascular structures.

❑❑ **What clinical indications predicate a renal nuclear scan?**

Evaluation of renovascular hypertension, renal transplant function and renal function can be assessed using a renal nuclear medicine study. Technitium-99m DTPA is a radiopharmaceutical agent used to obtain renal perfusion and function (glomerular filtration rate) information.

⬜⬜ What is the role of MRI in renal imaging?

The cross sectional (axial, coronal and sagittal) imaging capability of MRI is important in assessing origin of a mass in the vicinity of the kidneys. Renal, adrenal and liver masses can be accurately assessed, whereas CT or ultrasound may not provide the clear delineation of the site of origin. In the case where a renal abnormality is present, contrast enhanced CT is warranted, however if the patient has a history of contrast allergy or abnormal renal function, a MRI may be performed. Gadolinium may be safely administered in this situation.

⬜⬜ Describe the typical imaging findings of a Wilms' tumor.

A large (mean 12cm) mass arising from the renal cortex, displacing and distorting the pelvocalyceal system, with less contrast enhancement than the surrounding parenchyma. Uncommonly Wilms' tumors may have calcifications and may invade the adjacent vascular structures.

⬜⬜ What is the role of renal angiography?

Renal angiography is used to diagnose (renal artery stenosis) and provide treatment (angioplasty, embolize tumors prior to surgery to decrease their size and embolize traumatic injuries to the renal artery branches).

⬜⬜ Name the portions of the male urethra.

The anterior urethra is composed of the penile and bulbous segments. The posterior urethra consists of the membranous and prostatic segments.

⬜⬜ Which urinary tract stones are radiolucent on plain films?

Stones composed of cystine and urate are radiolucent.

⬜⬜ Which radiological test is the most sensitive for detecting urinary tract stones?

Helical CT performed without contrast is the most sensitive for detecting urinary tract stones.

⬜⬜ Are any of the urinary tract stones radiolucent on CT?

No. All compositions of urinary tract stones are visualized on CT.

⬜⬜ What is the advantage of assessing a possible urinary tract stone with CT vs. an intravenous pyelogram (IVP)?

Advantages include the speed of the exam (minutes compared to potential hours with IVP), assessing hydronephrosis and other complications associated with an obstructing stone, contrast material is not administered, therefore alleviating possible contrast reactions and the added benefit of assessing other entities which may be causing the patient's symptoms.

⬜⬜ In the region of the renal medulla, multiple, bilateral calcifications are present. What are the major diagnoses?

Renal tubular acidosis
Medullary sponge kidney
Hyperparathyroidism

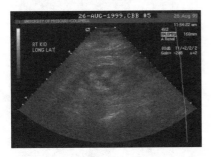

❑❑ **What is a staghorn calculus?**

A stone that fills the collecting system, forming a cast of the pelvis and calyces. Most are composed of struvite and associated with chronic renal infection. A staghorn calculus is associated with xanthrogranulomatous pyelonephritis.

❑❑ **Hydronephrosis/hydroureter are identified on an ultrasound. The patient has no history of compromised renal function. Which imaging study should be ordered next?**

A CT scan without and with contrast to evaluate for the cause of obstruction, such as an obstructing bladder stone or a bladder cancer obstructing the UVJ. However, if the renal function is compromised, alternatively a MRI may be obtained.

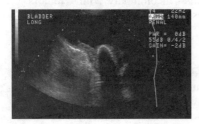

❑❑ **Name a few causes of ureteral obstruction.**

Prior stone, prior infection, pelvic neoplasm, retroperitoneal fibrosis or prior instrumentation.

❑❑ **A patient presents with decreasing renal function. An ultrasound shows multiple, bilateral large cysts. What is the diagnosis?**

Autosomal dominant polycystic kidney disease (ADPCKD). The ultrasound/CT findings are pathopneumonic with bilaterally large kidneys with multiple cysts. The mean age at diagnosis is 43 years old. ADPCKD is associated with cysts in the liver and pancreas and saccular berry aneurysms of the cerebral arteries. Renal insufficiency gradually develops.

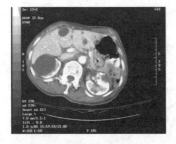

❑❑ **What is renovascular hypertension (RVH)?**

Elevated systemic hypertension due to an abnormality in the renal arterial system, impairing nephron perfusion. The causes of the abnormal renal arterial system are most commonly atherosclerosis, fibromuscular dysplasia and neurofibromatosis.

❑❑ **Which imaging studies evaluate for RVH?**

Angiography.
CT angiography/MR angiography.
Nuclear Medicine.
Ultrasound.
Renal vein sampling.

❑❑ **How does a Nuclear Medicine study evaluate for RVH?**

Technetium 99m-DTPA and MAG3 are radionuclide agents cleared by the kidneys. Patients with RVH may show a unilateral reduction in flow while function is preserved. This study may be performed in conjunction with an ACE inhibitor, such as captopril. The ACE inhibitor blocks efferent arterial vasoconstriction, resulting in a decrease in the GFR and ERPF. The study is considered suggestive of RAS if one of the kidneys GFR drops by 30% after captopril is administered.

❒❒ **What is the role of a renal captopril study in suspected RVH?**

The renal captopril study is a good screening test for those suspected of renal artery stenosis. However, patients with positive studies should undergo additional imaging, such as magnetic resonance angiography or renal angiography.

❒❒ **What single best non-invasive imaging test is used to confirm a renal mass is a cyst?**

Ultrasound characteristics of a simple cyst, a round or oval anechoic structure, imperceptible wall, smooth margins with the surrounding tissue and increased through transmission, can verify a cyst. Alternatively, if the patient is difficult to ultrasound, secondary to body habitus, a CT or MRI may be obtained

❒❒ **How can one characterize a simple renal cyst on CT?**

The findings are the same as ultrasound; however, the Houndsfeld numbers should be less than 20.

❒❒ **If a renal mass meets the criteria for a simple cyst on CT, but the Houndsfeld units are greater than 20, what is your differential diagnosis?**

The cyst either contains blood or proteinaceous material. In order to confirm that the finding is a cyst, an ultrasound may be obtained.

❒❒ **A patient presents with hematuria (microscopic or macroscopic), what is the best imaging test to evaluate the cause?**

Some institutions prefer intravenous pyelography, however a CT scan of the abdomen and pelvis may be more sensitive at picking up small cancers in the pelvocalyceal system. A nonenhanced, contrasted and delayed CT should be performed. The bladder should be carefully evaluated with contrast opacifying the majority of the structure.

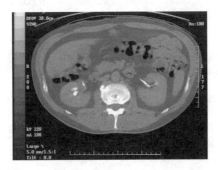 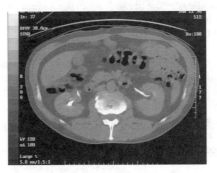

❒❒ **What conditions predispose a patient to developing renal cell carcinoma?**

Patients on long term dialysis and Von Hippel Lindau syndrome are predisposed to renal cell carcinoma.

❒❒ **Where does renal cell carcinoma typically metastasize?**

Renal cell carcinoma most commonly metastasizes to the lungs and bones. Lung lesions are typically a miliary pattern (innumerable nodules, each measuring 3 mm in size). The bone lesions are lytic and expansile.

❒❒ **What is the best imaging test to evaluate for vascular invasion of renal cell carcinoma?**

MRI with its multiplanar imaging capability will be able to assess for renal vein, IVC or right atrial tumor thrombus.

□□ **How can transitional cell carcinoma (TCC) be distinguished from a blood clot on ultrasound?**

TCC will have color flow on ultrasound and are immobile. Whereas blood clots are not vascular are mobile as the patient changes position, particularly in the bladder.

□□ **An echogenic, 2-cm renal mass is found on ultrasound. What imaging study should be performed next?**

If fat is found in the mass on CT, the diagnosis of an angiomyolipoma is confirmed. Fat is hypodense on CT and the Houndsfeld units should measure less than zero. Angiomyolipomas are benign lesions consisting of fat, smooth muscle and blood vessels. If they reach a large size they may hemorrhage, therefore they may be resected.

□□ **What renal transplant complications may occur immediately postoperative?**

Acute tubular necrosis.
Hyperacute rejection.
Renal artery/vein thrombosis.
Urine leak.

□□ **Acute tubular necrosis (ATN) is suspected in a renal transplant patient. What findings would you expect on the nuclear medicine renal scan?**

The classic findings of ATN are blood flow is preserved however poor function is present.

□□ **How can one tell the difference on nuclear renal scans between ATN and rejection?**

Subsequent renal scans show flow and function to improve in the setting of ATN, whereas flow and function continue to decrease with rejection.

□□ **What factors are evaluated on a renal transplant ultrasound?**

The kidney is identified, measured and the flow in the kidney is examined. The flow is evaluated with color and doppler imaging. The main renal artery and vein blood flow are evaluated. The resistive index should typically not exceed 0.80.

□□ **Fluid collections may accumulate around the transplanted kidney. Name the differential for the fluid collections immediately post op, three months and six months from surgery.**

Urinoma-one to two weeks post transplant
Hematoma-one to three weeks post transplant
Lymphocele-a few weeks to several months post transplant
Abscess-four to five weeks post transplant

□□ **What ultrasound findings are suggestive of rejection?**

Loss of the normal corticomedullary junction.
Decreased diastolic flow.

□□ **What ultrasound findings are suggestive of obstruction of the transplanted kidney?**

Either increasing dilatation of the renal collecting system on subsequent ultrasounds or significant dilatation of the collecting system may represent obstruction (ureteral stenosis or a blood clot). However, mild dilatation is often seen in normal transplants.

□□ **What is the normal appearance of the adrenal glands on CT?**

Each limb of the adrenal gland has straight or slightly convex borders, may measure up to 4 cm in length and should measure less than 10mm in thickness.

☐☐ **What imaging study is best to differentiate adrenal masses from upper pole renal masses?**

The multiplanar capabilities of MRI (coronal, sagital) make this modality the best choice in evaluating a renal vs. adrenal mass. Subtle fat planes between the renal mass and adrenal gland may be distinguished on a coronal or other planar imaging sequence.

☐☐ **What is the CT imaging characteristics of an adrenal adenoma?**

Adrenal adenomas are typically 3 cm or less, focal low densities with a smooth round margin. A CT performed with and without contrast at 5mm interval axial images provide optimal evaluation compared to the routine 10 mm axial images. The attenuation around zero Houndsfeld units or less confirms the diagnosis. If the adenoma is functioning, the contralateral gland may be suppressed and appear smaller.

☐☐ **What is the CT imaging characteristics of an adrenal carcinoma?**

Typically, adrenal carcinomas are large when imaged, due to the lack of symptoms. The large, suprarenal mass is heterogeneous with areas of necrosis and patchy areas of enhancement.

☐☐ **A pheochromocytoma is clinically suspected; however a CT of the abdomen and pelvis are normal. What imaging study may be done next to detect or confirm a pheochromocytoma?**

Iodine 131-labeled metaiodobenzyl guanidine (MIBG) is taken up by adrenergic tissue. The nuclear medicine study should scan the entire body looking for an extraadrenal primary tumor.

☐☐ **Describe the imaging characteristics of a pheochromocytoma on CT and MRI.**

Pheochromocytomas are usually greater than 3 cm at presentation. Heterogeneous contrast enhancement occurs on CT making differentiation from metastases difficult. Correlation with blood tests is required to establish the diagnosis. The use of intravenous contrast in-patients with pheochromocytomas, is controversial in the setting of a history of hypertensive episodes or if the patient has not had adequate adrenergic blockade. Pheochromocytomas have a characteristic appearance on MRI. On Tl weighted images pheochromocytomas are isointense to muscle and hyperintense to fat on T2 images. Gadolinium is safe to administer to these patients and intense enhancement occurs.

☐☐ **Describe the normal orientation of the kidneys.**

The lower poles are anterior and lateral in relation to the upper poles. The kidneys parallel the psoas muscles in orientation.

☐☐ **What is a dromedary hump?**

A normal variant. The spleen presses on the upper lateral aspect of the left kidney.

☐☐ **If a single kidney were seen in the abdomen on ultrasound, what differential would one consider?**

Congenital absence of a kidney.
Renal hypoplasia or atrophy.
An ectopic location, such as the pelvis.
Prior resection.
Nonfunctioning kidney (trauma or obstruction).

☐☐ **What is a horseshoe kidney?**

The lower poles of the kidneys fuse, creating a single band of tissue crossing the midline. The orientation of the kidneys is altered with the lower poles directed more medial and the collecting systems directed anterior. This condition is more predisposed to injury in trauma patients. The connecting tissue may or may not function.

○○ What is a retrocaval ureter?

Also known as a postcaval ureter or circumcaval ureter. The proximal right ureter curves medially, coursing behind the inferior vena cava, usually at the level of the fourth lumbar vertebral body.

○○ What is a duplicated collecting system and what is its significance?

Part or all of the collecting system and ureter may be duplicated. Partial duplications are rarely clinically significant. In a complete duplication, separate ureters drain the upper and lower collecting system. The upper pole ureter may insert into an ectopic location in the bladder creating a potential obstruction of the upper pole and the ureter from the inferior pole may reflux.

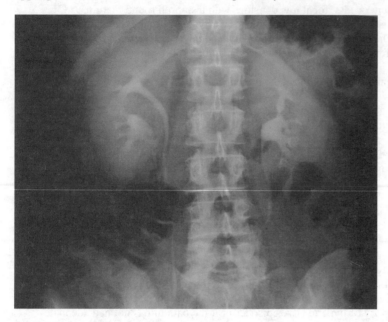

○○ What is the Weigert-Meyer rule?

When there is a complete duplication of the ureters, the lower pole ureter inserts craniolaterally into the bladder, and the upper pole ureter inserts medial and inferior in relation to the lower pole ureter.

○○ What is a cobra head abnormality?

This is seen on an IVP. This refers to a simple ureterocele, where the distal ureter inserts into the trigone, protruding into the bladder. The contrast in the bladder and in the ureter surrounds the thin wall of the ureterocele creating a lucency surrounded by opaque contrast.

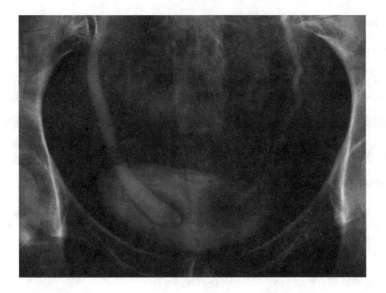

☐☐ Describe the imaging characteristics of an adrenal neuroblastoma on CT.

The mass is typically large, lobulated, crosses the midline and approximately half have stippled calcifications.

☐☐ What is an adrenal myelolipoma?

A hamartomatous lesion containing myeloid, fat and hematopoetic tissue. Size can range up to 30 cm and are inhomogenous on CT and ultrasound, due to their mixed components. The fat component provides an echogenic structure on ultrasound and a low density (Houndsfeld measurement less than zero) on CT.

☐☐ What are the most common causes of adrenal hemorrhage in pediatric and adult patients?

In neonates, the most common cause of adrenal hemorrhage is birth trauma, hypoxia or septicemia. Most cases are bilateral. In neonates, ultrasound is the imaging study of choice. In adults, trauma, anticoagulation and infection are the most common causes of hemorrhage. Typically, unilateral hemorrhage involving the right adrenal gland occurs in adults. CT is performed in adult patients evaluating for adrenal hemorrhage.

☐☐ What are the imaging characteristics of adrenal hemorrhage on ultrasound and CT?

Ultrasound initially images acute hemorrhage as hyperechoic and over time the blood becomes more hypoechoic and smaller. Noncontrast CT demonstrates the acute hemorrhage as hyperdense, in relation to the liver and spleen, becoming progressively hypodense with time. The adrenal glands are enlarged by the hemorrhage. Contrasted CT shows the adrenal hemorrhage as hypodense compared to the spleen and liver.

☐☐ Which imaging studies are used to evaluate acute scrotal pain?

Ultrasound and nuclear medicine.

☐☐ What are the ultrasound findings of testicular torsion?

Early torsion (less than 4 hours) may be normal on gray scale images. However, color imaging shows absence of flow to the affected testis. By twenty-four hours, the testicle may be hyper- or hypovascular on color images and enlarged with a heterogeneous echotexture on gray scale imaging.

☐☐ What are the nuclear medicine findings of testicular torsion?

Early torsion is photopenic, no flow, to the affected testis. In late torsion, the "ring sign" is present, indicating increased flow to the surrounding scrotal tissue and no flow to the actual testis.

❑❑ **What are the ultrasound and nuclear medicine findings in epididymitis?**

US: The epididymis is enlarged and hypervascular. If the testis is involved, increased blood flow will be present. A reactive hydrocele and skin thickening may be present.

Nuclear medicine: Increased flow to the epididymis and or testis.

❑❑ **What is the importance of differentiating an extra/intratesticular mass?**

The majority of intratesticular masses are malignant. Whereas, the extratesticular masses are benign.

❑❑ **Name several intratesticular masses.**

Primary and metastatic malignancies can involve the testicles. The vast majority of testicular neoplasms are primary. Most common germ cell tumors include seminomas, embryonal carcinoma, choriocarcinoma and teratomas. Common primaries, which may metastasize to the testicles, are lymphoma (the most common in-patients older than 60), prostate, leukemia and kidney.

❑❑ **Which zone of the prostate is the site of benign prostatic hypertrophy?**

The transitional zone is the site of origin (greater than 95%) of benign prostatic hypertrophy.

❑❑ **What is the percentage of prostate cancer arising from each zone?**

Peripheral zone 70%.
Central zone 10%.
Transitional zone 20%.

❑❑ **What is the indication for a voiding cystourethrogram (VCUG)?**

A VCUG should be performed after a first urinary tract infection in both boys and girls occurs. A VCUG is able to evaluate vesicoureteral reflux. In male patients, a VCUG is also suggested to evaluate the urethral anatomy (i.e., posterior urethral valves).

❑❑ **What are the advantages of a radionuclide cystogram compared to a fluoroscopic VCUG?**

The radionuclide cystogram is very sensitive for detecting reflux, due to continuous monitoring by the gamma camera. This modality is useful for follow up studies in-patients for known reflux. The disadvantage of the nuclear medicine study is the poor anatomic detail.

❑❑ **What is the difference between primary and secondary vesicoureteral reflux?**

Primary reflux is due to "immaturity" of the ureterovesical junction, allowing reflux to occur either during bladder filling or emptying. Secondary reflux is due to a functional abnormality of the ureterovesical junction, such as a ureterocele, or a bladder outlet obstruction.

❑❑ **What are the CT findings of pyelonephritis?**

Imaging studies, including CT is normal in 75% of cases. However, a contrast enhanced CT study may show wedge shaped areas of decreased density or renal enlargement. CT can rule out potential complications of pyelonephritis, such as abscess or scarring.

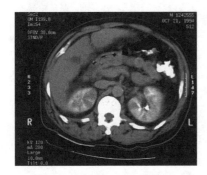 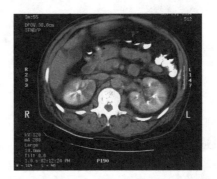

☐☐ What region of the kidney does a scar from reflux nephropathy occur?

The focal scar is typically polar, appearing as decreased parenchymal thickness. The scar overlies a blunted calyx.

☐☐ In a duplicated collecting system, hydronephrosis of the upper pole moiety is due to what entity?

The upper pole ureter inserts ectopically, and if associated with a secondary ureterocele, may obstruct.

BIBLIOGRAPHY

Adult and Pediatric Urology (3rd edition). Gillenwater JY, Grayhack JT, Howards SS and Duckett JW (eds.), Mosby, St. Louis, MO, 1996, p. 2061-2758.

American Journal of Hypertension 12 (1 Pt 1): 1-7, January 1999.

Barzon, L. and Boscaro, M.: Diagnosis and management of adrenal incidentalomas. J. Urol. 163:398-407, 2000.

Bauer SB. Anomalies of the kidney and ureteropelvic junction. In: Walsh PC, Retik AB, Vaughan ED, Wein AJ, eds. Campbell's Urology. Philadelphia: V@TB Saunders 1998.

Bearhs, O.H., Hanson, D.R., Hutter, R.V.P., Kenedy, B.J.: Manual for staging of cancer. 4th ed. Philadelphia: J.B. Lippincott 1992:181.

Beilby JA, Keogh EJ: Spinal cord injuries and anejaculation, Paraplegia 27:152, 1989.

Benson, MC, Olsson, CA: Continent urinary diversion. In Walsh PC, Retik AB, Vaughan ED, Wein AJ, eds: Campbell's Urology. 7th Ed. Philadelphia, W.B. Saunders Company, 1998, p. 3190.

Benson, MC, Olsson, CA: Continent urinary diversion. Urol Clin North Am 1999; 26:125-147.

Bihrle, R: The Indiana pouch continent urinary reservoir. Urol Clin North Am 1997; 24:773-779.

Blyth B, Snyder HM. Ureteropelvic junction obstruction in children. In: Krane RJ, Siroky MB and Fitzpatrick JM, eds. Clinical Urology. Philadelphia: JB Lippincott 1994.

Bosl, G.J., Motzer, R.J.: Testicular germ-cell cancer. N Engl J Med 1997, 337(4):242-53

Breneman JC, Donaldson SS and Hays DM. The management of pediatric genitourinary rhabdomyosarcoma. In: Vogelzang NJ, Scardino PT, Shipley WU and Coffey DS, eds. Comprehensive textbook of genitourinary oncology. Baltimore: Williams and Wilkins, 1996.

Brossner, C., Bayer, G., Madersbacher, S. Kuber, W., Klinger, C. and Pycha, A.: Twelve prostate biopsies detect signficant cancer volumes (> 0.5 ml). Br. J. Urol.; 85(6):705, 2000.

Bukowski, R.M. and Klein, E.A.: Management of adrenal neoplasms. In Comprehensive textbook of genitourinary oncology. Vogelzang, N.J., Scardino, P.T., Shipley, W.U. and Coffey, D.S. eds. Williams and Wilkins, 125-153,1996.

Buvat J and Lemaire A. Endocrine screening in 1022 men with erectile dysfunction: Clinical significance and cost-effective strategy. J Urol 1997; 158:1764-1767.

Campbells Urology (7th edition). Walsh PC, Retik AB, Darracott Vaughan Jr. E and Wein AJ (eds.), WB Saunders, Philadelphia, PA, 1998.

Carroll, P.: Ed. Testis cancer. Urol Clin North Am 1998, 23(3).

Carson CC. Management of penile prosthesis infection. Probi Urol 1993; 7:368-380.

Cassady JR, Hutter JJ Jr., and Whitesell LJ. Neuroblastoma: Natural history and current therapeutic approaches. In: Vogelzang NJ, Scardino PT, Shipley WU and Coffey DS, eds. Comprehensive textbook of genitourinary oncology. Baltimore: Williams and Wilkins, 1996.

Catalona, W.J., Urothelial tumors of the urinary tract, In Campbell's Urology, Ed: Walsh, P.C., Retik, A.B., Stamey, T.A.,and Vaughan, Jr., E.D., W.B.Saunder Company, Philadelphia, 1992, pp. 1094-1158.

CDC Surveillance Reports, Reported Tuberculosis in the United States, www.cdc.gov.

Cendron M, Elder JS, Duckett JW: Perinatal urology. In Gillenwater JY, Grayhack JT, Howards SS, Duckett JW (eds): Adult and Pediatric Urology, vol III, ed 3. St. Louis, Mosby-Year Book, Inc., 1996; pp 2075-2169.

Cheville JC. Classification and pathology of testicular germ cell and sex cord-stromal tumors. Urol Clin North Am 1999, 26(3):595-609.

Chodak, G.W., Keller, P., Scheonberg, H.W.: Assessment of screening for prostate cancer using digital rectal examination. J. Urol., 1989;141: 1136.

Clayman RV, McDougal EM, Figenshau RS. Endourology of the upper urinary noncalculous applications. In: Gillenwater JY, Grayhack JT, Howards SH, Duckett JW, eds. Adult and Pediatric Urology. St. Louis: Mosby 1996.

Clinical Pediatric Urology 3rd Edition, Panayotis P. Kelalis, Lowell R. King, and A. Berry Belman, 1992, volume 2, p.536

Clinical Urology, Krane, R.J., et al Eds., Philadelphia, JB Lippincott, 1994.

Complications or Urologic Surgery, Prevention and Management, Second Edition, Robert B. Smith and Richard M. Ehrlich, Copyright 1990, W.B. Saunders Company, Philadephia, pages 386 through 411.

Coplen, D.E., Snow, B.W., and Duckett, J.W.: Prune Belly Syndrome. In: Adult and Pediatric Urology. Edited by J. Y. Gillenwater, J. T. Grayhack,, S.S. Howards, and J.W. Duckett. St. Louis: Mosby, chapt. 49, p. 2297, 1996.

Cruz, DN, Huot, SJ: Metabolic complications of urinary diversions: an overview. Am J Med 1997; 102:477-484.

Current Opinion in Urology Volume 8 #2 – March 1998.

Davidson AJ. Hartman DS (eds): Radiology of the Kidney and Genitourinary Tract, 3rd ed. Philadelphia, W.B. Saunders, 1999.

deKernion, JB, Trapasso, JG: Urinary diversion and continent reservoir. In Gillenwater JY, Grayhack JT, Howards SS, Duckett JW, eds: Adult and Pediatric Urology. 3rd Ed. St. Louis, Mosby-Year Book, 1996, p. 1465.

Diamond DA, Gosalbez R: Neonatal Urologic Emergencies. In Walsh PC, Retik AB, Vaughn ED, Wein AJ (eds): Campbell's Urology, vol II, ed 7. Philadelphia, W.B. Saunders Company, 1998; pp 1629-1654.

Diamond M: Pediatric management of ambiguous and traumatized genitalia. J Urol 162(2):1021-1028, 1999.

Dunnick NR, McCallum RW, Snadler CM: Textbook of Uroradiology, 2nd ed. Baltimore, Williams and Wilkins, 1997.

Einhorn, L.H., Donohue, J.P.; Advanced testicular cancer: update for urologists. J Urol 1998, 160(6Pt 1):1964-9.

Eisenberger, CF, Schoenberg, M, Fitter, D, Marshall, FF: Orthotopic ileocolic neobladder reconstruction following radical cystectomy: history, technique and results of the Johns Hopkins experience, 1986-1998. Urol Clin North Am 1999; 26:149-156.

Elder JR, Hladky D, Selzmann AA: Outpatient nephrectomy for non-functioning kidneys. J Urol 154:712-715, 1993.

Feldman HA, Goldstein 1, Hatzichristou DG, Krane RJ and McKinlay JB. Impotence and its medical and psychosocial correlates. Results of the Massachusetts Male Aging Study. J Urol 1994; 151:54-46.

Fitzgerald, J, Malone, MJ, Gaertner, RA, Zinman, LN: Stomal construction, complications, and reconstruction. Urol Clin North Am 1997; 24:729-733.

Fowler JE, Koshy M and Strub M. Priapism associated with the sickle cell hemaglobinopathies: prevalence, natural history, and sequelae. J Urol 1991; 145:65-68.

Furness, P.D., Cheng, E.Y., Franco, I., and Firlit, C.F.: The Prune-Belly Syndrome: A New and SImplified Technique of Abdominal Wall Reconstruction. J. Urol.: 160: 1195, 1998.

Gillenwater, J.Y., Greyhack, J.T., Howards, S.S. and Duckett, J.W.: Eds. Adult and Pediatric Urology, 3rd Edition, Mosby-Year book Inc. St. Louis, MO 1996.

Goldstein I, Lue TF, Padma-Nathan H, Rosen RC, Steers WD and Wicker PA. Oral Sildenafil in the treatment of erectile dysfunction. N Engl J Med 1998; 338:1397-1404.

Gonzales, E.T., Jr.: Anomalies of the Renal Pelvis and Ureter. In: Kelalis, P.P., King, L.R., Belman, A.B.: (eds): Clinical Pediatric Urology, 3rd ed. Philadelphia: W.B. Saunders, 1992.

Gordon I: Ultrasonography in Uronephrology. In O'Donnell B, Koff SA)eds): Pediatric Urology, ed 3. Oxford, Butterworth-Heinemann, 1997; pp 41-64.

Gorelick JI, Goldstein M: Loss of fertility in men with varicocele, Fertil Steril 59: 613, 1993.

Gow, J.G., The current Management of Patinets with Genitourinary Tuberculosis. AUA Update Series, Lesson 26 Vol. XI, 1992.

Graves, F.T.: The anatomy of the intrarenal arteries and its application to segmental resection of the kidney. Brit. J. Surg. 2:132, 1955.

Gray, H.: Gray's Anatomy, the anatomical basis of medicine and surgery 38th ED., New York, Churchill Livingston, 1995.

Gray, SW, Skandalakis, JE. Embryology for Surgeons. WB Saunders, Philadelphia, 1972.

Greskovich, F.J. and Nyberg, L.M.: The Prune Belly Syndrome: A Review of Its Etiology, Defects, Treatment and Prognosis. J. Urol., 140: 707, 1988.

Guiney EJ: Emergency Room Problems. In O'Donnell B, Koff SA (eds): Pediatric Urology, ed 3. Oxford, Butterworth-Heinemann, 1997; pp281-285.

Gulml FA, Felsen D, Vaughan ED. Pathophysiology of urinary tract obstruction. In: Walsh PC, Retik AB, Vaughan ED, Wein AJ, eds. Campbell's Urology. Philadelphia: WB Saunders 1998.

Guyton, AC. Textbook of Medical Physiology, 8th edition. Philadelphia, PA. W.B. Saunders Co., 1991.

Haas, G.P., Triest, J., Pontes, E., and Trump, D.L. Nonsurgical treatment of adrenocortical cancer. In Principles and Practice of Genitourinary Oncology. Raghavan, D. Scher, H.I., Leibel, S.A. and Lange, P. eds. 1001-1006, Lippincott-Raven, 1997.

Hanno, P.M. Diagnosis of interstitial cystitis. Urol Clin N Am. 21(1):1, 63, 1994.

Hautmann, RE: The ileal neobladder to the female urethra. Urol Clin North Am 1997; 24:827-835.

Hedge, GA, Colby, HD, Goodman, RL. Clinical Endocrine Physiology. Philadelphia, PA, W.B. Saunders Co., 1987

Hendren, WH: Historical perspective of the use of bowel in urology. Urol Clin North Am 1997; 24:703-713.

Hendren, WH: Urinary undiversion: refunctionalization of the previously diverted urinary tract. In Walsh PC, Retik AB, Vaughan ED, Wein AJ, eds: Campbell's Urology. 7th Ed. Philadelphia, W.B. Saunders Company, 1998, p. 3247.

Kabalin, J.N. In: Walsh P.C., Retik, A.B., Vaughan, E.D., Jr., Wein, A.J., (eds): Campbell's Urology, 7th ed., Vol. I. Philadelphia, W.B. Saunders, 1998.

Kaefer, M, Retik, AB: The Mitrofanoff principle in continent urinary reconstruction. Urol Clin North Am 1997; 24:795-811.

Kass, E.J.: Megaureter., In: Kelalis, P.P., King, L.R., Belman, A.B.: (eds): Clinical Pediatric Urology, 3rd ed. Philadelphia: W.B. Saunders, 1992.

Katz, M.D. and Imperato-McGinley, J.: Adrenal Cancer: Endocrinology, Diagnosis and Clinical Staging. In Principles and Practice of Genitourinary Oncology. Raghavan, D. Scher, H.I., Leibel, S.A. and Lange, P. eds. 981-992, Lippincoft-Raven, 1997.

Kelalis, Panayotis P. , King Lowell R., and Belman, Barry A. eds, Clinical Pediatric Urology, 3rd ed., W.B. Saunders, Philadelphia, 1992.

Kidney Transplantation: Principles and Practice, Peter J. Morris Ed. 4th ed. 1994.

King, L.R.: Vesicoureteral Reflux, Megaurter and Ureteral Reimplantation. In: Walsh, P.C., Retik, A.B., Vaughan, E.D., Jr., Wein, A.J.: (eds) Campbell's Urology, 6th Ed.

Koch, M.O. and Smith, J.A. Surgical management of adrenal tumors. In Principles and Practice of Genitourinary Oncology. Raghavan, D. Scher, H.I., Leibel, S.A. and Lange, P. eds. 993-1000, Lippincoft-Raven, 1997.

Kogan, B.A.: Disorders of the Ureter and Ureteropelvic Junction. In: Tanango, E.A., McAnich, J.W.: (eds.) Smith's General Urology, 14th ed. Norwalk: Appleton and Lange, 1995.

Kogan, S., Hadziselimovic, F., Howards, S.S., Snyder, H.M. and Huff, D.: Pediatric Andrology. In: Adult and Pediatric Urology. J.Y. Gillenwater, J.T. Grayhack, S.S. Howards and J.W. Duckett, eds. Mosby Year Book, Inc., St. Louis, pp 2623-2674, 1996.

Koo, H.P. and Bloom, D.A.: Laparoscopy for the nonpalpable testis. Seminars in Laparoscopic Surgery, 5: 40-46, 1998.

Korman, H.J., Watson, R.B., and Soloway, M.S., Bladder Cancer: Clinical Aspects and Management, 1996 Monographs in Urology, Ed: Stamey, T.S., 17:6, 1996, pp. 81-110.

Koziol, J.A. Epidemiology of interstitial cystitis. Urol Clin N Am. 21(1):1, 7, 1994.

Kramer, S.A.: Vesicoureteral Reflux. In: Kelalis, P.P., King, L.R., Belman, A.B.: (eds): Clinical Pediatric Urology, 3rd ed. Philadelphia: W.B. Saunders, 1992.

Lancet 353 (9149): 282-6, January 23, 1999.

Langman's Medical Embryology 6th Edition, T.W. Sadler, 1990, p. 260-296.

Lee PA: Fertility in cryptorchidism: does treatment make a difference? Endocrinol Metab Clin North Am 22:479, 1993.

Levy, David A., Resnick, Martin I. Laparoscopic Pelvic Lymphadenectomy and Radical Perineal Prostatectomy: A Viable Alternative to Radical Retropubic Prostatectomy. Journal of Urology, Volume 151, Page 905, 1994.

Licht MR, Lewis RW, Wollan PC and Harris CD. Comparison of RigiScan and sleep laboratory nocturnal penile tumescence in the diagnosis of organic impotence. J Urol 1995; 154:1740-1743.

Malone, MJ, Izes, JK, Hurley, LJ: Carcinogenesis: the fate of intestinal segments used in urinary reconstruction. Urol Clin North Am 1997; 24:723-728.

Manyak, M.J., Hinkle, G.H., Olsen, J.O., Chiaccherini, R.P., Partin, A.W., Piantadosi, S., Burgers, J.K., Texter, J.H., Neal, C.E., Libertino, J.A., Wright, G.L., Jr., and Maguire, R.T.: Immunoscintigraphy with indium-111-capromed pendetide: evaluation before definitive therapy in patients with prostate cancer. Urology 54(6):1058. 1999.

McDougal, WS: Use of intestinal segments and urinary diversion. In Walsh PC, Retik AB, Vaughan ED, Wein AJ, eds: Campbell's Urology. 7th Ed. Philadelphia, W.B. Saunders Company, 1998, p. 3121.

Meyers, R.P., Practical pelvic Anatomy Pertinent to radical retropubic prostatectomy. AUA Update Series XIII, Lesson 4, 1994.

Henly, DR, Farrow, GM, Zincke, H: Urachal Carcinoma: Role of conservative surgery. Urol, 42: 635-639, 1993.

Hinman, F., Jr.: Atlas of Urologic Surgery, 2nd Ed., Philadelphia: WB Saunders, 1998.

Hoffman, Daniel M., Resnick, Martin I. Return of Perineal Prostatectomy, MediGuide to Urology, Volume 6, Issue 3, 1993.

Horgan JD, Smith AD. Endopyclotomy and Pyeloplasty. In: Krane RJ, Siroky MB and Fitzpatrick JM, eds. Clinical Urology. Philadelphia: JB Lippincott 1994.

Husmann DA, Levy JB, Cain MP, et al: Micropenis: Current Concepts and Controversies. In AUA Update Series. Lesson 10, vol XVII. Houston, American Urological Association, 1998; 74-79.

International Union Against Cancer, TNM Classification of Malignant Tumours, Ed: Sobin, L.H., and Wittekind, CH., Wiley-Liss, New York, 1997, pp. 187-190.

Johnson, DE, Hodges, GB, Abdul-Karim, FW et al: Urachal Carcinoma. Urol, 26: 218-221, 1985.

Journal of Vascular Surgery 29 (4): 617-24, April 1999.

Narayan P, Konety BR. Surgical treatment of female urethral carcinoma. Urol. Clin. North Amer. 19(2): 373-382, 1992.

New England Journal of Medicine. 338(3):161-5, 1998 Jan 15.

Nieh, PT: The Kock pouch urinary reservoir. Urol Clin North Am; 24:755-772.

Noh P.H., Cooper C.S., Winkler, A.C., et al: Prognostic Factors for Long-Term Renal Function in Boys with Prune-Belly Syndrome. J. Urol., 162: 1399, 1999.

Novick, A.C. and Howards, S.S.: The Adrenals. In Adult and Pediatric Urology. Gillenwater, J.Y, Grayhack, J.T., Howards, S.S. and Duckett, J.W. eds., Mosby Publishing, 3rd edition, 587-616, 1996.

Novick AC, Streem SB. Surgery of the kidney. In: Walsh PC, Retik AB, Vaughan ED, Wein AJ, eds. Campbell's Urology. Philadelphia: " Saunders 1998.

Oates RD, Lipshultz LI: Fertility and testicular function in patients after chemotherapy and radiotherapy, Adv Urol 10:52, 1989.

Parsons, C.L. and Parsons, J.K. Interstitial cystitis. In: Female Urology, Shlomo Raz, 2nd ed., Saunders, 1996.

Parton, A.W. U.J. Carter, H.B., Pearson, J.D., Chan, D.W., Epstein, J.I., Walsh, P.C. Journal of Urology, Letter to the Editor, Volume 172, 1994. Journal of Urology, Volume 152, Page 172

Parton, A.W., U.J., Carter, H.B. Pearson, J.D., Chan, D.W., Epstein, J.I., Walsh, P.C. The Use of Prostatic Specific Antigen, Clinical Stage and Gleason's Score to Predict Pathological Stage in Men With Localized Prostate Cancer. Journal of Urology, Volume 150, Page 110, 1993.

Paul Peters, M.D.: "Ball Ping Hammer " appearance of the duplicated collecting system. Personal communication.

Pediatric Urology. Eds., O'Donnell, B., Koff, S.A. Pub. Butterworth Heinemann. 1997.

Pisansky, T., et al: An EnhancedPrognostic System for Clinically Localized Carcinoma of the Prostate. Cancer, 79: 2154-2161, 1997.

Penn I, Transplant Proceedings. 15:1079, 1983.

Presti, J.C., Chang, J.J., Bhargava, V., Shinohara, K.: The optimal systematic prostate biopsy scheme should include 8 rather than 6 biopsies: results of a prospective clinical trial. J. Urol., 163(1):163, 2000.

Primer on Transplantation, Norman and Suki, eds. 1998.

Pryor JP, Hendry WF: Ejaculatory duct obstruction in subfertile males: analysis of 87 patients, Fertil Steril 56:725, 1991.

Radiology 212 (2): 378-84, August 1999.

Ramos, Christian G., Gustavo Carvalhal, Gustavo F. Smith, S. Meager, Douglas E., Catalona, William J.; Retrospective Comparison of Radical Retropubic Prostatectomy and 125-Iodine Brachytherapy for a Localized Prostate Cancer. J. Urology, Volume 161, No. 4, April 1999, pages 1212 through 1215.

Redman, J.F. In: Raghavan, D., Scher, H.I., Leibael, S.A., Lange, P. (eds): Principles and Practice of Genitourinary Oncology. Philadelphia, Lippincott-Raven, 1997.

Reoperative Urology – Cohen & Resnik 1995.

Resnik MI, Kursh ED. Extrinsic obstruction of the ureter. In: Walsh PC, Retik AB, Vaughan ED, Wein AJ, eds. Campbell's Urology. Philadelphia: WB Saunders 1998.

Retik, A.B., and Peters, C.A.: Ectopic Ureter and Ureterocele. In: Walsh, P.C., Retik, A.B., Vaughan, E.D., Jr., Wein, A.J.: (eds) Campbell's Urology, 6th Ed.

Ritchie, J.P.: Testicular Neoplasms. In Walsh P, Retik A, Vaughan E, Wein A Eds. Campbell's Urology 7th Ed. Philidelphia, WB Saunders, 1998 p2411.

Rob D. H., Blascoe, J.C., Grim, Peter D., Kenny, Gerald M., Sylvester, John E., Hoke, David C., Landin, K., Cavanagh, W. Interstitial Iodine—125 Radiation Without Adjuvant Therapy, The Treatment of Clinically Localized Prostate Cancer, Volume 80, Page 442, 1997.

Sarosdy, M.F., Immunotherapy of superficial bladder carcinoma, AUA Update Series, Lesson 29, Volume XIV, 1995, pp. 234-9.

Schaeffer AJ. Infections and Inflammations of the Genitourinary Tract. In: Walsh PC, Retik AB, Vaughan ED, Wein AJ, eds. Campbell's Urology. Philadelphia: YY'B Saunders 1998.

Schaeffer AJ. Urinary Tract Infections. In: Gillenwater JY, Grayhack JT, Howards SH, Duckett JW, eds. Adult and Pediatric Urology. St. Louis: Mosby 1996.

Shokeir AA. The diagnosis of upper urinary tract obstruction. European Urology Update Series 1999:3. BJU 1999; 83:893.

Siroky Mike B. , Edelstein, Robert A., and Krane Robert J. eds. , Manual of Urology 2nd. Ed., Lippincott Williams and Wilkins, Philadelphia, 1999.

Smith's General Urology (14th edition). Tanagho EA, McAninch JW (eds.), Appleton & Lange, Norwalk, CT, 1995.

Snyder HM III, D'Angio GJ, Evans AE and Raney RB. Pediatric Oncology. In: Walsh PC, Retik AB, Vaughan ED and Wein AJ, eds. Campbell's Urology, 7th ed Philadelphia: W.B. Saunders Company, 1998.

Splinter, T.A., and Scher, H.I., Adjuvant and neoadjuvant chemotherapy for invasive (T3-T4) bladder cancer, In Comprehensive Textbook of Genitourinary Oncology, Ed:Vogelzang, N.J., Scardino, P.T., Shipley, W.U., Cofffey, D.S., and Miles, B.J., Williams and Wilkins, Baltimore, 1996, pp. 464-471.

Stamey, T.A., Yang, N., Hay, A.R., McNeal, J.E., Freiha, F.S., Redwine, E.: Prostate-specific antigen as a serum marker for adenocarcinoma of the prostate. N. Engl. J.. Med. 1987;317:909.

Stamm WE. Treatment of Acute Uncomplicated Urinary Tract Infection. In: Bergan T, ed. Urinary Tract Infections

Stampfer, DS, McDougal, WS, McGovern, FJ: Metabolic and nutritional complications. Urol Clin North Am 1997; 24:715-722.

Stephens, FD. Congenital malformations of the Urinary Tract. Praeger, New York, 1983.

Studer, UE, Zingg, EJ: Ileal orthotopic bladder substitutes: what we have learned from 12 years experience with 200 patients. Urol Clin North Am 1997; 24:781-793.

Tolkoff-Rubin NE, Rubin RH. Urinary Tract Infection in the Renal Transplant Recipient. In: Bergan T, ed. Urinary Tract Infections. Basel: Karger 1997.

Turek PJ, Lipshultz LI: Immunologic infertility, Urol Clin North Am 21:447, 1994.

Valicenti, R.K., et al: Effect of Higher Radiation Dose on Biochemical Control After Radical Prostatectomy for pT3NO Prostate Cancer. Int. J. Rad. Oncol. Biol. Phys, 42(3)501-506, 1998.

Vates TS and Steinberg GD. Testicular, sacrococcygeal, and other tumors. In: Vogelzang NJ, Scardino PT, Shipley WU and Coffey DS, eds. Comprehensive textbook of genitourinary oncology. Baltimore: Williams and Wilkins, 1996.

Vaughan, E. D., Blumenfeld, J. D.: The Adrenals. In Campbell's Urology. Walsh, P.C. Retik A.B., Vaughan, E.D. and Wein A.J.eds. W.B. Saunders Company, 7th ed., 2915-2972, 1998.

Vaughn, ED, Jr., Blumenfeld, JD. The Adrenals in Campbell's Urology, 7th edition. Walsh, PC, et al (eds.). Philadelphia, PA. W.B. Saunders Co., 1998.

Vogelzang, N.J., Scardino, P., Shipley, W.U., Coffey, D.S.: eds. Comprehensive Textbook of Genitourinary Oncology, Williams & Wilkins Press 1996.

Vogelzang, N.J. et al, Eds.: Comprehensive Textbook of Genitourinary Oncology 2nd Ed., Philadelphia: Lippincott Williams and Wilkins, 1999.

Walsh, P.C., Retick, A.B., Vaughn, E.D., Jr., Wein, A.J.: Cambell's Urology, Sixth Edition, W.B. Saunders, Copyright 1992, pages 1194 through 1221.

Walsh, P.C., Retik, A.B., Stamey, T.A., Vaughan, E.D., Jr.,: Campbell's Urology, 7th Edition,W.B. Saunders Co., 1998, pp. 2055-2069.

Wein, A.J. and Broderick, G.A. Interstitial cystitis: current and future approaches to diagnosis and treatment. 21(1):1, 153, 1994.

Weiss, RE and Fair, WR: Urachal anomalies and urachal carcinoma. In AUA Update Series, Vol XVII, Lesson 38, 1998, American Urological Association.

Wilimas JA, Greenwald CA and Rao BK. Wilms' Tumor. In: Vogelzang NJ, Scardino PT, Shipley WU and Coffey DS, eds. Comprehensive textbook of genitourinary oncology. Baltimore: Williams and Wilkins, 1996.

Williams, O, Vereb, MJ, Libertino, JA: Noncontinent urinary diversion. Urol Clin North Am 1997; 24:735-744.

Williamson, Michael R. and Smith, Anthony Y., Fundamentals of Uroradiology, W.B. Saunders, Philadelphia, 2000.

Woodard J.R. and Zucker, I.: Current Management of the Dilated Urinary Tract in Prune Belly Syndrome. Urol. Clin. N. Amer., 17: 407, 1990.

Woodard, J.R., and Smith, E. A.: Prune-Belly Syndrome. In: Campbell's Urology. Edited by P.C. Walsh, A.B. Retick, E.D. Vaughan, and A.J. Wein. Philadelphia: W. B. Saunders Co., chapt. 62, p. 1917, 1998.

World Health Organization: A double-blind trial of clomiphene citrate for the treatment of idiopathic male infertility, lnt J Androl 15:299, 1992.

Young, RH: Pathology of carcinomas of the urinary bladder in Comprehensive Textbook of Genitourinary Oncology, Vogelzang, NJ, Scardino, PT, Shipley, WU and Coffey, DS (Eds), Lippincott Williams & Wilkins, Philadelphia, PA, 2000.

The authors wish to thank Dr. Thomas Borden and Dr. Ace Powers for providing some of the radiographs and Joseph Montoya for his help in preparing the radiograph photos. Additionally the authors would like to thank Dr. Paul Peters for his recognition of the "Ball ping" hammer classification of the duplicated collecting system.